T0257943

Encyclopedia of Parkinson's Disease: Diagnosis

Volume III

Encyclopedia of
Parkinson's Disease: Diagnosis
Volume III

Edited by **Kate White**

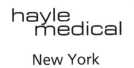

New York

Published by Hayle Medical,
30 West, 37th Street, Suite 612,
New York, NY 10018, USA
www.haylemedical.com

Encyclopedia of Parkinson's Disease: Diagnosis
Volume III
Edited by Kate White

International Standard Book Number: 978-1-63241-191-4 (Hardback)

Printed in the United States of America.

Contents

Preface

The purpose of the book is to provide a glimpse into the dynamics and to present opinions and studies of some of the scientists engaged in the development of new ideas in the field from very different standpoints. This book will prove useful to students and researchers owing to its high content quality.

This book on Parkinson's disease provides latest information pertaining to topics associated with this disease, including research, early biomarkers for the diagnostics, and latest applications of brain imaging to analyze Parkinson's disease. Researchers have currently started to focus on the non-motor symptoms of this disease, which are poorly identified and insufficiently treated by clinicians and have a considerable effect on the quality of life of the patient and mortality and include autonomic, sensory and gastrointestinal symptoms, and cognitive impairments. Detailed discussion of the use of imaging tools to analyze disease mechanisms is also given, with stress on the abnormal network organization in Parkinsonism. Deep brain stimulation management is a paradigm-shifting therapy for this disease and dystonia as well as essential tremor. Novel approaches of early diagnostics, treatments and training programs have greatly enhanced the lives of people suffering from this disease in the latest years, significantly decreasing symptoms and delayed disability. This comprehensive book consists of information contributed by renowned veteran scientists from across the globe.

At the end, I would like to appreciate all the efforts made by the authors in completing their chapters professionally. I express my deepest gratitude to all of them for contributing to this book by sharing their valuable works. A special thanks to my family and friends for their constant support in this journey.

Editor

Part 1

Biomarkers for Preclinical Diagnosis of PD

Diagnosis of Parkinson's Disease by Electrophysiological Methods

Elena Lukhanina, Irina Karaban and Natalia Berezetskaya
Department of Brain Physiology, A.A. Bogomoletz Institute of Physiology,
Parkinson's Disease Treatment Centre, Institute of Gerontology,
Kiev,
Ukraine

1. Introduction

Effective differential diagnosis of Parkinson's disease (PD) needs in informative indices that objectively reflect the functional state of the extrapyramidal system. And also, when evaluating an efficacy of antiparkinsonian therapy, it is essential to have both, qualitative and quantitative characteristics, permitting to correct treatment and predict a disease course. One of informative diagnostic method in PD is surface (interference) electromyography. As know, a nigrostriatal dopamine deficit results in disturbances of the central supraspinal control over the muscle tonic activity and voluntary movements (Valls-Solé & Valldeoriola, 2002). Electromyographically, the extrapyradimal insufficiency shows itself by a high level of bioelectrical activity of muscles at rest, changes of motor unit conduction velocity and synchronization (Farina et al., 2004; Semmler & Nordstrom, 1999). The traditional methods to evaluate surface electromyograms (EMGs) are based on amplitude and spectral analysis. However, myoelectric signals are nonlinear by its nature (Nieminen & Takala, 1996). A surface EMG is formed by the summation of a number of single muscle fiber action potentials. Therefore different world clinics have been searching for new relevant methods based on nonlinear time-series analyses of EMG to quantify the motor features of the disorder in PD (Del Santo et al., 2007; Meigal et al., 2009). Some other novel EMG characteristics, such as dimensionality based on fractal analysis or higher order statistics of EMG distribution have also proved to be sensitive to neuromuscular status (Swie et al., 2005).

Although the cardinal symptoms of the disease are movement disorders the manifestations of PD also comprise a variety of diverse abnormalities including disturbance of sensory gating and cognitive decline (Lewis & Byblow, 2002). Several authors suggested that movement disorders in PD might be also developed because of dysregulation of sensory processing that affects sensorimotor integration (Abbruzzese & Berardelli, 2003). This is an important issue because one of the proposed key functions of basal ganglia is the gating of sensory input for motor control (Kaji, 2001). Numerous studies have demonstrated marked changes in the somatosensory (Rossini et al., 1998), acoustic (Teo et al., 1997;) and visual (Sadekov, 1997) evoked potentials in PD patients. Evaluation of brain evoked potentials may have potential in the assessment of the severity of PD. In contemporary neurophysiology, studies of the central mechanisms underlying the organization of motor function and its impairments increasingly involve analysis of endogenous cortical event-related potentials, a set of potentials which includes contingent negative variation (CNV). The CNV extent depends on the level of attention, motivation, and volitional effort (Deecke, 2001). The magnitude of this potential is known to decrease in diseases accompanied by motor disorders, including PD (Aotsuka et al., 1996; Pulvenmuller et al., 1996). CNV has been shown to display significant increases after administration of levodopa in patients with Parkinson's disease, suggesting a role for the central dopaminergic system in its generation (Oishi et al., 1995).

Although electrophysiological methods objectively reflect motor and sensory dysfunctions, they are still used rather rarely in the clinical evaluation of PD. We carried out systematic and detailed research of surface EMG characteristics in PD patients in comparison with age-matched healthy subjects, paying the special attention on the correlation associations between EMG parameters and subitems of the Unified Parkinson's Disease Rating Scale (UPDRS). Amplitude and spectral features, statistics of distribution, fractal dynamics of the EMG signals were investigated. Separate research was dedicated to the study of EMG characteristics of clinically healthy kinsmen of the patients suffering from PD in order to detect latent symptoms of extrapyramidal insufficiency that can be considered genetic determinants of the risk of development of the above disease. Since the question of the relationship the early and late phases of CNV with the mechanisms controlling motor functions in PD has received inadequate study we conducted such research in patients with this disease. With the purpose of evaluation of the brain inhibitory processes in PD patients the study of cortical evoked potentials upon paired-click auditory stimulation was performed. The results of these investigations are presented below.

2. Surface electromyography

Surface EMG is a simple and noninvasive method that permits to estimate the severity of symptomatology in patients and also may help to exposure of the hidden manifestations of the disturbed muscles activity on the presymptomatic stage of the neurodegenerative process (Kryzhanovsky et al., 2002; Lukhanina et al., 2010). In PD patients the EMG characteristics of the tonic and phasic shoulder muscle activities at rest, during voluntary contraction and under tonic muscle strain were studied. In kinsmen of the patients, suffering from PD, EMGs in the resting state and under conditions of two functional tests (retention of load and retention of arms in the elevated and outstretched state) were recorded.

2.1 Amplitude and spectral analysis of EMGs in patients with Parkinson's disease
One of the informative EMG sign of extrapyramidal insufficiency appears to be the resting EMG amplitude values that reflect the muscle ability for relaxation. Spectral analysis of resting EMGs is used for assessing the burst muscle discharges with a frequency of 4-8 Hz reflecting parkinsonian tremor. Amplitude values of the EMGs recorded during the voluntary muscle contraction serve to calculate the phasic activation coefficient. This coefficient clearly reflects the competitive relationships between the tonic and phasic processes. Study of the reflex agonist/antagonist muscle involvement under tonic strain is valid for establishing coordinating muscle relationships.

2.1.1 Methods

Studies were performed in two groups: 48 patients with PD, 1.5-3.5 Hoehn-Yahr scale (23 men and 25 women, mean ± SE age 62.2 ± 1.6, range 49-75 years) and 42 age-matched healthy controls (20 men and 22 women, mean ± SE age 65.8 ± 1.43, range 58-74 years). All of them were right-handed persons. The study patients, who regularly underwent treatment at the Parkinson's Disease Centre of Institute of Gerontology, gave their written informed consent to participate in this investigation. They had 4-13-year history of an idiopathic PD and received an antiparkinsonian medication (an individual dose 0.250-12g of levodopa/carbidopa, daily). All patients were studied in the OFF state. For the quantitative evaluation of levodopa therapy 20 patients (in which the clinical "ON-OFF" phenomenon was verified) were studied also in the ON state, one hour after an intake of the single individual dose of levodopa/carbidopa. The motor activity of PD patients was evaluated in ON state, according to sections II-III of the UPDRS.

For each subject, we recorded the surface EMG from the flexors and extensors (mm. biceps and triceps brachii) of the right and left arms. The subject lay on his back, with the arms lying on the horizontal surface. The EMGs were recorded using four bipolar skin electrodes (0.5x1.0 cm) with an interelectrode distance constant of 1.5 cm. Bioelectrical potentials were amplified with a band pass of 10 Hz - 10 kHz. The amplified analogue signals were fed to a computer, which digitized them at a sampling rate of 1000 Hz and then stored the data for further measurements. The time of each recording was 10 sec. EMG recordings were made:

1. At a resting state, being cautious that the subject is relaxed.
2. During a voluntary m. biceps brachii contraction started after a command to bend the arm at the elbow, fingers touching the shoulder. The sound signal served as a command to initiate arm bending, and it was simultaneously registered on EMG. An electrical contact enclosure marked the start of arm lifting, being recorded simultaneously with the EMG on a free channel.
3. During a tonic m. biceps brachii strain under weight holding (2 kg) in the hand, with arm lifted upward and stretched forward, for 5 sec.

In resting EMG recordings, the average and maximal EMG amplitudes were calculated to evaluate the muscle ability for relaxation. An artefact-free section on the EMG record was selected by the experimenter. The single EMG wave amplitude was defined as the difference between the values of upper and lower peaks. The oscillations with no less than 2 µV amplitude were considered. The resting average EMG amplitude was calculated based on minimum 100 measurements. The maximum amplitude value was calculated on the same EMG section. The amplitude distribution histograms were constructed.

The resting EMG recordings were also used for assessing the burst muscle discharges For this purpose, the Fourier spectrum diagrams for the low frequency area were constructed. In doing this, part of the data with negative EMG amplitude meanings were discarded. Data with the positive EMG amplitude meanings underwent a Butterworth digital sinus low pass filtering with a band pass of 0-20 Hz As a result, the envelope of EMG amplitude was formed, which then served as the data array for fast Fourier transformation. The data for each lead were divided into several successive sections, each containing 512 points, which underwent the fast Fourier transformation. The obtained spectra were averaged, and the envelope of EMG amplitude frequency with a maximal power was determined (Fig 1). The statistical significance of the frequency peak was determined by means of constructing the 95% confidential intervals (M ± 2 S.D).

The EMG recordings made during the voluntary m. biceps brachii contraction served to calculate the phasic activation coefficient (PhAC), from a formula :

$$PhAC = (AVCa-ARa)/AVCa \qquad (1)$$

where AVCa is the average EMG amplitude on a section with most marked changes in the muscle activity under voluntary contraction, and ARa is the average amplitude of resting EMG. In the conditions of low tonic muscle activity at rest the phasic muscle activation during voluntary movement is facilitated and the PhAC value is close to 1. On the contrary, when the resting tonic activity increases, the PhAC falls.

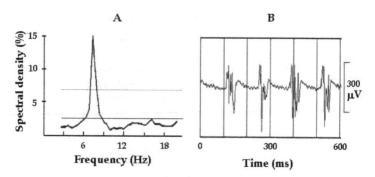

Fig. 1. The spectrogram of the power of EMG envelope frequency with 95% confidence intervals (A) and the corresponding resting EMG pattern of m. biceps brachii in a patient with Parkinson's disease (B). Peak deviation on the spectrogram reflects the frequency of the rhythmic burst muscle discharges.

The functional test with weight holding served for study of the reflex agonist and antagonist involvement during tonic muscle strain. We calculated the coefficients of reflex involvement of the muscles of the opposite arm, which characterized "distant" synergies. The coefficients of reflex involvement, respectively for the m. biceps brachii and m. triceps brachii of the opposite upper limb were obtained by calculation of the ratio of the mean amplitude recorded from the m. biceps (or triceps) on the resting side and mean amplitude recorded from the m. biceps on the side of retention of a load; the latter value was taken as 100%. In the norm, the value should not exceed 15%. An increase in this index is indicative of abnormal intensification of muscle coordinative interactions; if the coefficient of reflex involvement value exceeds 50%, such a disorder is qualified as gross.

Statistical analysis of the obtained data was performed using Statistic 8 software. Dispersion analysis ANOVA and a non-parametric two-tailed Mann-Whitney criterion were used in the course of comparison of the values observed in the different groups of the tested persons. Data obtained from the same patients before and after Levodopa treatment were compared using two-tailed paired t-test. The nonparametric Spearman test was used to evaluate possible correlation between above EMG parameters and subitems of UPDRS. Differences were considered to be significant at $P < 0.05$.

2.1.2 Results and discussion

In the group of age-matched healthy subjects, the EMG amplitude of the shoulder flexors and extensors during muscle relaxation showed low values (Fig 2, Controls 1, 2). The average EMG amplitude values for mm. biceps and triceps brachii varied across the subjects within 3-12 μV and the maximal amplitude values within 4-34 μV. For the whole group of healthy subjects, mean ± SE average amplitude did not exceed 5.9 ± 0.2 μV and mean ± SE maximal amplitude was no more 12.8 ± 2.3 μV (Table 1).

	Healthy controls (n = 42)	PD patients (n = 48)
Average EMG amplitude (μV)		
m. biceps dexter	5.3±0.8	19.5±3.8 ***
m. biceps sinister	5.5±0.7	21.4±7.4 ***
m. triceps dexter	5.9±0.2	13.1±1.7 *
m. triceps sinister	5.4±0.8	12.5±3.1
Maximal EMG amplitude (μV)		
m. biceps dexter	12.5±2.1	74.0±17.9 ***
m. biceps sinister	12,8±2.3	73.8±15.6 ***
m. triceps dexter	11.9±1.3	60.1±7.4
m. triceps sinister	12.3±2.1	61.9±12.0

Table 1. Resting EMG amplitudes of shoulder muscles in healthy controls and patients with Parkinson's disease. Notes: values are Mean ± Standard Error; n - number of subjects in each group; *, *** significant difference compared to healthy controls according to Mann-Whitney test, $p< 0.05$ and $p< 0.001$, respectively.

There were no statistical differences in EMG amplitude values between men and women. A significant positive correlation ($p<0.05$) was found for the resting activities of the antagonist muscles of the upper extremities in the age-matched healthy subjects (Table 2). The use of the envelope EMG construction technique demonstrated the presence of rhythmic burst muscle discharges in those cases where they were badly visualized on the EMG. Low amplitude burst discharges were occasionally identified in healthy subjects with the help of this technique (Fig 2, Control 2). Of EMG recordings taken from flexors and extensors on both sides in 42 persons of the control group, 11 recordings (6.5%) made in eight subjects displayed the burst discharges, with a mean ± SE frequency of 6.1 ± 0.3 Hz. The maximal amplitude of burst discharges in control subjects did not exceed 11-18 μV (mean ± SE = 14.3 ± 1.1 μV).

Healthy controls		PD patients, OFF state		PD patients, ON state	
right side	left side	more impaired side	less impaired side	more impaired side	less impaired side
0.42**	0.40**	0.27	0.33*	- 0.26	0.32*

Table 2. Correlation coefficients between average EMG amplitudes of the antagonist shoulder muscles (mm. biceps and triceps brachii) at rest in healthy controls and PD patients. * significant correlation, $p< 0.05$; ** is . $p< 0.01$.

In the group of PD patients, we observed a significant increase in the resting EMG amplitudes, which was ascribed to muscle relaxation disturbances. The mean average amplitude values for various study muscles, estimated for a whole PD group, were 2-3 times greater compared to control values, and the mean maximal amplitude values were approximately 5-6 times greater (Table 1). In some patients, average amplitude from a more impaired side reached 44-123 μV and maximal amplitude - 210-508 μV

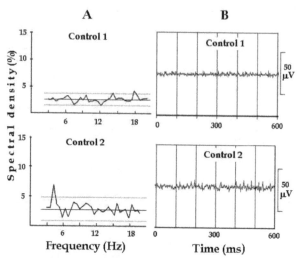

Fig. 2. The spectrograms of the power of EMG envelope frequency with 95% confidence intervals (A) and the corresponding resting EMG patterns of m. biceps brachii (B) in healthy controls (Control 1 and 2) Peak deviation on the spectrogram reflects the frequency of the rhythmic burst muscle discharges. Control 1: the absence of the burst muscle activity. Control 2: low amplitude burst muscle discharges with a frequency of 4 Hz in a healthy control subject.

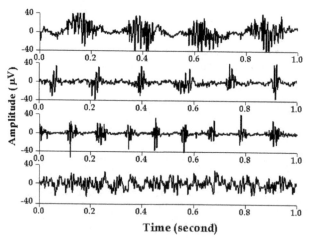

Fig. 3. Typical examples of EMGs registered in the resting state from three patients with the akinetic-rigid trembling form of Parkinson's disease (three upper records) and a patient with the akinetic-rigid form of this disease (low record).

Of interest is the fact that PD patients did not show a significant correlation between resting activities of the antagonist mm. biceps and triceps brachii on the dominant side, as has been true in the cases of the right and left sides in healthy subjects (Table 2). On the EMGs taken from PD patients with the akinetic-rigid-trembling form of the disease burst muscle discharges occurred as a rule with a frequency of 4-8 Hz. The mean ± SE frequency of the burst discharges was 5.2 ± 0.2 Hz. They had high amplitude (Fig.3). The maximal amplitude of burst discharges varied from 30 to 508 μV (mean ± SE = 89.8 ± 15.6 μV). Of special note, no significant correlation was found between resting EMG amplitude values and the occurrence of burst muscle discharges.

When comparing the data in OFF-state and ON-state, we observed a noticeable decrease in amplitude values. Mean ± SE average EMG amplitude of different muscles decreased to 8.2 ± 1.9 – 12.3 ± 5.1 μV and mean ± SE maximal amplitude decreased to 20.1± 5.3 – 32.1± 7.1 μV In this respect, the amplitude histograms made for the same patient during both states were very illustrative (Fig.4).

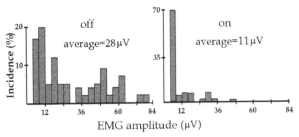

Fig. 4. The decrease of resting EMG amplitude values (calculated from peak to peak) of m. biceps brachii in a PD patient after intake of single dose of levodopa/carbidopa. OFF: the histograms of distribution of EMG amplitude values during the off-medication state; ON : one hour after drug intake. The bin of histograms is 4 μV.

But the treatment with levodopa did not result in the normalization of correlations between resting activities of the antagonist shoulder muscles (Table 2). Following a single dose of levodopa/carbidopa the number of cases displaying burst discharges with a frequency of 4-8 Hz decreased. In some patients the rhythmic discharges disappeared, as is shown in Figure 5, top records. In the other patients who displayed discharges after a dose of levodopa, an increase occurred in the discharges frequency (Fig. 5, lower records).

EMGs recorded during the performance of voluntary arm bending were found to differ considerably in healthy subjects and PD patients. In the healthy subjects, we clearly distinguished an onset of muscle phasic activation on the EMG (Fig. 6, Control). Means ± SE of average EMG amplitude of the mm. biceps brachii during their voluntary contraction was 49 ± 8 μV from the right and 44 ± 2 μV from the left, the maximal amplitude – 189 ± 31 μV and 137 ± 30 μV, respectively. In view of the low resting EMG amplitude value in healthy subjects, the coefficient of phasic activation in most cases was equal to 0.7-0.9; mean ± SE was 0.77 ± 0.04.

In contrast, in the PD patients it was often difficult to locate a site on the EMG at which the muscle phasic activation started because of increased resting tonic muscle activity and a very delayed rise in EMG amplitude after the delivery of a command to move (Fig. 6, PD). During peak voluntary flexor contraction, some patients showed a noticeable reduction of

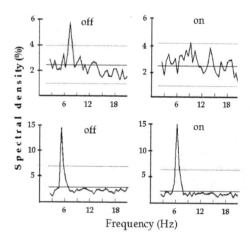

Fig. 5. Changes in the rhythmic (4-7 Hz) burst muscle discharges in patients with Parkinson's disease after the intake of an individual single dose of levodopa/carbidopa. The spectrograms of the power of EMG envelope frequency in two patients in an off-medication state (OFF) and one hour after drug intake (ON). After the drug intake, burst muscle discharges disappeared in one patient, while their frequency somewhat increased in another patient. For other notes see Fig. 1.

EMG amplitude, while other patients had the same meanings as healthy subjects. The coefficient of phasic activation of a voluntarily contracting mm biceps brachii in PD patients was generally decreased to 0.1-0.6 and, sometimes (when amplitude values at rest exceeded those that were observed during phasic activation), even had negative values; mean ± SE was 0.42 ± 0.08. The magnitude of the phasic activation decrease showed a distinct dependence on the side which was most affected. Reduction of the coefficient of phasic activation in the OFF patient group compared to healthy individuals was statistically significant (p<0.01).

Disturbance of coordinative muscle interactions was one more typical feature of the EMG recorded in Parkinson's patients. This was manifested in increased reflex involvement of the muscles of the opposite arm (distant synergy) at tonic tension of the m. biceps brachii at one of the sides within the period of retention of a load. In this group, the mean values of the coefficients of reflex involvement for the m. biceps brachii and m. triceps brachii of the opposite side exceeded 50%. As was already mentioned, these phenomena should be considered a gross disturbance of coordinative interactions. In control group the mean values of the coefficients of reflex involvement were 20-26%.

The dose of levodopa/carbidopa in PD patients produced a decrease in resting muscle activity parallel to an increase, more often, to normal values (0.8-0.9) of the coefficient of phasic activation during voluntary contraction of flexors. With regard to the reflex activation of the agonist and antagonist muscles during weight holding, a noticeable reduction of the coefficients of reflex involvement was only observed in some of the patients who took levodopa/carbidopa treatment. In seven patients, after medication even more marked enhancement developed in the agonist or antagonist muscles, and was registered during the performance of the functional test.

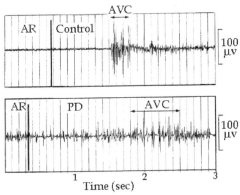

Fig. 6. The phasic activation of m. biceps brachii dexter during voluntary movement in healthy control and off-medication patient with Parkinson's disease. Two sections of native EMGs in a healthy 64-year old subject (Control) and in a 53-year old patient (PD). The vertical thick lines designate the moment of experimenter's command. The horizontal lines over EMGs designate the periods, at which the amplitude measurements of maximal muscular activity during voluntary contractions (AVC) were taken. The resting EMG amplitudes (AR) were measured during 5 s prior to command presentation.

The described quantitative EMG parameters added fundamentally to the clinical motor characteristics of PD patients and correlated selectively with definite UPDRS subitems. Thus, the most significant increases in the resting average and maximal EMG amplitude and decreases in the coefficient of phasic activation were observed in patients whose part III UPDRS scores exceeded 50. At the same time, the greatest involvement of the reciprocal muscles during the functional test was noted in patients with high part II UPDRS scores on the upper extremity daily activity. These patients also, had the greatest dyskinesia (disability) scores. We established the following statistically significant correlations (see Table 3). The resting muscle amplitudes from the more affected side correlated positively with the upper extremity rigidity and general motor scores. We found negative correlations between the phasic activation coefficient of m. biceps brachii from the more affected side and the upper extremity rigidity and general motor scores. The antagonist muscle involvement during the tonic strain holding a weight correlated positively with the handwriting, cutting food, dressing score and dyskinesia (disability) score. Levodopa intake did not influence essentially on the correlations between the reflex muscle involvement and UPDRS scores.

We found the present computer EMG analysis to be a sensitive tool for the objective evaluation of PD symptoms and to quantify the efficacy of levodopa therapy. One of the most useful EMG signs of extrapyramidal insufficiency appears to be the resting EMG amplitude value. In PD, the resting EMGs in the OFF state were characterized by the splashes of high muscle activity in contrast to the flat EMGs seen in age-matched healthy subjects. The average resting EMG amplitude was 2-3 times and the maximal amplitude was 5-6 times greater in PD patients than in the control group. Of interest are our data indicating the statistically significant correlation between levels of resting activity in the antagonist muscles (m. biceps and triceps brachii) in healthy subjects and the lack of such a correlation in PD patients on the most affected side. These findings appear to be an objective EMG manifestation of the disorganisation of the brain's neuronal excitatory-inhibitory processes and the loss of functional balance between the structures which regulate muscle tone, all of which are due to a neostriatal dopamine deficit (DeLong, 1990).

EMG indices		Upper extremity rigidity score (point 22)	Motor score (points 18-31)	Handwriting, cutting food, dressing score (points 8-10)	Dyskinesia (disability) score (point 33)
Average amplitude of m. biceps at rest	ON	0.51 *	0.50 *	ns	ns
	OFF	ns	0.67 **	ns	ns
Phasic activation coefficient of m .biceps during voluntary contraction	ON	-0.49 *	-0.60 **	ns	ns
	OFF	ns	-0.64 **	ns	ns
M. biceps involvement under tonic strain of m. biceps of the opposite arm	ON	ns	ns	0.55 *	0.52*
	OFF	ns	ns	0.52 *	ns
M. triceps involvement under tonic strain of m. biceps of the opposite arm	ON	ns	ns	0.57 **	0.48*
	OFF	ns	ns	0.53 *	0.51*

Table 3. Significant correlations of EMG indices with the UPDRS scores studied in 20 PD patients in which the clinical "ON-OFF" phenomenon was verified. Data on the EMG indices and the upper extremity rigidity score for a more impaired side are presented. *- $p<0.05$; ** - $p<0.01$; "ns "- not statistically significant ($p\geq0.05$).

A distinguishing feature of the bioelectrical muscle activity at rest in PD patients was the presence of burst muscle discharges with a rhythm of 4-8 Hz. It should be noted that no significant correlation was found between resting EMG amplitude value and the occurrence of burst muscle discharges. This fact is consistent with the viewpoint that muscle rigidity and tremor at PD do not constitute symptoms which influence one another, and that different pathophysiological mechanisms underlie their origin (Furukawa et al., 1991; Otsuka et al., 1996).

The brain systems, regulating the tonic and phasic muscle activities, were shown to be antagonistically interrelated: the activation of the phasic processes is accompanied by an inhibition of the tonic impulses and, vice versa, the enhancement of tonic impulsation hampers the phasic activity (Houk, 1979). In PD, due to an increased tonic muscle activity at rest, increment in EMG amplitude during phasic activation was reduced relative to the norm, and, in addition, a decrease in the active contraction amplitudes occurred in some of the patients. As a consequence, the phasic activation coefficient of the voluntarily contracting m. biceps brachii of the patients was generally reduced to 0.1-0.6 and even had negative values, while in healthy subjects the value of the phasic activation coefficient was in most cases 0.7-0.9. Our study data suggest that phasic activation coefficients represent a sufficiently informative index that may be used to quantify phasic muscle activity in PD.

Involvement of the agonist and antagonist muscles appeared to be useful for establishing cooriditating muscle relationships. We demonstrated significantly ($p<0.05$) greater activation of the agonist and antagonist muscles during m. biceps brachii tonic strain in PD patients compared to age-matched healthy subjects. The present findings confirm the results of other investigators who consider this fact to be a consequence of increased excitation in the motor centers, caused by dopaminergic control failure (Kryzhanovsky et al, 2002).

When examining the action of an individual dose of levodopa/carbidopa in PD patients with ON-OFF phenomenon, we observed distinct positive drug effects in the following EMG parameters: average and maximal EMG amplitudes at rest; the number of cases with registered rhythmic burst muscle discharges of 4-8 Hz; value of the phasic activation coefficient during voluntary muscle contraction. However, levodopa therapy didn't appear to be effective in terms of the normalization of coordinating agonist - antagonist muscle relationships, either at rest and during holding a weight. In some of patients on levodopa/carbidopa, we even observed an enhancement of the activation of agonist and antagonist muscles during above functional test. We believe that such an increased coactivation of the agonist and antagonist muscles is an objective indicator of risk for developing levodopa-induced dyskinesia in PD patients. According to the literature data, the latter is the result of hypersensitivity of the dopamine receptors in the nigrostriatal system or of a disturbed balance between the degrees of activation of D1 and D2 dopamine receptors (Jenner, 1994).

2.2 Statistics of EMG distribution in patients with Parkinson's disease

The histograms of distribution of EMG amplitude values at rest are informative characteristic of muscle activity (Meigal, 2009). The histogram sharpness and statistical EMG parameters, such as range, variance and kurtosis reflect the magnitude of bioelectrical muscle signals and the level of motor unit synchronization.

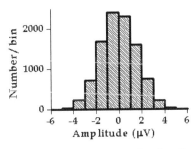

Fig. 7. Example of the histogram of resting EMG amplitudes distribution in healthy subject.

An artifact-free EMG recordings (no less than 10 seconds in duration) from the flexors and extensors (mm. biceps and triceps brachii), registered in 33 patients with PD and 24 age-matched healthy subjects at rest, were analyzed by the computer programs "Origin 8" and "Statistic 8". EMG in healthy subjects was characterized by low amplitude, flat symmetric histogram (fig. 7) and small values of range, variance and kurtosis (table 4). Range did not exceed 20 μV, variance – 7 and kurtosis – 0.4. In patients with the akinetic-rigid form of the disease, the amplitude of EMG signals was considerably increased because of impossibility of entire muscle relaxation. The mean values of EMG statistical parameters, estimated for this PD group, were significantly (p<0.001) augmented as compared to control. In some patients range amounted to 66 μV, variance – 56 and kurtosis – 1.4 (table 4).

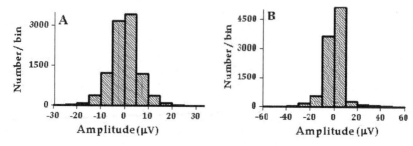

Fig. 8. Examples of the histograms of resting EMG amplitudes distribution in a patient with akinetic-rigid form of Parkinson's disease (A) and a patient with akinetic-rigid- trembling form of this disease (B).

Groups of the tested persons	Statistical parameters		
	Range (μV)	Variance	Kurtosis
Patients with akinetic-rigid-trembling form of the disease n=20	112.75 ± 16.80 *** (24.48 – 381.62)	147.20 ± 44.38 ** (6.91 – 950.63)	4.32 ± 0.51 *** (1.04 – 12.98)
Patients with akinetic-rigid form of the disease n=13	36.81 ± 3.96 *** (21.16 – 66.18)	20.26 ± 4.26 *** (7.89 – 56.16)	0.58 ± 0.14 *** (0.07 – 1.40)
Control group of age-matched healthy subjects n=24	11.18 ± 0.71 (7.08 – 16.46)	2.30 ± 0.31 (0.70 – 5.14)	-0.17 ± 0.03 (-0.10 to -0.30) n = 10 0.18 ± 0.04 (0.01 – 0.33) n = 14

Table 4. Statistical characteristics of EMG in patients with Parkinson's disease and age-matched healthy subjects. EMG characteristics in patients were taken at the side where morbid affection was more expressed; in healthy persons such characteristics were taken at the side where higher values were observed. ** p <0.01, *** p <0.001 compared to control group. n is number of subjects in each group. In brackets the range of indices in different tested persons is presented.

Patients with the akinetic-rigid-trembling form of PD had the highest values of the EMG statistical parameters. The histograms of EMG amplitude distribution had a sharp peak (fig. 8, B). In some patients of this PD group range reached 382 µV, variance – 951 and kurtosis – 13 (table 4). Correlation analyses revealed statistically significant connection of kurtosis with scores of the point 20 of UPDRS, estimating intensity of tremor of the hand, on which EMG was registered. A coefficient of nonparametric Spearman rank-order correlation between these indices was 0.46 (p<0.01). This fact is in accordance with the point of view (Meigal, 2009) that kurtosis well reflects synchronization of motor units responsible for the origin of burst muscle discharges.

2.3 Fractal dynamics of EMGs in patients with Parkinson's disease

Fractal analysis is a new method for biomedical signal processing. Nonlinear analysis techniques are necessary to understand the complexity of the EMG. Study of fractal dynamics of EMG data is based on detrended fluctuation analysis and calculation of Hurst exponent. The Hurst exponent is used as a measure of the long term memory of time series, i.e., the autocorrelation of the time series. (Talebinejad et al., 2010).

Fractal dynamics of EMG signals was studied in 33 patients with akinetic-rigid-trembling form of PD (mean ± SE age 62.1 ± 2.6, range 48-77 years), 30 age-matched healthy subjects (mean ± SE age 65.4 ± 1.9, range 57-78 years) and 20 persons of middle age (mean ± SE age 48.3 ± 1.49, range 45-58 years). EMGs were recorded from m. biceps brachii at the side, where morbid affection was more expressed, at rest no less than 10 seconds in duration.

The rescaled range was calculated for time series. The first step was calculation of the mean. Then mean-adjusted series were created and the cumulative deviate series were calculated from the formula:

$$y(k) = \sum_{i=1}^{k}(z_i - \overline{z})$$
(2)

Where $\overline{z}$ is the mean and $z(i)$ is the value from time series. Then the row of values y (k), k = 1,...N was divided into the segments of length n, and within the limits of each segment the equalization of stright, approximating the sequence of $y(k)$, was defined by least squares method. It is considered that approximation of y_n (k) is the local trend. Further a standard deviation was created from the formula:

$$F(n) = \sqrt{\frac{1}{N}[(y(k) - y_n(k)]^2}$$
(3)

Dependence lg $F(lg$ $n)$ was further built, the angle of slope of approximating line was determined and the value of Hurst index was estimated (Stanley et al., 1999).

We identified three different patterns of surface EMG signals according to fractal dimension (Fig 9, 10): with one, two and three scaling regions, every of which is characteristic by own local exponent. In healthy subjects, the fractal dimension with two exponents was most frequently observed, in 60% among persons of middle age and in 50% among elderly individuals. One exponent was observed in 20% in both groups of healthy subjects and three exponents – in 20% and 30% in middle age and elderly, respectively. In patients with akinetic-rigid-trembling form of PD the fractal dimension of surface EMG signals with three exponents was most characteristic (64%). One exponent did not occur in PD patients (Fig. 11).

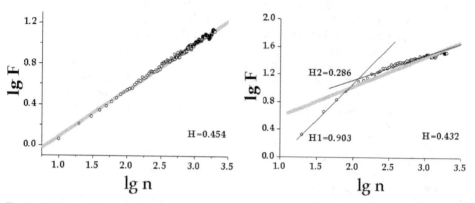

Fig. 9. Patterns of fractal dimension of the surface EMG signals with one and two exponents. Thick line is general exponent, thin lines are local exponents. H is general Hurst index; H1, H2, H3 are values of local Hurst indices.

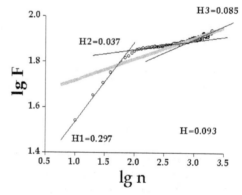

Fig. 10. Pattern of fractal dimension of the surface EMG signals with three exponents. Thick line is general exponent, thin lines are local exponents. H is general Hurst index; H1, H2, H3 are values of local Hurst indices.

Another difference concerned the value of general Hurst index (H). In persons of middle age mean value of H was 0.47 ± 0.02 (range 0.32 – 0.71) and in elderly – 0.44 ± 0.02 (range 0.33 – 0.57). In PD patients mean value of H was significantly ($p<0.01$) lower as compared to elderly subjects – 0.31 ± 0.03 (range 0.09 – 0.49). In PD patients, the value of Hurst index of the third scaling region (H3) in patterns with three exponents also significantly differed from H3 in healthy subjects. H3 was 0.30 ± 0.06 in middle-aged persons, 0.39 ± 0.05 in elderly and 0.14 ± 0.05 in patients with PD ($p<0.05$). It is of interest that the tendency to negative correlation between H and motor scores of part III UPDRS was observed in patients with PD ($r = -0.35$, $p =0.05$).

Our data showed essential alterations in short and more long-range EMG correlation properties in patients with akinetic-rigid-trembling form of PD. The mean value of H1/H3 in patterns with three exponents in the group of PD patients came up to 27.2 ± 9.5 that significantly (p<0.001) differed from same value in elderly subjects (2.7 ± 0.5). Negative correlation between H1 and H3 (r = -0.67, p<0.01) was revealed in PD patients.

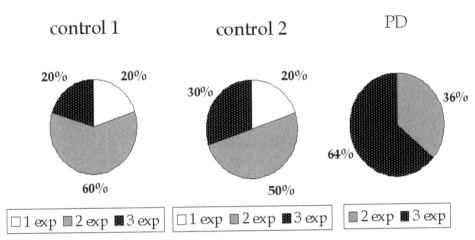

Fig. 11. Comparison of the incidence of different patterns of surface EMG signals fractal dimension (with one, two or three Hurst exponents) in persons of middle age (control 1), elderly subjects (control 2) and patients with Parkinson's disease (PD).

Overall, the present investigation has demonstrated the following distinctive features of surface EMG signals fractal dimension in patients with akinetic-rigid-trembling form of PD: 1) correlation behavior of the resting EMG time series in patients was more complex compared to healthy subjects and often suggested three scaling regions; 2) the value of Hurst exponent was significantly lower in patients, its value may descend to 0.1 - 0.2 that indicates a time series with negative autocorrelation (e.g. a decrease between values will probably be followed by an increase); 3) considerable degradation of short and longer range correlation properties, that, perhaps, is associated with the loss of integrated physiological responsiveness at this disease (Goldberger et al., 2002).

2.4 EMG characteristics of clinically healthy kinsmen of the patients with Parkinson's disease

According to modern concepts, the genetic factor plays a considerable role in the development of Parkinson's disease. Modifications in several genetic loci responsible for the development of this disease have been identified. The considerable role of the genetic factor for the propensity to Parkinson's disease has been confirmed by the data of epidemiological studies. The frequency of development of this disease in kinsmen of Parkinsonian patients is two to seven times higher than that in persons of the control groups (Elbaz et al., 1999). Symptoms of functional insufficiency of the extrapyramidal system can be identified very early, namely several decades prior to possible onset of the development of the clinical form of Parkinson's disease (Berg et al., 2002). Prevention or deceleration of the development of this disease can be provided by the detection of the early, presymptomatic stage of the neurodegenerative process and identification of informative "biomarkers" of PD (Illarioshkin, 2008). We studied surface EMG in clinically healthy kinsmen of the patients suffering from PD in order to detect latent symptoms of extrapyramidal insufficiency that can be considered genetic determinants of the risk of development of the above disease. The task of our study included estimation of the frequency of occurrence of muscle activity disorders in kinsmen of the patients, characterization of correlations between the appearance symptoms of extrapyramidal insufficiency and age of the tested persons, and formulation of recommendations for individuals belonging, from the aspect of risk of development of PD, to a risk group.

We examined two groups of persons. The first group consisted of 37 clinically healthy kinsmen/kinswomen of patients suffering from PD (children, brothers, and sisters; 22 women and 15 men aged 30 to 56; mean age 45.6 ± 1.5 years). The second group (control) included 30 healthy young and middle-aged persons (19 women and 11 men; age nearly corresponding to that of persons of the first group , i.e., from 34 to 58 years, mean age 46.9 ± 2.2 years. All examined persons gave informed consent to be involved in the study. We recorded surface EMG at rest using superficial bipolar electrodes fixed on the flexor and extensor of the elbow joint (m. biceps brachii and m. triceps brachii, respectively); an electroneuromyograph NeuroMPF (Russia) was used. The detailed description of method is presented in section 2.1.1.

In 9 (24%) clinically healthy kinsmen of PD patients symptoms of functional insufficiency of the extrapyramidal system were evident. They demonstrated the mean amplitude value of 5.4-12.4 μV, maximal amplitude value of 25-93 μV, and the mean power of EMG oscillations reached 0.85- 1.8 mV/sec. In control group the mean amplitude value varied from 3.4 to 5.0 μV, maximal amplitude varied from 5.6 to 20.6 μV and the mean power of EMG oscillations did not exceed 0.02-0.71 mV/sec. Higher values of the intensity of electrical muscle activity in kinsmen of PD patients positively correlated with their age; it should be noted that, in this respect, age older than 45 years can be considered to be critical. The number of elder (older than 45 years) subjects with values of the mean power of EMG oscillations higher than the mean value of this parameter in persons of control group exceeded significantly the number of elder persons with low values of the mean power of EMG oscillations ($p < 0.05$, χ^2 criterion). The correlation coefficient between the age of the tested persons and the value of mean power of EMG oscillations was 0.40 ($p < 0.05$).

In 6 (16%) kinsmen of PD patients short burst-like discharges consisting of two to three oscillations generated with a frequency of 5-10 Hz were observed within the resting EMG (Fig. 12). As a rule, the amplitude of these potentials did not exceed 52 μV.

For more detailed investigation we used statistics of EMG distribution, namely such parameters as range, variance and kurtosis. Range and variance reflect the extent of bioelectrical muscle signals. Kurtosis characterizes motor unit synchronization. We supposed that statistical methods might appear effective for exposure of pathological signs of muscle activity. In control group of healthy middle-aged persons the extreme value of resting EMG amplitude range was 20 μV, variance – 7 and kurtosis – 0.4. The parameters of range, variance and kurtosis were considered going out outside a norm, if they exceeded the extreme values of these indices in the control group. We found 16 (43 %) kinsmen of patients with PD, who had high statistical parameters of EMG signals. In 14 kinsmen (38 %) range and variance were augmented compared to the extreme values of these indices in the control group. In 11 kinsmen (29 %) kurtosis had higher values than normal, presumably, reflecting enhanced synchronization in activity of motor units (Table 5).

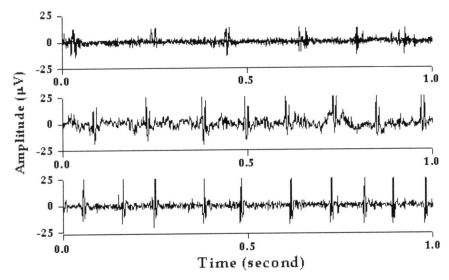

Fig. 12. Types of burst-like muscle discharges with frequency 6, 8 and 10 Hz recorded in three kinsmen of patients suffering from Parkinson's disease.

Statistical parameters	Number of tested persons
Range [22.46 – 113.61 µV] Variance [8.23 – 112.32] Kurtosis [0.43 – 16.30]	9 (24 %)
Range [24.22 – 28.33 µV] Variance [8.08 – 13.55]	5 (14 %)
Kurtosis [0.67; 0.70]	2 (5 %)
Total	16 (43 %)

Table 5. Incidence of resting EMG statistical parameters, going out outside a norm, in kinsmen of patients with Parkinson's disease. In square brackets the range of indices in different persons is presented.

The data obtained in our work agree with findings of other authors who emphasized that data obtained using EMG techniques are of a high informative value in the diagnostics of subclinical manifestations of weakening of the supraspinal control (Robichaud et al., 2009), and that the genetic factor responsible for the propensity for development of the extrapyramidal insufficiency is rather important (Elbaz et al., 1999; Illarioshkin, 2002).

A single common pathogenetic factor, namely conformational modifications of some cellular proteins at a post-translational stage of their synthesis, underlies most neurodegenerative diseases, including PD. Due to the existence of powerful compensatory and detoxication systems in cells, such units are capable of successfully "overcoming" abnormal protein substrates for many years (Sherman & Goldberg, 2001). Delayed manifestation of clinical symptoms of the above disease is a feature of "conformational" pathologies of the brain. Latent pathological process can run course up to 30 years (Kryzhanovskii et al., 1995). The rate of pathological modifications in nerve cells within the presymptomatic period of PD is relatively low, but neuronal death is intensified significantly with transition to the stage of manifestation of this disease (Antonini et al., 1998). In relation to the above data, it is quite obvious that early diagnostics of the existence of latent extrapyramidal insufficiency is of exceptional importance. To prevent manifestations of PD in persons belonging to the risk group with respect to the development of parkinsonism, certain basic recommendations should be taken into account. They included a description of the rational daily routine, a recommended dietary intake with an increased content of vitamin B6 (pyridoxine, which is the main catalyzer in the synthesis of dopamine), and also a list of the drugs whose long-term administration should be avoided. Among the latter drugs are therapeutic agents whose administration leads either to depletion of the regulatory function of the dopaminergic system or to an increase in the functional activity of this system. Among such agents are haloperidol, the indole reserpine, fluoxetine (Prozac), metoclopramide (Cerucal), clozapine, and Cordarone, as well as derivatives of phenothiazine and butyrophenol, and also lithium preparations.

3. Investigation of contingent negative variation

Endogenous cortical movement-related reaction contingent negative variation (CNV) is a sensitive indicator for the objective evaluation of the severity of PD and quantifying the efficacy of antiparkinsonian therapy. Many authors identify two phases in CNV: an early phase, the Bereitschaftpotential, and a late phase, the negative slope (Filipovic et al., 1997). It has been suggested that these are generated by different brain structures: the cerebellar efferent system is more involved in generating the Bereitschaftpotential, while the basal ganglia are more involved in generating the negative slope (Ikeda et al., 1997). The question of the relationships between each of these phases and higher integrative processes and the mechanisms of direct motor control have received insufficient study. The aims of the present work were to study the extent to which the early and late phases of CNV depend on motor and mental functions and to determine what effect have neurotrophic agents on CNV. Tasks to be addressed were: 1) identification of the individual characteristics of the early and late phases of CNV in patients with PD as compared with subjects of similar age; 2) identification of correlation the measures of the two phases of CNV with clinical characteristics of the PD patients; 3) investigation the effect of the brain-derived peptide drug cerebrolysin on the amplitude characteristics of CNV in PD.

3.1 Methods

Studies were performed using 28 healthy subjects (13 male, 15 female, age 48–73 years, mean age 60.9 ± 1.2 years) and 56 patients with idiopathic PD (23 male, 33 female, age 45–74 years, mean age 61.3 ± 1.1 years). Patients were in stages 1.5–3.0 (2.2 ± 0.1) H-Y (international classification of Hoehn and Yaht, 1967). Patients received basic antiparkinsonism treatment with levodopa-containing agents (levodopa/carbidopa). Individual daily doses of levodopa were 250–750 mg. All subjects were right-handed.

Monopolar recordings were made of CNV from intermediate leads: frontal (Fz), central (Cz), and parietal (Pz). The indifferent electrode was located on the earlobe. The ground electrode was located on the left forearm. During studies, subjects were in a relaxed, calm state with the eyes closed. Bioelectrical signals were passed to an amplifier with a bandpass of 0.08–15 Hz and then to a computer hard disk. CNV was recorded using two sound stimuli of different intensities with a 1-sec interval: the ready signal was at 50 dB HL and the trigger signal was at 80 dB HL. The subject pressed a key in response to the trigger signal. Analysis was performed using computer programs. The sampling frequency was 200 Hz. The analysis time was 3.1 sec, the first 400 ms being a record of the baseline electroencephalogram. Mean initial activity was determined from an artefact-free part of the electroencephalogram trace. Averaging of 30 trials yielded: 1) the duration of CNV measured as the time interval between the start of the negative deviation from the baseline after the ready stimulus and the moment of presentation of the trigger stimulus (ms); 2) the areas of Bereitschaftpotential and negative slope, between the baseline and the negativity curve of the corresponding region $S = (\Sigma Ai) \times \Delta t$ (mV·ms), where Ai is the amplitude of the negative deviation from the initial level at a sampling frequency of 200 Hz and Δt is a time interval of duration 5 ms; 3) the mean amplitudes of Bereitschaftpotential and negative slope defined by $A = \Sigma Ai/n$ (µV). The program also allowed calculation of the simple sensorimotor reaction time (the mean latent period of pressing the key in response to the trigger signal).

Motor symptomatology was assessed quantitatively in patients with PD in points using the unified scale UPDRS. The total score was measured in each of three dimension scales: I (impairments in thought, mood), II (decreased daily activity, impairment of hygiene activities); and III (disturbances of motor function, including bradykinesia, rigidity, and tremor) using four-point subscales for each symptom. General cognitive status of the PD patients was characterized using the standard quantitative scale Mini Mental State Examination (MMSE). The overall assessment of mental functions in normal patients yielded 30 points. Decreases in the total score to less than 25 were regarded as a sign of early dementia.

The state of coordinatory muscle interactions was studied in 29 patients with PD (aged 47–72 years) by assessing the level of reciprocal involvement of the triceps brachii antagonist muscle (the extensor muscle of the shoulder) on functional loading of the biceps brachii muscle (the flexor of the shoulder) on the right side. EMGs were recorded using bipolar skin electrodes (0.5×1.0 cm^2) with a constant interelectrode distance of 1.5 cm. Bioelectrical signals were passed to the amplifiers of a Medikor MG440 (Budapest) electromyography with a bandpass of 10 Hz to 10 kHz. Functional loading on the biceps brachii muscle was applied by holding a load of 2 kg on the elevated and forward extended arm for 5 sec. With the patient in the calm, relaxed state and during holding of the load, at least 100 measurements were processed using the computer program to determine the mean EMG amplitude in the triceps brachii at rest (Ar) and loading (Al), the coefficient of reciprocal involvement of the antagonist muscle was calculated as $Al/(Ar + Al)$. This coefficient had a value of 0.5 when the amplitude on loading showed no change. If the amplitude decreased, then coefficient of reciprocal involvement had values of less than 0.5, while increases yielded coefficient of reciprocal involvement values of greater than 0.5.

The effects of cerebrolysin on measures of CNV were studied in 21 patients with PD that were taking antiparkinsonian therapy, which was not changed during one month before cerebrolysin treatment and under the whole cerebrolysin course (intravenously 10 ml, during 10 days). Before and after cerebrolysin treatment we studied clinical scores of UPDRS and CNV.

Data obtained in healthy subjects and patients with PD were compared using the non-parametric Mann–Whitney test. Data obtained in individual patients before and after administration of cerebrolysin were analyzed using the t- test for pairwise dependent variables. Correlations between the amplitudes of the two phases of CNV, the UPDRS and MMSE scales, and the levels of reciprocal involvement of antagonist muscles were identified by calculating the correlation coefficient by the non-parametric Spearman method (rS). Relationships were regarded as moderate at $0.3 \leq rS \leq 0.5$ and considerable at $rS > 0.5$. Differences were taken as significant at $p < 0.05$.

3.2 Results
3.2.1 Characteristics of the early and late phases of CNV in healthy subjects and patients with Parkinson's disease

Repeat studies in individual subjects showed that CNV had the most stable characteristics in the central medial lead (Cz), so data obtained from this lead were analyzed in detail. CNV in healthy subjects could usually be discriminated into two phases: an early phase (Bereitschaftpotential) 505–728 (596.3 ± 12.1) ms before the trigger signal and a late phase (negative slope) apparent as an additional negative deviation 170–365 (230.2 ± 15.4) ms before the trigger signal (Fig. 13). However, the second phase was not always clearly evident; in this situation CNV consisted of an initial drop-off followed by a uniform negative deviation from baseline lasting to the trigger signal. In these cases, the second half of CNV was analyzed as the second phase. In healthy subjects, the mean amplitudes of Bereitschaftpotential and negative slope were 9.0 ± 1.1 and 10.6 ± 1.0 µV respectively, with areas of 2.8 ± 0.4 and 3.2 ± 0.2 mV·ms (Table 6). Unlike healthy subjects, CNV in many patients was poorly evident; in some, no negativity at all developed between the ready and trigger signals (Fig. 14). Statistical analysis of the data revealed significant decreases in the mean amplitudes and areas of both phases of CNV in patients with PD as compared with healthy subjects (Table 6). In addition, patients showed an increase in the simple sensorimotor reaction time for pressing the key in response to the trigger signal, from 240.9 ± 13.7 ms in healthy subjects to 299.6 ± 17.3 ms ($p < 0.05$).

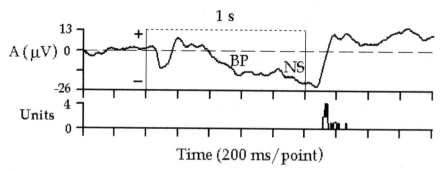

Fig. 13. Characteristic record of contingent negative variation (CNV) in healthy subject aged 64 years. A is the amplitude, µV. BP is the early phase and NS' is the late phase of CNV. Vertical lines show the moments of presentation of the warning and trigger signals, with an interval of 1 sec. Positivity is shown by upward deviations from the baseline and negativity by downward deviations. Low trace is simple sensorimotor reaction times for pressing the key after presentation of the trigger signal. Units show the number of keypresses.

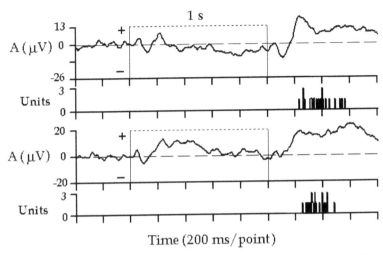

Fig. 14. Example traces of contingent negative variation (CNV) in two patients with Parkinson's disease aged 65 and 54, years. CNV in the first patient was poorly expressed, and the second patient showed no negative deviation. For further details see caption to Fig. 13.

Group	Area of early phase, mV·ms	Mean amplitude of early phase, μV	Area of late phase, mV·ms	Mean amplitude of late phase, μV
Healthy, n = 28	2,8 ± 0,4	9,0 ± 1,1	3,2 ± 0,2	10,6 ± 1,0
Patients, n = 53	1,8 ± 0,2 *	5,7 ± 0,4 *	1,7 ± 0,1 *	6,5 ± 0,5 *
p	< 0,01	< 0,01	< 0,001	< 0,01

Table 6. Differences in measures of the two phases of contingent negative variation in the median central lead (Cz) in healthy subjects and patients with Parkinson's disease. n is the number of subjects in the group.* is significant difference between patients with PD and healthy subjects (non-parametric Mann–Whitney test).

3.2.2 Correlation between the amplitudes of the early and late phases of CNV and characteristics of the patients with Parkinson's disease

Correlation analysis revealed moderately significant relationships between the amplitudes of the two phases of CNV and point scores for individual subscales on the UPDRS. Table 7 shows that the mean amplitudes of Bereitschaftpotential and negative slope were negatively related (rS = -0.31 and rS = -0.3 respectively, $p < 0.05$) to the total point score on UPDRS subscale II, which reflects decreases in the activities of daily living (impairments of hygiene habits, cutting and holding food, difficulty dressing and walking). It was interesting to note that there was a selective negative correlation (rS = -0.32, $p < 0.05$) between the magnitude of negative slope and symptoms on subscale II such as gait freezing, while Bereitschaftpotential showed no significant relationships of this type. There were no significant correlational relationships between measures of the two phases of CNV and the total score on UPDRS subscale III, reflecting intrinsic motor functions, or with clinical point scores for rigidity, tremor, or bradykinesia.

Clinical scale points	Mean amplitude of early phase	Mean amplitude of late phase
Total points on UPDRS subscale II; n=56	rS = -0,31 *	rS = -0,30 *
Points on UPDRS subscale II; item 14 (gait freezing); n=56	rS = -0,24	rS = -0,32 *
Coefficient of reciprocal involvement between antagonist muscles; n=29	rS = -0,58 **	rS = -0,51 **
Total score on MMSE (mental functions); n=28	rS = 0,47 *	rS = 0,47 *
Points on MMSE item 4 (memory); n=28	rS = 0,56 **	rS = 0,46 *

Table 7. Relationships between the amplitudes of the two phases of contingent negative variation in the median central lead (Cz) and clinical point scores in patients with Parkinson's disease. n is number of investigated persons. rS is the Spearman correlation coefficient.. * is p<0.05; ** is p<0.01.

The existence of a link between measures of the two phases of CNV and the state of coordinatory muscle interactions was addressed by studying the relationship between the amplitude characteristics of CNV and the extent of reciprocal impairments between antagonist muscles in patients with PD by calculating the coefficient of reciprocal involvement. Bereitschaftpotential and negative slope were completely absent in those patients in whom the coefficient of reciprocal involvement was high (0.67–0.8), which is evidence for an abnormal increase in the reciprocal involvement of the extensor muscles in the operation of the flexor muscles. Conversely, low coefficient of reciprocal involvement was associated with maximal amplitudes for both phases of CNV. The negative correlations between the extent of reciprocal muscle involvement and the amplitudes of Bereitschaftpotential and negative slope were significant ($rS = -0.58$ and $rS = -0.51$ respectively, $p < 0.01$). Comparison of the parameters of CNV and quantitative measures on the MMSE scale revealed an identical moderate positive relationship ($rS = 0.47$, $p < 0.05$) with the magnitudes of both phases and the state of mental functions in patients with PD (Table 7). The strongest relationship was between Bereitschaftpotential and point 4 of the MMSE scale, which reflects memory ($rS = 0.56$, $p < 0.01$).

3.2.3 Effects of cerebrolysin on measures of CNV in patients with Parkinson's disease

The results of the present study showed that the course of cerebrolysin treatment combined with levodopa has the positive therapeutic effect, such as: a significant decrease of the part I, II and III UPDRS scores. A decrease of the UPDRS part I scores (improvement in thought, mood) and part II scores (that is an increase of daily activity and ability of more full value selfattendance) was the most expressed. Significant increase of the CNV amplitude value and duration well reflected the enhancement of the brain activity (Table 8).

Time of investigation	Duration of CNV (ms)	Mean amplitude of CNV (µV)	UPDRS part I scores	UPDRS part II scores	UPDRS part III scores
Before CER	423.1 ± 43.3	3.1 ± 0.9	5.6 ± 0.7	14.2 ± 1.3	40.4 ± 3.4
After CER	600.6 ± 38.5*	6.8 ± 1.4***	3.5 ± 0.7***	11.3 ± 1.4***	32.9 ± 3.2*

Table 8. Change of contingent negative variation (CNV) and UPDRS scores in Parkinson's disease patients after cerebrolysin (CER) treatment. Footnotes: * - the significant change after cerebrolysin treatment, $p < 0.05$; *** - $p < 0.001$ (paired t-test).

3.3 Discussion

The results showed that patients with PD, as compared with healthy subjects, had significant decreases in the amplitudes and areas of both the early and late phases of CNV. We established that one significant factor decreasing both phases of CNV in patients with parkinsonism is impairment of coordinatory muscle interactions. Thus, the more significant the coordinatory impairment, apparent as an increase in the reciprocal involvement of the antagonist muscle during functional tests, the smaller the values of Bereitschaftpotential and negative slope in patients (rS = –0.58 and rS = –0.51 respectively; $p < 0.01$). As shown by the present data, a further significant factor affecting both phases of CNV was the state of mental functions. The positive correlation between Bereitschaftpotential amplitude and point 4 on the MMSE scale, characterizing memory (rS = 0.56, $p < 0.01$), was the most marked. This suggests that CNV can be regarded not only as a correlate of the initiation and preparation of motor structures for performing an action, but also as a neurophysiological component of mental functions. This point of view is in good agreement with published data showing sharp reductions in CNV in Alzheimer's-type dementia (Zappoli et al.,1991). The suggestion (Ikeda et al., 1997), that the nigrostriatal dopaminergic system has a greater role in generating the late phase than the early phase of CNV is supported by our finding of the existence of a selective negative correlation ($p < 0.05$) between the magnitude of negative slope and the severity of symptoms such as gait freezing; there was no such correlation for Bereitschaftpotential. The symptom of "gait freezing" does not correlate with rigidity or bradykinesia (Bartels et al., 2003), is significantly decreased by levodopa (Schaarsma et al., 2003) and depends on the functional state of the globus pallidus: stimulation of its internal zone (the main source of the efferent output of the whole of the striopallidal complex) effectively eliminates the phenomenon of "gait freezing" (Katayama et al., 2000). The results of the present study enlarge the perspectives in application of cerebrolysin and are in agreement with literature data on the efficacy of cerebrolysin in neurological practice. Thus, it was shown that cerebrolysin might be useful in patients with senile dementia of the Alzheimer type (Ruther, al., 2002). The positive therapeutic effect of the brain-derived peptide drug cerebrolysin can be connected with its ability to increase the expression of BBB-GLUT1 and MAP2 genes, that improves the transport of the glucose through blood-brain barrier and keeps the cytoskeleton wholeness accordingly (Boado, 2001). Cerebrolysin can also reduce the glutamate induced excitotoxicity (Hutter-Pair, al., 1998).

Obtained data proof that CNV appears to be a good tool for the evaluation of the medication efficiency. The parameters of CNV well reflected the improvement of the functional state of the patients after the course of cerebrolysin treatment.

4. Cortical evoked potentials upon paired-click auditory stimulation

It has been previously reported in clinical and experimental studies that movement disorders in PD largely occur due to the imbalance of inhibitory and excitatory processes in motor cortical and subcortical neuronal circuits following a nigrostriatal dopamine deficit (Ridding et al., 1995). A paired-pulse paradigm is usually used to study postexcitatory inhibition effect related to sensory gating mechanisms and synaptic processes in neurotransmitters release (Chu et al., 2009). There are two mechanisms that might explain paired-pulse inhibition phenomena. The first mechanism is the decrease in release probability of excitatory neurotransmitters from terminals of afferent axons (Szabo et al., 2000). Another possible mechanism of the decrement of the second response on paired stimulation is connected with synaptically released GABA from terminals of inhibitory interneurons (Chu & Hablitz, 2003). As the paired-pulse facilitation, paired-pulse inhibition is considered to be a form of a short-term synaptic plasticity. The investigation of cortical evoked potentials to paired-pulse sensory stimulation may provide additional information about mechanisms of neurological disturbances in PD.

The aim of this study was to investigate the postexcitatory inhibition of the N1/P2 complex of the cortical evoked potentials on auditory paired-click stimulation in patients with PD in comparison with age-matched healthy subjects. Our second goal was to evaluate the influence of neurotrophic drug cerebrolysin on postexcitatory cortical inhibition.

4.1 Methods

Studies were performed in two groups. The first group included 58 PD patients, with the severity of the disease corresponding to 1.5 - 3.0 of Hoehn M.M. and Yahr M.D. (1967) scale (28 men and 30 women, mean ± SE age 61.5 ± 1.1, range 45 - 74 years). The second group was control and consisted of 22 age-matched healthy subjects (10 men and 12 women, mean ± SE age 61.4 ± 1.1, range 48 - 73 years).

The study was approved in advance by the Ethical Committee of the Institute of Gerontology and was in accordance with the Declaration of Helsinki. The patients regularly underwent treatment at the Parkinson's Disease Centre of the Institute of Gerontology and gave written informed consent to participate in this study. The diagnosis of Parkinson's disease was determined according to the UK Bank Criteria (Hughes A. et al., 1992). The patients had from 2 to 22 year individual histories of idiopathic PD and were taking antiparkinsonian therapy at individual dose of 187.5 - 750 mg of levodopa / carbidopa daily. Besides levodopa / carbidopa, the patients were using other antiparkinsonian medication: selegiline, pramipexol, amantadine. The neurological status of PD patients was evaluated with Unified Parkinson's Disease Rating Scale (UPDRS; Fahn S. and R. Elton., 1987; Holloway R.G. et al., 2004) in the "ON" state 1 hour after levodopa / carbidopa intake. Mini Mental State Examination (MMSE) was used to study general cognitive status of the PD patients.

Auditory evoked potentials were recorded in the PD patients in their "OFF" state in the morning, after they were free from levodopa treatment and other antiparkinsonian medications for at least 12 hours. During registration of evoked potentials the subjects were sitting comfortably in a semi-reclined armchair in a quiet room with closed eyes. Cortical auditory evoked potentials were recorded at the vertex (Cz) referenced to a linked-ear electrode. The ground electrode was placed at the left wrist. The impedance of the electrodes was less than 10 kΩ. The electrode signal was amplified using a bandpass filter (0.53 - 30 Hz), digitised with 200 Hz sampling rate and stored for further analysis.

The pattern for double stimulation consisted of paired auditory clicks with 500, 700, 800, 900, 1100 and 2000 ms interstimulus intervals. The identical parameters (duration of 0.15 ms and intensity of 80 dB HL - hearing level) were used for the preceding conditioning click and following test click. Pairs of clicks were delivered once every 7 s for each interstimulus interval. Previous studies have shown that stimulation at faster frequencies can lead to a decrement in the cortical evoked potentials. A 2000 - 3000 ms electroencephalography epoch was recorded for each trial, including a 300 ms pre-stimulus baseline. The recording time depended on interstimulus intervals. The epochs contaminated with blinks or other artefacts were excluded from the data and twenty acceptable artefact-free trials were averaged for each interstimulus interval and used for further analysis. In electroencephalography recordings upon paired stimulation, amplitudes of N1-P2 complex (peak to peak) in the first (A1) and the second (A2) responses were measured. The amplitudes of the components N1 and P2 were estimated in the 60 – 150 ms and 120 - 220 ms ranges of time, respectively. The percent of paired-pulse inhibition of the N1-P2 complex was calculated using the formula: $(A1-A2)/A1 \times 100$. The effects of cerebrolysin on the postexcitatory inhibition of the N1/P2 complex of the cortical evoked potentials on auditory paired-click stimulation were studied in 21 patients with PD that were taking antiparkinsonian therapy, which was not changed during one month before cerebrolysin treatment and under the whole cerebrolysin course (intravenously 10 ml, during 10 days).

The results were analyzed statistically. Comparisons between PD patients and control groups were made using a non-parametric two-tailed Mann-Whitney criterion. Data obtained from the same patients before and after cerebrolysin treatment were compared using two-tailed paired t-test.

4.2 Results
4.2.1 Investigation of the postexcitatory inhibition following paired stimulation
The postexcitatory cortical inhibition in response to auditory stimulation studied with a paired-pulse paradigm was significantly reduced in patients with PD compared to control subjects. Amplitudes of N1-P2 complexes following the second stimulus of a pair at interstimulus intervals of 500, 700 and 900 ms were greater in PD patients. The mean values of paired-pulse inhibition in the group of PD patients were decreased to 29.8 ± 4.8 % (p<0.01), 25.4 ± 3.2 % (p<0.001) and 15.1 ± 2.6 % (p<0.001) for intervals 500, 700 and 900 ms respectively as compared to these values (54.1 ± 4.2 %; 49.8 ± 2.3 % and 42.9 ± 2.7 %) in the group of age-matched controls (Table 9).

The mean amplitude of N1-P2 complex elicited by a single (first) auditory stimulus in the group of PD patients was 16.2 ± 0.8 µV which was less than in age-matched subjects (18.5 ± 1.6 µV) but this difference was not statistically significant (p>0.05).

4.2.2 The influence of cerebrolysin treatment on the postexcitatory inhibition
A distinct positive effect of the course of cerebrolysin treatment on the postexcitatory cortical inhibition at paired-click stimulation was observed in the group of 21 PD patients. A noticeable shift of the paired-pulse inhibition value for 700, 800 and 900 ms intervals towards the values of the healthy control was found (Table 10, Fig 15).

Investigated groups	Inhibition in % of the second N1-P2 complex at interstimulus intervals			Averaged
	500 ms	700 ms	900 ms	
Age-matched control	54.1 ± 4.2	49.8± 2.3	42.9 ± 2.7	48.0 ± 2,1
PD patients	29.8 ± 4.8 *	25.4 ± 3.2 **	15.1± 2.6 **	21,4 ±2,4 **

Table 9. Inhibition of the second N1-P2 complex of cortical auditory evoked potentials at paired-click stimulation in age-matched control group and patients with Parkinson's disease (Mean ± SE).
* - P<0.01; ** - P<0.001 compared to control subjects (nonparametric Mann-Whitney test).

Time of investigation	Averaged value of paired-pulse inhibition (%) at interstimulus intervals (ms)			
	700	800	900	Averaged data
Before cerebrolysin	29.9 ± 3.9	26.7 ± 3.4	17.1 ± 3.1	24.6 ± 2.3
After cerebrolysin	38.1 ± 3.2	37.1 ±3.3	27.5 ± 4.1	34.2 ± 2.9
P (paired t-test)	<0.01	<0.001	<0.05	<0.001

Table 10. The influence of the course of cerebrolysin treatment on the postexcitatory inhibition following paired-click auditory stimulation in patients with Parkinson's disease (Mean ± SE).

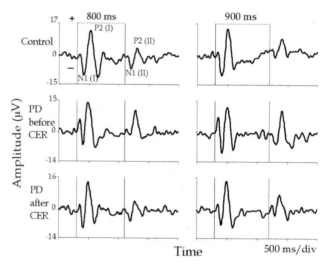

Fig. 15. Cortical auditory evoked potentials at paired auditory stimulation with interstimulus intervals of 800 and 900 ms in healthy control and patient with Parkinson's disease (PD) before and after the course of cerebrolysin (CER). N1(I), P2(I) – the components of cortical evoked potentials on the first conditional stimulus and N1(II), P2(II) – on the second test stimulus. Vertical solid bars on the records correspond to the onset of auditory signals.

4.3 Discussion

The main result of this study showed that PD patients had significantly reduced paired-pulse inhibition of the N1/P2 component of evoked potentials in the auditory cortex for interstimulus intervals of 500, 700 and 900 ms compared to the healthy age-matched subjects. Possible explanation of the reduced cortical inhibition in PD is the functional deficiency of inhibitory interneurons caused by depletion of dopaminergic innervation in the cerebral cortex (Gaspar et al., 1991). As already established (Krnjevic et al., 1966), afferent volleys after initial excitatory postsynaptic potentials (EPSPs) result in inhibitory postsynaptic potentials (IPSPs). A system of GABAergic interneurons, which can be activated by direct and indirect stimulation, may play the major role in the genesis of these IPSPs (Hanajima & Ugawa, 2000). The synaptic release of GABA is regulated by presynaptic GABA receptors of the B-type (Chu & Hablitz, 2003). There is also strong evidence that dopamine regulates inhibitory transmission at the synapses between pyramidal cells and interneurons by activating D1-like receptors located on the presynaptic terminals of GABAergic axons (Gonzalez-Islas & Hablitz, 2001). Dysfunction of cortical interneurons in PD also might be a result of noradrenergic denervation and monoamine terminal loss (Marie et al., 1995), as some investigations showed that cortical GABAergic interneurons can be excited via alpha-adrenoreceptors (Kawaguchi & Shindou, 1998).

Another possible explanation of the reduced inhibition in the auditory cortex in patients with PD may be the loss of dopaminergic transmission in the basal ganglia and the dysfunction of the caudal pallidum that sends its direct projections to the inferior colliculus, medial geniculate nucleus and temporal cerebral cortex (Shammah-Lagnado et al., 1996). The basal ganglia appear to "gate" sensory inputs at various levels and activation of basal ganglia outputs (entopeduncular nucleus and substantia nigra pars reticulate) is able to inhibit sensory responses (Boecker et al., 1999).

Our findings allow to suppose that drugs, which are able to activate cerebral inhibitory GABAergic system, can be useful in medication of PD. Phenibut (noofen) belongs to such drugs (Marshall & Foord, 2010). Application of noofen in complex therapy of PD appeared effective for the improvement of cognitive functions, enhancement of emotional state and increase of social adaptation of the PD patients (Karaban et al., 2006).

This study demonstrated that course of cerebrolysin treatment promotes normalization of the inhibitory brain processes. The positive effect of cerebrolysin indicates that neurotrophic drugs can also be useful in complex antiparkinsonian therapy for advance of the ability of the brain to provide normal inhibition.

5. Conclusion

The present investigation has shown that the surface EMG data add essential information to the clinical characteristics of PD patients. We found that separate EMG indices correlated, in a specific manner, with certain UPDRS sub-items, which could result in a better understanding of the pathogenesis of clinical PD symptoms. Motor disorders in PD (part III UPDRS scores) were found to be predominantly associated with disturbances in regulation of the tonic and phasic muscle activities. At the same time, disorders of the upper extremity daily activity (points 8-10 of UPDRS) and the dyskinesia (disability) (point 33 of UPDRS) are largely conditioned by the disturbance of reflex coordinating relationships between the muscles in PD. EMG analysis seems to be a useful tool for levodopa therapy adjustment and for predicting the course of disease.

In this study critical values of normal statistics of surface EMG distribution at rest were defined. Evaluation of statistical parameters of the EMG signals, to our opinion, appeared to be effective for the detection of signs of the disturbed muscle activity. Range and variance reflect the extent of bioelectrical muscle signals. Kurtosis characterizes motor unit synchronization. These EMG characteristics assist to detect latent symptoms of extrapyramidal insufficiency in clinically healthy kinsmen of the patients suffering from PD that can be considered genetic determinants of the risk of development of the above disease. Formulation of recommendations for individuals belonging to a risk group is of exceptional importance to prevent manifestations of PD.

Novel EMG characteristic is fractal dynamics of EMG data based on detrended fluctuation analysis and calculation of Hurst exponent. Fractal dimension studies the non-linear properties of EMG. The present investigation has demonstrated distinctive features of surface EMG signals fractal dimension at rest in patients with akinetic-rigid-trembling form of PD: 1) fractal dimension in PD patients is more complex compared to healthy subjects; 2) the value of Hurst exponent is significantly less in patients; 3) there is the considerable degradation of short and longer range correlation properties of EMG signals in PD. Fractal analysis has proved to be sensitive to neuromuscular status and may have potential in the assessment of the severity of PD

Evaluation of brain evoked potentials provides additional information about the mechanisms of neurological disturbances in PD. The results obtained in the present study produce evidence for significant relationships between both the early and late phases of movement-related potential CNV and the neurophysiological mechanisms supporting coordinatory muscle interactions and mental functions, including the simultaneous activity of numerous specific and non-specific brain structures (motor cortex, supplementary motor cortex, prefrontal cortex, cerebellar and thalamic projections). The existence of a selective negative correlation between the magnitude of the late CNV phase and the severity of symptoms such as "gait freezing" suggests a great role of efferent system of the basal ganglia in generating this phase of CNV. The investigation of cortical evoked potentials at paired-pulse sensory stimulation shows that inhibitory processes are deficient in PD patients. The findings may suggest that drugs, being the derivates of GABA, can be useful in treatment of PD. The parameters of CNV and the value of postexcitatory cortical inhibition at paired-click sensory stimulation well characterize the state of brain activity. Together with other neurophysiological parameters the brain evoked potentials might be a good tool for quantifying the efficacy of medication of PD patients.

6. References

Abbruzzese, G. & Berardelli, A. 2003. Sensorimotor integration in movement disorders. Mov. Disord., Vol. 18, pp. 231-240.

Antonini, A., Leenders, K. L. & Eidelberg, D. 1998. [11C]raclopride-PET studies of the Huntington's disease rate of progression: relevance of the trinucleotide repeat length. Ann. Neurol., Vol. 43, No. 2, pp. 253-255.

Aotsuka, A., Wheate, S. J., Dranke, M. E., Jr. & Paulson, G. W. 1996. Event-related potentials in Parkinson's disease. Electromyogr. Clin. Neurophysiol., Vol. 36, No. 4, pp. 215-220.

Bartels, A. L., Balash, Y., Gurevich, T., Schaafsma, J. D., Hausdorff, J. M. & Giladi N. 2003. Relationship between freezing of gait (FOG) and other features of Parkinson's:

FOG is not correlated with bradykinesia. J. Clin. Neurosci., Vol. 10, No. 5, pp. 584 - 588.

Berg, D., Roggendorf, W., Schroder, U. et al.. 2002. Echogenicity of the substantia nigra: association with increased iron content and marker for susceptibility to nigrostriatal injury. Arch. Neurol., Vol. 59, No. 6, pp. 999-1005.

Boado, R.J. 2001. Amplification of blood-brain barrier GLUTI glucose transporter gene expression by brain-derived peptides. Neurosci. Res, Vol. 40, No. 4, pp. 337-342.

Boecker, H., Ceballos-Baumann, A., Bartenstein, P., Weindl, A., Siebner, H.R., Fassbender, T., Munz, F., Schwaige,r M. & Conrad, B. 1999. Sensory processing in Parkinson's and Huntington's disease: investigations with 3D H(2) (15) O-PET. Brain, Vol. 122 (Pt 9), pp. 1651-1665.

Chu, Z., Hablitz, J.J. 2003. GABA (B) receptor-mediated heterosynaptic depression of excitatory synaptic transmission in rat frontal neocortex. Brain Res., Vol. 959, pp. 39-49.

Chu, J., Wagle-Shukla, A., Gunraj, C., Lang, A. E. & Chen R. 2009. Impaired presynaptic inhibition in the motor cortex in Parkinson disease. Neurology, vol. 72, No. 9, pp. 842–849.

Deecke, L. 2001. Clinical neurophysiology of Parkinson's disease. Bereitschaftpotential and contingent negative variation. Adv. Neurol., Vol. 86, pp. 257–271.

DeLong, M.R. 1990. Primate models of movement disorders of basal ganglia origin. Trends Neurosci., Vol. 13, pp. 281-286.

Del Santo, F, Gelli, F.,Mazzocchio, R. & Rossi, A. 2007. Recurrence quantification analysis of surface EMG detects changes in motor unit Synchronization induced by recurrent inhibition. Exp. Brain Res, Vol. 178, pp. 308-315.

Elbaz, A., Grigoletto, F., Baldereschi, M. et al. 1999. Familial aggregation of Parkinson's disease: a population-based case-control study in Europe. EUROPARKINSON Study Group. Neurology, Vol. 52, No. 9, pp. 1876-1882.

Fahn, S., Elton, R. & members of the UPDRS Development Committee. 1987.Unified Parkinson's disease rating scale. In: Recent developments in Parkinson's disease, Fahn, S., Marsden, C.D., Calne, D.B., & Goldstein, M., editors, Vol. 2, pp. 153-163, 293-304, NJ Macmillan Health Care Information, Florham Park.

Farina, D., Merletti, R. & Enoka, R.M. 2004. The extraction of neural strategies from the surface EMG. J. Appl. Physiol, Vol. 96, pp. 1486-1495.

Filipovic, S. R., Covickovic-Sternic, N., Radovic, V. M., Dragasevic, N., Stoyanovic-Svete, M. & Kostic, V. S.. 1997. Correlation between Bereitschaftpotential and reaction time measurements in patients with Parkinson's disease. Measuring the impaired supplementary motor area function? J. Neurol. Sci., Vol. 147, No. 2, pp. 177 - 183.

Furukawa, Y., Kondo, T., Nishi, K., Yokochi, F. & Narabayashi, H. 1991. Total biopterin levels in the ventricular CSF of patients with Parkinson's disease: a comparison between akineto-rigid and tremor types. J Neurol Sci,, Vol. 103, pp. 232-237

Gaspar, P., Duyckaerts, C., Alvarez, C., Javoy-Agid, F., & Berger B. 1991 Alterations of dopaminergic and noradrenergic innervations in motor cortex in Parkinson's disease. Ann. Neurol., Vol. 30, pp. 365-374.

Goldberger, A. L., Amaral, L.A.N., Hausdorff, J.V., Ivanov, P.Ch., Peng, C.-K. & Stanley, H.E. 2002. Fractal dynamics in physiology: alterations with disease and aging. Proc. Natl. Acad. Sci. USA, Vol. 99, Suppl. 1, pp. 2466-2472.

Gonzalez-Islas, C. & Hablitz, J.J. 2001. Dopamine inhibition of evoked IPSCs in rat prefrontal cortex. J. Neurophysiol., Vol. 86, pp. 2911-2918.

Hanajima, R. & Ugawa, Y. 2000. Intracortical inhibition of the motor cortex in movement disorders. Brain Dev., Vol. 22, Suppl. 1, pp. 132-135.

Holloway, R.G., Shoulson, I., Fahn, S. et al. 2004. Parkinson Study Group. Pramipexole *vs* levodopa as initial treatment for Parkinson's disease: a 4-year randomized controlled trial. Arch. Neurol., Vol. 61, pp. 1044-1053.

Houk, J.C. 1979. Regulation of stiffness by skeletomotor reflexes. Ann. Rev. Physio.l, Vol. 41, pp. 99-114.

Hughes, A.I., Ben-Shlomo, Y., Daniel, S.E. & Lees, A.I. 1992. What features improve the accuracy of clinical diagnosis in Parkinson's disease: a clinico-pathologic study. Neurology, Vol. 42, pp. 1142-1146.

Hutter-Paier, B., Grygar, E., Fruhwirth, M., Temmel, I. & Windisch, M. 1998. Further evidence that Cerebrolysin protects cortical neurons from neurodegeneration in vitro. J. Neural. Transm., Vol. 53, pp. 363-372.

Ikeda, A., Shibasaki, H., Kaji, R., Terada, K., Nagamine, T., Honda, M. & Kimura, J. 1997. Dissociation between contingent negative variation (CNV) and Bereitschaftspotential (BP) in patients with parkinsonism. Electroencephalogr. Clin. Neurophysiol., Vol. 102, No. 2, pp. 142 - 151..

Illarioshkin, S. N. 2002. Conformational Disease of the Brain [in Russian], Yanus-K, Moscow.

Illarioshkin, S. N. 2008. Molecular basis of Parkinson's disease, in: Parkinson's Disease and Motor Disorders, pp. 8-17, Handbook for Physicians Based on Proceedings of I National Congress, Moscow.

Jenner, P. 1994. The contribution of dopamine receptor subtypes to the therapeutic actions and side-effects of anti-parkinsonian drugs. In: Beyond the Decade of the Brain, Stern, M.B., editor, pp. 131-156, Wells Medical Limited Chapel Place, Royal Tunbridge Wells, Kent.

Kaji, R., Urushihara, R., Murase, N., Shimazu, H. & Goto, S. 2005. Abnormal sensory gating in basal ganglia disorders. J. Neurol. 2005, Vol. 252, Suppl 4, 1V/13-1V/16.

Karaban, N., Lukhanina, E. P., Melnik, N. A. & Berezetskaya, N. M. 2006. Influence of course treatment with Noofen on motor activity, cognitive functions and emotional state in patients with Parkinson's disease. Ukrainskiy Vestnik Psihonevrologii, vol. 14, No. 46, pp. 26–30.

Katayama, Y., Kasai, M., Oshima, H., Fukaya, C. & Yamamoto T. 2000. Effects of anterodorsal pallidal stimulation on gait freezing (Kinesia paradoxa) in Parkinson's disease. Stereotact. Funct. Neurosurg., Vol. 74, No. 3-4, pp. 99-105.

Kawaguchi, Y. & Shindou, T. 1998. Noradrenergic excitation and inhibition of GABAergic cell types in rat frontal cortex. J. Neurosci., Vol. 18, pp. 6963-6976.

Krnjevic, K., Randic, M. & Straughan, D.W. 1966. Nature of a cortical inhibitory process. J. Physiol., Vol. 184, pp. 49-77.

Kryzhanovskii, G. N., Karaban', I. N., Magayeva, S. V. et al. 2002. Parkinson's Disease [in Russian], Meditsina, Moscow.

Lewis, G.N. & Byblow, W.D. 2002. Altered sensorimotor integration in Parkinson's disease. Brain, Vol. 125, pp. 2089-2099.

Lukhanina, E.P., Karaban', I.N., Chivliklii, M.A., Pil'kevich, N.A. & Berezetskaya, N.M. 2010. Electromyographic manifestations of hereditary signs of extrapiramidal insufficiency. Neurophysiology, Vol. 42, No 1, pp. 39-49.

Marie, R.M., Barre, L., Rioux, P., Allain, P., Lechevalier, B. & Baron J.C. 1995. PET imaging of neocortical monoaminergic terminals in Parkinson's disease. J. Neural. Transm. Park. Dis. Dement. Sect., Vol. 9, pp. 55-71.

Marshall, F. H. & Foord, S. M. 2010. Heterodimerization of the GABAB receptor-implications for GPCR signaling and drug discovery. Advances in Pharmacology, vol. 57, C, pp. 63–91.

Meigal, A.I., Rissanen, S., Tarvainen, M.P., Karjalainen, P.A., Iudina-Vassel, I.A., Airaksinen, O. & Kankaanpää, M. 2009. Novel parameters of surface EMG in patients with Parkinson's disease and healthy young and old controls. J. Electromyogr. Kinesiol, Vol. 19, pp e206-e213.

Nieminen, H. & Takala E.P. 1996. Evidence of deterministic chaos in the myoelectric signal. Electromyogr. Clin. Neurophysiol, Vol. 36, pp. 49-58.

Oishi, M., Mochizuki, Y.C. Du. & Takasu T. 1995. Contingent negative variation and movement-related cortical potentials in parkinsonism. EEG Clin. Neurophysiol., Vol. 95, No. 5, pp. 346–349.

Otsuka, M., Ichiya, Y., Kuwabara, Y., Hosokawa, S., Sasaki, M., Yoshida, T., Fukumura, T., Masuda, K. & Kato, M. 1996. Differences in the reduced 18F-Dopa uptakes of the caudate and the putamen in Parkinson's disease: correlations with the three main symptoms. J. Neurol. Sci., Vol. 136, pp. 169-173.

Pulvermuller, F., Lutzenberger, W., Muller, V., Mohr, B., Dichgans, J. & Birbaumer, N. 1996. P3 and contingent negative variation in Parkinson's disease. EEG Clin. Neurophysiol., Vol. 98, No. 6, pp. 456–467.

Ridding, M.C., Inzelberg, R. & Rothwell, J.C. 1995. Changes in excitability of motor cortical circuitry in patients with Parkinson's disease. Ann. Neurol., Vol. 37, pp. 181-188.

Robichaud, J. A., Pfann, K. D., Leurgans, S. et al. 2009. Variability of EMG patterns: a potential neurophysiological marker of Parkinson's disease? Clin. Neurophysiol., Vol. 120, No. 2, pp. 390-397.

Rossini, P.M., Filippi, M.M. & Vernieri, F. 1998. Neurophysiology of sensorimotor integration in Parkinson's disease. Clin. Neurosci., Vol. 5, pp. 121-130.

Ruether, E., Alvarez, X.A., Rainer, M. & Moessler, H. 2002. Sustained improvement of cognition and global function in patients with moderately severe Alzheimer's disease: a double-blind, placebo-controlled study with the neurotrophic agent Cerebrolysin. J. Neural. Transm., Suppl., Vol. 62, pp. 265-75.

Sadekov, R.A. 1997. Evoked potentials in parkinsonism. Zh. Nevropatol. Psikhiatr. Im. S. S. Korsakova, Vol. 97, pp. 64-65.

Schaafsma, J. D., Balash, Y., Gurevich, T., Bartels, A.. L., Hausdorff, J. M. & Giladi N. 2003. Characterization of freezing of gait subtypes and the response of each to levolopa in Parkinson's disease. Eur. J. Neurol., Vol. 10, No. 4, pp. 391 - 398.

Semmler, J.G. & Nordstrom, M.A. 1999. A comparison of cross-correlation and surface EMG techniques used to quantify motor unit Synchronization in humans. J. Neurosci. Methods, Vol. 90, pp. 47-55.

Shammah-Lagnado, S.J., Alheid, G.F. & Heimer, L. 1996. Efferent connections of the caudal part of the globus pallidus in the rat. J. Comp. Neurol., Vol. 376, pp. 489-507.

Sherman M. Y. & Goldberg A. L. 2001. Cellular defenses against unfolded proteins: a cell biologist thinks about neurodegenerative disease. Neuron, Vol 29, No. 1, pp. 15-32.

Stanley, H.E., Amaral, L.A.N., Goldberger, A.L., Havlin, S., Ivanov P.Ch. & Peng, C.-K. 1999. Statistical physics and physiology: monofractal and multifractal approaches. Physica, Vol. 270, p. 309.

Swie, Y. W., Sakamoto, K. & Ahimizu, Y. 2005. Chaotic analysis of electromyography signal at low back and lower limb muscles during forward bending posture. Electromyogr. Clin. Neurophysiol, Vol. 45, pp. 329-342.

Szabo, B., Wallmichrath, I., Mathonia, P. & Pfreundtner, C. 2000. Cannabinoids inhibit excitatory neurotransmission in the substantia nigra pars reticulate. Neuroscience, Vol. 97, No. 1, pp. 89–97.

Talebinejad, M., Chan, A.D. & Miri, A. 2010. Fatigue estimation using a novel multi-fractal detrended fluctuation analysis-based approach. J. Electromyogr. Kinesiol, Vol. 20, № 3, pp. 433-439.

Teo, Ch., Rasco, L., Al-Mefty, K., Skinner, R.D., Boop, F.A. & Garcia-Ril,l E. 1997. Decreased habituation of midlatency auditory evoked responses in Parkinson's disease. Mov. Disord., Vol. 12, pp. 655-664.

Valls-Solé, J. & Valldeoriola, F. 2002. Neurophysiological correlate of clinical signs in Parkinson' s disease. Clin. Neurophysiol., Vol. 113, pp. 792-805.

Zappoli, R., Versari, A., Arnetoli, G., Paganini, M., Muscas, G. C., Arneodo, M. G., Gangemi, P. F. & Bartelli M. 1991. Topographic CNV activity mapping, presenile mild primary cognitive decline and Alzheimer - type dementia. Neurophysiol. Clin., Vol. 21, No. 5-6, pp. 473-483.

2

Early Marker for the Diagnosis of Parkinson's Disease

Silvia Marino, Pietro Lanzafame, Silvia Guerrera,
Rosella Ciurleo and Placido Bramanti
IRCCS Centro Neurolesi "Bonino-Pulejo"
Messina
Italy

1. Introduction

Parkinson's disease (PD) is a progressive disorder with a relentless neuronal cell loss in several brain areas and nuclei notably in the substantia nigra (SN). The course of this neuronal loss is still unclear and may be highly variable in different PD patients and at different phases of the disease.

At present, no treatment has proven to influence this progressive course of the disease by protecting neurons or by postponing cell death.

One potential reason for the lack of neuroprotective effects of various agents, which have been highly effective in animal experiments, is the fact that the neurodegenerative process has already substantially proceeded when the diagnosis is established on the basis of widely accepted diagnostic criteria for PD: when the patients fulfill the clinical criteria of PD, 60–70% of neurons of the SN are degenerated and the striatal dopamine content is reduced by 80%, suggesting that the remaining neurons of the SN are also altered.

The "preclinical" phase may give the incorrect impression of patients exhibiting no clinical signs or symptoms of the incipient disease. Conversely, it is known that motor signs develop insidiously and minor signs of asymmetric hypokinesia may be detected years before the diagnosis of PD can be established. In addition, non-motor symptoms such as mood disorders, olfactorial, vegetative, sensory or neuropsychological signs may be noticed by the patients or physicians in advance of motor signs reflecting the dysfunction of dopaminergic or non-dopaminergic neurons.

Therefore, the term "early" or "prediagnostic" phase of PD would more appropriately characterize this stage of the disease. The clinical impression of autonomic, olfactorial and affective symptoms preceding motor signs of PD are in line with the findings demonstrating that neuronal alteration, with regard to Lewy body formation, occurs first in the dorsal vagal nucleus, the olfactory bulb, the raphe and coeruleus nuclei before entering the SN.

According to neuropathological findings, it is suggested that approximately 10% of subjects older than 60 years are in the "prediagnostic" phase of PD. These subjects exhibit the pathological hallmarks of PD, like Lewy bodies and neuronal loss at the SN, without showing the motor signs during life time that allow the diagnosis of PD. In only 10% of this group with so-called "incidental Lewy body disease", neuronal loss will proceed reaching the degree where motor symptoms are distinct enough to allow the diagnosis of PD.

It would be of great interest with respect to research and treatment to identify those subjects at risk i) to initiate neuroprotective treatment earlier, giving them a better base to act and ii) to define the causes of more rapid neuronal loss and disease progression in those patients with "incidental Lewy body disease" who will cross the threshold of critical neuronal loss at the SN and develop PD.

The duration of the early or prediagnostic period remains unknown. The duration of this phase of PD was estimated to last from a few years up to several decades before the first symptoms are noticed by the patients.

Several procedures have been proposed to identify subjects in early ("prediagnostic") stages of PD. In the following we present some instrumental approaches to identify patients in the early stages of PD.

One set of simple behavioural tasks that may provide insight into the neural control of response suppression uses saccadic eye movements to investigate and quantify motor impairments in PD. The study of ocular movements has been increasingly used to detect subtle pathological modifications, caused by a wide variety of neurological diseases.

A recent method, a new vision-based, nonintrusive, eye tracker, previously described in de novo PD patients (Marino et al., 2007), was proposed as a possible tool for supporting the diagnosis of PD in association with levodopa test, as an add-on to the Unified Parkinson Disease Rating Scale (UPDRS) score (Marino et al., 2010).

In addition, conventional MR Imaging (cMRI), as well as different advanced MRI techniques, including magnetic resonance spectroscopy (MRS), magnetization transfer imaging (MTI), diffusion-weighted and diffusion tensor imaging (DWI/DTI) are helpful to distinguish PD from atypical or secondary PD, especially in early stage of disease where a differentiation of these conditions is not easy.

Objective olfaction tests, such as olfactory-evocated potentials or functional magnetic resonance imaging, can be used to assess the severity of olfactory dysfunction, an early clinical feature of PD, its correlation with cerebral changes, and then the risk of developing PD in asymptomatic subjects.

2. Analysis of pursuit ocular movements in Parkinson's disease by using a video-based eye tracking system

Patients with PD characteristically have difficulty initiating movements (akinesia). When movements are initiated, they are of low velocity (bradykinesia) and reduced amplitude (hypokinesia). In addition, patients with PD are unable to sustain repetitive motor action. When they attempt to open or close the hand rapidly or tap the foot on the ground, the movement rapidly decreases in amplitude and slows in speed until it ceases. This disability is easily appreciated in the progressive micrographia of the handwriting of PD patients.

Research in the past 30 years has established that PD impairs control of eye movements. Voluntary saccades, such as self-paced, predictive and remembered saccades, are hypometric, multistep, of reduced velocity and of increased duration. Visually guided saccades are normal. Advanced PD is known to be associated with reduced ocular smooth pursuit gain (Bares et al., 2003; Lekwuwa et al., 1999). This has been explained in terms of advanced PD affecting other structures outside the basal ganglia.

A recent study (Marino et al., 2007) described a new eye movement measurement and analysis system which was developed for generating a set of visual stimuli paradigms and which is able to measure, analyze and record the resulting horizontal eye movements.

Oculomotor movements are controlled by many brain areas including the cerebral cortex, basal ganglia, brain stem and cerebellum. PD is a condition of degeneration of dopaminergic neurons in the substantia nigra pars compacta, resulting in progressive basal ganglia dysfunction. Because important eye movement pathways travel through the basal ganglia, aspects of oculomotor movement control should be impaired by the disease progression. This study showed that deficit in Pursuit Ocular Movements (POM) also occurs in patients with non-advanced PD and is closely correlated with clinical stage and motor scores.

The authors used a vision-based non-intrusive eye tracker. The developed interface provides the patients a visual stimulation. This system was able to measure, analyze and record the resulting horizontal eye movements.

The subjects were seated at 60 cm from the scene monitor, in front of the camera, on a chair which could be raised or lowered so that the subject's eyes were at the same height as the PC monitor, when the visual stimulus was administered on. The subjects were asked to perform the test three times.

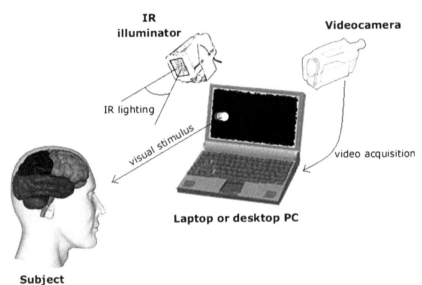

Fig. 1. Video-based eye-tracking functional scheme: subject looks at the screen (laptop or desktop PC) and all mechanical and electronic supports help to perform a real-time acquisition of eye movements.

The results of the study confirm that POM are clearly impaired in patients with de novo PD. The same authors (Marino el al., 2010) studied the POM by using the same vision-based non-intrusive eye tracker, in patients with suspected PD, before and after L-Dopa administration.

All patients had a positive test demonstrated by the improvement of UPDRS motor subscore, after L-Dopa administration, and as a new finding, by the improvement of POM.

A plausible explanation is that the improvement of horizontal eye displacement gain was induced by the dopaminergic action of L-Dopa. Some newly diagnosed PD patients have been shown to improve POM after L-Dopa treatment and this suggested the possibility of dopaminergic control of ocular movements, particularly smooth pursuit and saccades.

The POM methodology could be considered as a not invasive, objective and repetitive method (and these conditions could be an advantage with respect to only UPDRS examination) to support the clinical evaluation.

This method could be considered as a possible tool for supporting the diagnosis of PD in association with levodopa test, as an add-on to the UPDRS score. These results showed that this vision-based eye tracker can be used as reliable indices of disease severity in early and suspected PD patients.

3. Diagnosis of Parkinson's disease by using MR techniques

PD in its early stages can easily be mistaken for any number of disorders. Indeed PD is most likely to be confused with various Atypical Parkinsonian Disorders (APDs) such as Progressive Supranuclear Palsy (PSP), Multiple-System Atrophy (MSA), especially the Parkinson variant of MSA (MSA-P), and Corticobasal Degeneration (CBD).

A differentiation of these clinical entities, each characterized by completely different natural histories, may be challenging, particularly in the early stages of the disease, where overlapping clinical signs lead to a high rate of misclassification. However, a differentiation between APDs and PD, that may make easier early diagnosis, is crucial for determining the prognosis and choosing a treatment strategy.

Magnetic Resonance Imaging (MRI) plays an important role in the differential diagnosis in PD. Conventional MRI (cMRI) and advanced MRI techniques, including proton magnetic resonance spectroscopy, diffusion-weighted and diffusion tensor imaging and magnetization transfer imaging, are helpful to distinguish PD from atypical or secondary PD.

3.1 Magnetic Resonance Spectroscopy

MRS is a non-invasive technique that can be used to measure the concentrations of different low-molecular weight chemicals. The technique is based on the same physical principles as MRI, i.e. the detection of energy exchanges between external magnetic fields and specific nuclei within atoms. MRS is the more modern version of Nuclear Magnetic Resonance which over the past five decades has evolved from a technique used in chemistry to determine the structure of molecules to a method with which to probe the metabolism of cells, tissues, intact animals and humans (Allen, 1990; Avison et al., 1986).

MRS has been demonstrated in vivo for different nuclei, including ^1H, ^{31}P, ^{13}C, ^{15}N, ^{19}F and ^{23}Na. While most of these nuclei are very difficult to detect, ^1H and ^{31}P are available in the human brain in significant concentration and have the appropriate physical configuration to be detected by MRS. For instance, ^{31}P-MRS has been the first to be applied to medicine in vivo, and can be used to evaluate brain energy metabolism by directly and non-invasively measuring of Adenosine Triphosphate (ATP), Phosphocreatine (PCr) or Inorganic Phosphate (Pi) concentrations. While ^{31}P-MRS was the first spectroscopic technique to be applied in vivo, the main nucleus studied today in neurospectroscopy is ^1H, which provides information on markers of neurons, myelin, energy metabolism and other metabolically active compounds.

^1H-MRS detects very small differences in the frequencies of proton resonances from comparatively large volumes (1 ml or more) of brain tissue. The frequency of the resonance is affected by its local chemical environment, while the amplitude reflects its concentration. As such, ^1H-MRS is able to provide a measurement of certain proton-containing chemical markers. Proton spectroscopy presents the problem that metabolites at millimolar concentration must be detected in the presence of a background water signal that is present at about 100 molar. For this reason solvent-suppression techniques have been combined with localization schemes to produce spatially localized solvent-suppressed spectra. The two most commonly used localization methods are STEAM and PRESS. These methods can be implemented as single-voxel and multi-voxels methods. With the single voxel localization, the signal is acquired from a single brick-shaped volume of various sizes (minimum volume 2-3 cm³). The multi-voxel or MR spectroscopic imaging (MRSI) or Chemical Shift Imaging (CSI) approach generates individual spectra from multiple voxels at the same time (minimum volume 0.5-1 cm³). Single-voxel spectroscopy detects the signal from a single region during one measurement, whereas MRS imaging, using additional phase-encoding pulses, obtains the signal from multiple regions at the same time and provides the information of spatial distribution of major cerebral metabolites. The spatial information in MRI is done in 2-D for one or more slices and can generate low-resolution images for each metabolite by integration of the MR signals from each voxel (Ross & Bluml, 2001). The possibility to acquire the spectra from 2D multi-voxel allows to study the metabolite distribution of a large area of the brain with the advantage of identifying more anatomical and functional details. Most importantly, collecting data from many different adjacent regions simultaneously reduces the potential for systemic errors that can affect sequential measurements and thus results in more accurate repeated studies.

The metabolites detectable with ^{1}H-MRS include the prominent resonances of N-acetylaspartate (NAA), choline-containing compounds (Cho), creatine + phosphocreatine (Cr), myo-inositol (mI), lactate (Lac), and a variety of other resonances that might not be evident depending on type and quality of spectra as well as on the pathological condition (Figure 2) (Bonavita et al., 1999; Lin et al., 2005).

NAA, which resonates at 2.02 parts per million (ppm), represents the largest proton metabolic concentration in the human brain after water. Indeed the concentration of NAA reaches on the order of 10 μmol/g. NAA is widely interpreted as a neuronal marker and implicated in several neuronal processes, mitochondrial functioning and osmoregulation. NAA synthesis occurs in mitochondria and requires acetyl-CoA and L-aspartic acid as substrates. NAA has been proposed to serve as a mitochondrial shuttle of acetyl-CoA used for fatty acid synthesis. NAA undergoes dramatic increase during brain development and significant decrease during lesion progression in various neurodegenerative diseases, suggesting an important, unknown role in brain metabolism (Clark, 1998).

The Cho peak (3.2 ppm) represents a combination of several choline-containing compounds, including free Cho, phosphorylcholine and glycerophosphorylcholine, and to a small extent acetylcholine. Free Cho acts as a precursor to acetylcholine, while glycerophosphorylcholine is a product of breakdown of membrane phosphatidylcholine and acts as an osmoregulator. The concentration of Cho is relatively low on the order of 0.5 to 1.5 μmol/g and can be altered in normal aging and many focal inflammatory diseases. The Cho peak is often viewed as a marker of membrane turnover or inflammation in ^{1}H MRS studies.

The concentration of total Cr is estimated on the order of 8 to 9 μmol/g and is approximately 20% higher in human gray matter than white matter. In ^{1}H-MRS, the resonance at 3.03 ppm represents total Cr and PCr supplies phosphate for conversion of ADP to ATP in creatine kinase reaction. Indeed these metabolites buffer the energy use and energy storage of cells. The level of total Cr mainly remains constant in many neuronal

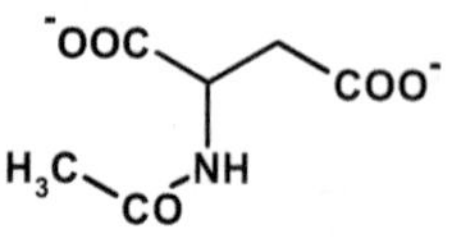

N-Acetylaspartate (NAA)

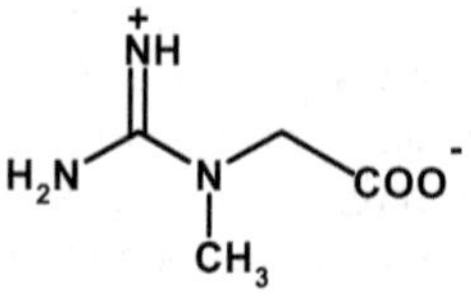

Creatine (Cre)

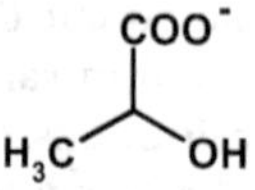

Lactate (Lac)

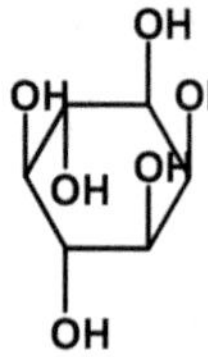

Myo-inositol (mI)

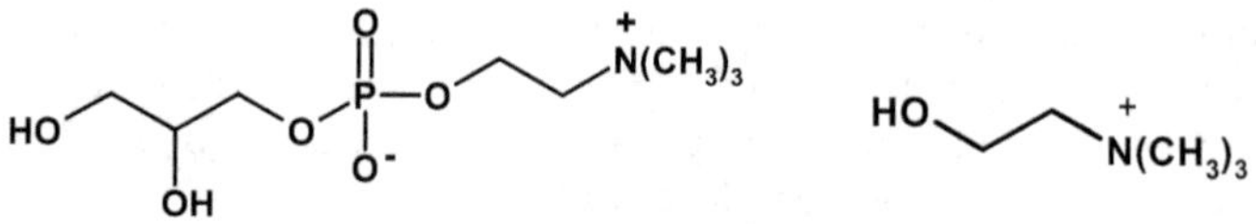

Choline - containing compounds (Cho)

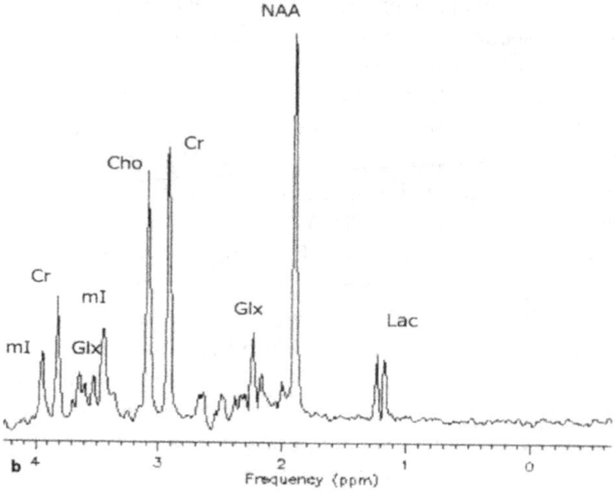

Fig. 2. Chemical structure of main cerebral metabolites detected by ^{1}H-MRS.

diseases. Thus, total Cr is often used as an internal reference (i.e., a denominator in metabolite signal ratio).

The mI (3.56 ppm) has been recognized as a cerebral osmolyte or an astrocyte marker due to its cellular specificity based on cell culture studies. mI is also been known as a breakdown product of myelin and precursor of inositol polyphosphate, an intracellular messenger. The concentration of mI is on the order of 5–10 μmol/g while one of its isomers, syllo-inositol, has substantially lower concentrations of on the order of less than 1 mol/g in the brain and remains relatively consistent in many diseases.

The Lac (1.3 ppm) is an end product of anaerobic glycolysis, thus increase in Lac concentrations often serves as an index of altered oxidative metabolism, i.e., in ischemia, hypoxia, and cancer. The concentration of Lac is on the order of about 1 μmol/g in normal aerobic conditions. Increases of Lac in the brain are often accompanied by decreased intracellular pH and high-energy phosphates. The proposed role of Lac is a source of energy for neurons and the transport of Lac plays an essential role in the concept of metabolic coupling between neurons and glia.

The concentration changes of all metabolites detected by ^{1}H-MRS and ^{31}P-MRS could help to evaluate PD subjects in the "preclinical" stages, especially in early differential diagnosis.

^{1}H-MRS of striatal structures might differentiate PD from APDs by virtue of reduced NAA/Cr ratios in MSA but not PD. ^{1}H-MRS showed reduced NAA/Cr ratios in the lentiform nucleus in six of seven MSA-P cases, whereas normal levels of putaminal NAA were found in eight of nine PD subjects (Davie et al., 1995).

As compared to normal controls, in patients with PSP, CBD, and MSA, but not in those with PD, significant reduction of the NAA/Cr ratio in the frontal cortex was found (Abe et al., 2009). Patients with CBD showed significant reduction of the NAA/Cr ratio in the frontal cortex and putamen as compared to patients with PD and MSA. Patients with PSP showed a significant reduction of the NAA/Cr ratio in the putamen as compared with patients with PD and MSA. Patients with CBD showed clear asymmetry in the putamen as compared to controls and other patients (Abe et al., 2009). By application of ^{1}H-MRSI statistically significant difference in regional patterns of the NAA/Cr and NAA/Cho ratios between patients with PD and those with CBD and between patients with PD and those with PSP was found (Tedeschi et al., 1997).

Other ^{1}H-MRS examinations didn't show significant difference between the PD patients and the control subjects (Tedeschi et al., 1997), also in the striatum (Holshouser et al., 1995), in the putamen and globus pallidus (Federico et al., 1997), and in occipital lobe (Bowen et al., 1995). The NAA/Cho and NAA/Cr ratios were significantly reduced in the putamen and globus pallidus of MSA and the PSP patients, in which neuronal loss involves, compared with the control subjects (Federico et al., 1997). In another study Federico at al. showed that NAA/Cho peak ratio was significantly reduced in MSA and in PSP patients compared to PD patients and to control. Moreover the NAA/Cr peak ratio was significantly reduced in MSA, in PSP and in PD patients also compared to controls, but only in MSA compared to PD patients (Federico et al., 1999).

Normal ^{1}H-MRS data could suggest the clinical diagnosis of PD, whereas low striatal levels of NAA could suggest the diagnosis of MSA or PSP.

However, further MRS studies have shown reduced NAA/Cr and NAA/Cho ratios in the lentiform nucleus not only in APD, but also in PD (Clarke & Lowry, 2001; Firbank et al., 2002).

Technical factors such as MRS technique including different echo- time and relaxation-time, voxel sizes, field strength and pulse sequences used in the different studies, may be responsible for some of the variation of results seen in the published literature on ^{1}H-MRS for the differential diagnosis of neurodegenerative parkinsonism (Clarke & Lowry, 2001; Firbank et al., 2002). The development of ^{1}H-MRS at higher magnetic field strengths may lead ^{1}H-MRS to a more important role as imaging tool in the differential diagnosis of parkinsonian disorders.

^{1}H-MRS of the brain with high magnetic field at 3 Tesla has many advantages that, with respect to the well-established and technologically advanced 1.5 Tesla ^{1}H-MRS, include better signal to noise ratio (SNR) and increased spectral, spatial and temporal resolution,

allowing the acquisition of high quality, easily quantifiable spectra in acceptable imaging times (Di Costanzo et al., 2007).

The increase SNR associated with higher magnetic fields permits shorter imaging times for a given spatial resolution, higher resolution for a given imaging time or the combination of both.

The spectral resolution is linearly correlated with the field strength and is about twice at 3 Tesla as compared to 1.5 Tesla. Clinical 1.5 Tesla scanners equipped with ^{1}H-MRS packages allow the quantification of NAA, Cho, Cr and lactate at long echo-time, and further metabolites, such as mI and glutamate-glutamine (Gxl), at short echo-time. mI is a strongly coupled system and resonates at four chemical shift positions. At 1.5 Tesla, only the singlet component at 3.57 ppm is detected. However, at 3 Tesla this resonance is resolved into its components at 3.55 and 3.61 ppm. Therefore by increasing of spectral resolution and SNR, the quantification precision of mI is significantly better at 3 Tesla relative to 1.5 Tesla (Srinivasan et al., 2004).

Despite shorter T2 relaxation times and increased field inhomogeneity, the chemical shift doubling at 3 Tesla yields better spectral resolution. This is reflected by improved baseline separation of Cho and Cr, which are only 0.2 parts per million (ppm) apart, and by slightly better resolution of Glu/Gln region, between 2.05 and 2.5 ppm, at shorter TE.

Higher field strengths also lead to a flatter baseline that contributes to more reliable estimation of peak area and, hence, more precise quantification, in addition to a more accurate identification of each metabolite.

This has been shown by a recent study applying multiple regional single voxel ^{1}H-MRS including putamen, pontine basis and cerebral white matter at 3 Tesla in 24 patients with MSA compared to 11 PD patients and 18 controls. Significant NAA/Cr reductions have been shown in the pontine basis of both patients with MSA-C (cerebellar ataxia variant of MSA) and MSA-P, while putaminal NAA/Cr was only reduced in the patients with MSA-P. Eight of the 11 MSA-P patients compared to none of the PD and control group were classified correctly by combining individual NAA/Cr reductions in the pontine basis and in the putamen. These results suggest that combined assessment of NAA/Cr in the pontine basis and putamen may be effective in differentiating MSA-P from PD in terms of the high specificity of reduced NAA/Cr in the pontine basis or in the putamen in patients with MSA-P (Watanabe et al., 2004).

Moreover, in these studies, the metabolite concentrations were expressed in terms of semiquantitative ratios such as NAA/Cr, NAA/Cho, Cho/Cr and mI/Cr. In relative quantification, one of the metabolite peaks measured is used as the concentration standard and serves as the denominator of the peak ratios. As a result, the total number of quantifiable metabolites is decreased by one. Furthermore, alterations in the peak ratio do not necessarily reflect a change in the concentration of the numerator. The alteration may be caused by change in the concentration of the numerator, the denominator, or both or may be due to changes in relaxation behavior. The assumption that the concentration of certain reference metabolites (e.g. total creatine, choline) remains constant may be incorrect under normal conditions, as well as in many pathologic states. It is therefore advisable to obtain concentration expressed in standard units (such as millimoles per kilogram wet weight) by applying absolute quantification.

Combined ^{31}P- and ^{1}H-MRSI at 3 Tesla measuring absolute adenosine diphophosphate (ADP), ATP, Cr and PCr concentrations in two well-defined cohorts of patients with early and advanced PD has been performed to evaluate brain energy metabolism (Hattingen et al., 2009). In the putamen and midbrain of both PD groups compared to control was found a bilateral reduction of high-energy phosphates such as ATP and PCr as final acceptors of energy from mitochondrial oxidative phosphorylation. In contrast, low-energy metabolites such as ADP and Pi were within normal ranges. Patients with early Parkinson's Disease, with clearly lateralized motor symptoms, exhibited a significant reduction of putamen high-energy phosphates in the less affected hemisphere with a less pronounced dopaminergic cell loss. Therefore, mitochondrial dysfunction is a rather early occurring and subsequently persistent event in the pathophysiology of dopaminergic degeneration in PD. These data strongly support the hypothesis that mitochondrial dysfunction is involved early in pathogenesis of PD and it may be used as early marker for this pathology.

In vivo MRS is increasingly utilized for the study of neurochemistry and cerebral energy metabolism in PD. Particularly, the recent technical advances of in vivo MRS including the availability of higher magnetic fields permitting improved spectral and spatial resolution, the development of a reliable method for absolute metabolite quantification, the development of various spectroscopic methods to enhance metabolite signal identification, and the application of combined ^{31}P- and ^{1}H-MRS can be use to examine the changes in neurochemical profile non–invasively and to achieve a differential diagnosis of PD versus other forms of parkinsonism, especially in early stages of disease when signs and symptoms of different forms of parkinsonism have greater overlap. However, several multicentre trials using a larger sample of patients, absolute quantification of tissue metabolite concentrations and a standardized technique are required to fully determine the place of MRS in early clinical differential diagnosis.

3.2 Conventional Magnetic Resonance

In the early disease stages the clinical separation of atypical parkinsonism disorders (APD)s from PD carries a high rate of misdiagnosis. An early differentiation between APD and PD, each characterized by completely different natural histories, is crucial for determining the prognosis and choosing a treatment strategy.

The principles of MR imaging are based on the ubiquitous presence of hydrogen in body tissues and the spin of the hydrogen atom proton, which induces a small magnetic field. In general, T2- weighted sequences are sensitive to changes in tissue properties, including tissue damage, due to changes of the transverse magnetization or T2 decay. Neurodegenerative processes characterized by cell loss, increased age-related deposition of iron or other paramagnetic substances, and by astroglial reaction and microglial proliferation may lead to signal changes in affected brain areas, like the basal ganglia or infratentorial structures, in neurodegenerative parkinsonism (Duguid et al., 1986; Gupta et al., 2008; Hirsch et al., 2007; Wilms et al., 2007).

Because cMRI is believed to be usually normal in patients with PD, while it frequently shows characteristic abnormalities in patients with APD, cMRI images takes a major part in excluding underlying pathologies such as vascular lesions, multiple sclerosis, brain tumors, normal pressure hydrocephalus, bilateral striopallidodentate calcinosis, and other potential, but rare, causes of symptomatic parkinsonism such as Wilson disease, manganese-induced parkinsonism, or different subtypes of neurodegeneration associated with brain iron accumulation.

At 1,5 T, patients with advanced PD, and sometimes those with APD, may show distinct abnormalities of the substantia nigra, including signal increase on T2-weighted MR images, smudging of the hypointensity in the substantia nigra towards the red nucleus or signal loss

when using inversion recovery MRI (Brooks, 2000; Rutledge et al., 1987; Savoiardo et al., 1994).
Biochemical studies have reported increased iron content in the substantia nigra pars compacta (SNc) in PD, with changes most marked in severe disease, suggesting that measurement of nigral iron content may provide an indication of the pathologic severity of the disease (Youdim et al.,1990). Iron accumulates in the brain as a function of age, primarily in the form of ferritin and particularly in oligodendrocytes, but also in neurons and microglia. The adult brain has a very high iron content, particularly in the basal ganglia. Brain iron concentration is highest in the globus pallidus, substantia nigra, red nucleus, caudate, and putamen. Abnormally elevated iron levels are evident in various neurodegenerative disorders, including PD where there is evidence of increased iron in the substantia nigra (Dexter et al.,1989; Sofic et al.,1988). Signal changes on T2-weighted images in the basal ganglia as well as in infratentorial structures have been reported for all APDs at 1.5 T, where they have been used as a differentiating criterion from PD. Furthermore, estimation of transverse relaxation in patients with PD, using a 1.5 Tesla whole body imaging system, showed shortened T2 values in substantia nigra, caudate and putamen in PD patients as compared to healthy controls (Antinoni et al., 1993). These data do suggest a potential utility of these measurements as a biomarker of disease progression.

3.3 Magnetization Transfer Imaging
Standard MR imaging detects signal only from hydrogen nuclei (protons) that are "mobile" (contained within a liquid); if a hydrogen atom is part of a molecule that is large and cannot move about freely, the signal from that hydrogen atom decays too quickly to be seen using a clinical MR imaging scanner. Such protons are found in large molecules (macromolecules), such as those of cell membranes and myelin. The mobile protons are in constant motion, however, and come into regular and intimate contact with the macromolecular protons, and the spin state (the proton magnetization state, which is measured with MR imaging) of the mobile protons can exchange with that of the macromolecular protons. This exchange of magnetization forms the basis of magnetization transfer imaging (Horsfield, 2005). Magnetization transfer is a physical phenomenon that results from interactions and exchanges between magnetized protons in water that are unrestricted in their molecular motion and those that are restricted because of their association with macromolecules. The latter have a much shorter T2 relaxation time and broader resonance, which makes it possible to selectively saturate their magnetization with an appropriate off-resonance pulse. The acquisition of two images, one obtained with the magnetization transfer saturation pulse turned on and the other with it turned off, can be used to generate a magnetization transfer ratio (MTR) image in which the signal intensity of each voxel is determined by the percent magnetization transfer in that voxel.
A MTR image is calculated from a pair of images acquired in an identical way, except that one has extra off-resonance RF pulses applied, which saturates the macromolecular magnetization pool. The MTR is calculated for every corresponding pair of pixels in the two images. If the intensity of the pixel in the image without saturation pulses is M0 and the corresponding intensity in the image with saturation pulses is Ms, the MTR is as follows:

$$MTR = [(M0 - Ms)/M0] * 100\%$$

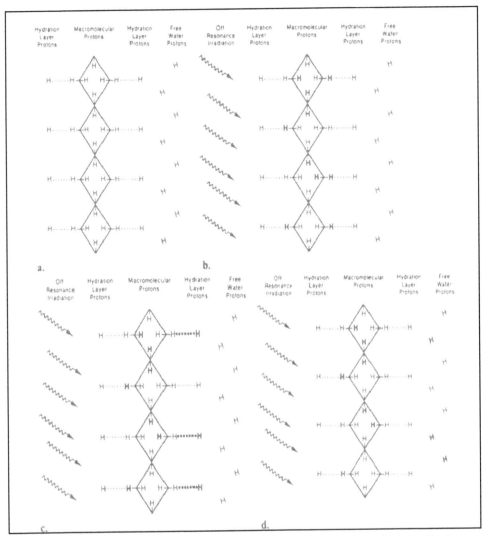

Fig. 3. Diagrams illustrate magnetization transfer, that is, the exchange of longitudinal magnetization between restricted protons associated with rigid macromolecules and free water protons. (a)Diagram shows macromolecular protons (H), including hydration layer protons and free water protons. (b) Off-resonance irradiation (arrows) saturates the immobile macromolecular protons (unsatured protons are designated H, while satured are designated H). (c) Saturation is transferred to hydration layer protons (…H). (d) Satured protons diffuse into the free water proton pool and decrease the signal from this pool.

Misregistration can occur if the subject moves between the two scans, but the M0 and Ms images must be in register; otherwise, artifacts appear at the edges of features in the calculated MTR image, with false MTR values. It is best to acquire the two images in an interleaved way (Barker et al., 1996; Inglese at al., 2001) although it is possible to register them after acquisition. Two forms of data analysis have been used extensively for MTR images: region of interest (ROI) and histogram analysis. ROI analysis may be useful for elucidating the degree of tissue damage within individual lesions seen on T2-weighted scans or within anatomic regions associated with particular symptoms. ROI analysis, however, can be subject to operator bias, because the placement of regions is normally done manually. This could be overcome by first registering scans to an anatomic template and using ROIs defined on the template image. With MTR histogram analysis, a histogram of pixel MTR values is formed from the whole of the brain parenchyma; thus, focal damage and more widespread diffuse tissue damage are reflected in changes to the shape of the histogram, with a general shift toward lower MTR values as the density of macromolecules is reduced with demyelination or axonal loss. Extraction of the brain parenchyma, using the same procedures that are used in atrophy measurements, is a necessary preprocessing step. After normalization (to remove any effect of the absolute brain size), the MTR histogram can be characterized by several simple statistics, such as the histogram peak position, the peak height, and the average MTR. The employment of off-resonance irradiation was first proposed by Wolff and Balaban (Wolff & Balaban, 1989), who found that use of an off-resonance radio-frequency preparation pulse could generate excellent tissue contrast in images of rabbit kidney, and they referred to the technique as "magnetization transfer contrast." The initial magnetization transfer occurs between the macro-molecular protons and the transiently hound hydration layer protons. The efficiency of this interaction is directly related to the number of irradiation sites (hydrogen bonds) and their mobility. The utilization of magnetization transfer was extended to clinical imaging, including its use with gradient-echo imaging and MR angiography (Wolff et al.,1991; Pike et al., 1992). A decrease in the MTR, which reflects a reduction in the exchange of magnetization of protons that are tumbling freely and those that are bound to macromolecules, is evidence of demyelination in cerebral white matter. MTR imaging is sensitive to both microscopic and macroscopic pathology and provides quantitative data on the extent of myelin loss in MS.

By using MTI, abnormalities of the basal ganglia and SN have been reported in patients with PD, MSA and PSP. One study (Eckert et al., 2004) investigated the potential of MT imaging in the differential diagnosis of neurodegenerative parkinsonism, including 37 patients with different parkinsonian syndromes and 20 age-matched controls. The main finding in this study was a change in the MTR in the globus pallidus, putamen, caudate nucleus, SN, and white matter in PD, MSA, and PSP patients, matching the pathologic features of the underlying disorder. MTR were significantly reduced in the putamen in MSA patients compared with PD patients and healthy controls, as well as in the SN in patients with PSP, MSA, and PD. Another study (Yonca et al., 2007) determined the role of MTR in the early period of 33 patients with PD, comparing the findings with those in 30 normal healthy volunteers. Signal intensity measurements were obtained from 15 anatomic regions: SNc, substantia nigra pars reticulate (SNPR), red nucleus, dentate nucleus, cerebellum, pons, globus pallidus, putamen, caudate nucleus, thalamus, internal capsule posterior horn, forceps major, forceps minor, genu, and splenium of corpus callosum. Results showed a significant decrease of MTR in the SNc, SNPR, red nucleus, and pons compared with normal healthy volunteers. No significant decrease in MTR were found at supratentorial paraventricular white matter and cerebellum, which may be attributed the duration of the disease.

Perhaps in the initial stages of PD, supratentorial paraventricular white matter is not influenced by the disease. The decrease of MTR at SNc, SNPR, red nucleus, and pons in PD patients can be attributed to neurodegeneration (Tambasco et al., 2003)).

These studies show that MTR analysis may be a useful technique for PD diagnosis and decrease in MTR probably begins previously than the clinical onset of the disease.

3.4 Diffusion-Weighted Imaging

DWI imaging visualizes the random movement of water molecules in the tissue by applying diffusion-sensitizing gradients to assess changes in diffusion magnitude and orientation of water molecules in tissue. Quantification of the diffusivity is achieved by applying diffusion-sensitizing gradients of different degrees in 3 orthogonal directions and calculating the apparent diffusion coefficient (ADC) for each direction. The ADC is very dependent on the direction of diffusion encoding.

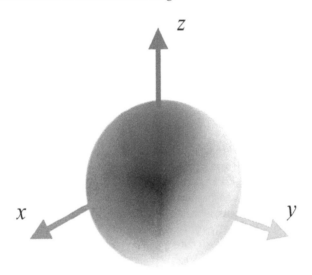

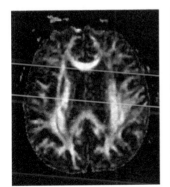
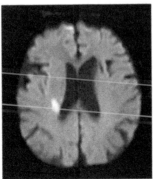
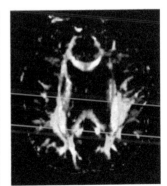

Fig. 4. Image-based visualization of diffusion tensor data. Top: Sphere representing directional color encoding. Second row: 2D images of image based visualization (from left: FA image, mean diffusivity image, and color-encoded image).

The random translational motion (diffusion) of water molecules in tissue is restricted by the highly organized architecture of fiber tracts in the central nervous system. Neuronal loss and gliosis disrupt this architecture, resulting in an increase of diffusivity and ADC. The complex neuronal architecture with its organization in fiber bundles that are surrounded by dense myelin sheaths leads also to a distinct anisotropy of water diffusion, which is facilitated along the direction of fiber tracts and restricted perpendicular to the fibers.

The degree of anisotropy can be quantified by applying diffusion-sensitizing gradients in at least 6 directions, which permits calculation of fractional anisotropy (FA). Decreased FA values represent tissue degeneration due to normal aging or due to pathologic reasons such as neurodegeneration. Both diffusivity and FA can be combined to form the so-called diffusion tensor, which indicates direction and extent of diffusivity with the help of a vector (Hagmann et al., 2006; Le Bihan, 2003; Schocke et al., 2004). The central nervous system (CNS) is highly organized in numerous tracts of myelinated fibre bundles, whereby the movement of the water molecules is restricted perpendicular to these fibre bundles. The resulting anisotropic diffusion is quantified by the FA, which is determined by diffusion-sensitised gradients in at least six directions. Both the diffusivity and the FA form the diffusion tensor (Le Bihan, 2003).

Widespread cerebral changes are observed in advanced stages of PD, suggesting that PD is a multisystem disorder.

Recently, several studies pointed out the capability of the histogram analysis of the apparent diffusion coefficient computed from diffusion-weighted images and of the mean diffusivity and FA computed from DTI to reveal brain-tissue damage in early clinical stages of neurodegenerative diseases. A recent study including 27 patients with de novo drug-naïve PD hypothesized that global measurements of brain volume and structure, such those possible with SIENAX software (part of FSL 4.0 http://www.fmrib.ox.ac.uk/fsl/) and histogram analysis of DTI could reveal subtle tissue changes in the early clinical phase of PD (Tessa et al., 2008). Accordingly, a group of patients with drug-naive de novo PD and a group of 16 healthy controls, were investigated with SIENAX and DTI. Results showed no significant differences for total brain, GM, and WM volumes and histogram-derived mean diffusivity metrics between controls and the whole group of patients with PD or any subgroup of patients with PD. As compared with controls, patients with PD as a whole and patients with the akinetic-rigid type showed an increase of the twenty-fifth percentile of the FA histogram. In patients with the akinetic-rigid type, there also was a trend toward an increase of the mean and fiftieth and seventy-fifth percentiles, and a reduction of the skewness of the FA histogram. This finding is consistent with the hypothesis that subtle GM loss is present in patients with PD since the early clinical phases and that this feature is more pronounced in patients with akinetic-rigid type. Another recent study including only patients with newly diagnosed PD used high-resolution DTI at 3 Tesla to evaluate rostral, middle, and caudal ROIs within the SN on a single slice of the midbrain and this study found that PD patients could be completely separated from the control group based on reduced FA values in the caudal ROI of the SN, such that further confirmatory studies seem to warrant. By using statistical parametric mapping analysis of DT imaging, changes in FA were found in the frontal lobes, including the supplementary motor area, the presupplementary motor area, and the cingulum in non demented PD patients relative to controls, whereas VBM analysis in the same patients revealed no volume loss (Karagulle

Kendi et al., 2008). These results confirm that the neurodegenerative process extends beyond the basal ganglia in PD (Tessa et al., 2008).

Olfactory impairment, which is common in PD and often predates clinical diagnosis, may be a useful biomarker for early PD. One study (Rolheiser et al., 2011) compared newly diagnosed PD patients with a matched control group using both olfactory testing and diffusion tensor imaging of the substantia nigra and anterior olfactory structures. Fourteen PD patients with stage 1-2 of Hoehn & Yahr were matched to a control group by age and sex. All subjects completed the University of Pennsylvania Smell Identification Test, as well as a series of MRI scans designed to examine diffusion characteristics of the olfactory tract and the substantia nigra. Olfactory testing revealed significant impairment in the patient group. Diffusion tensor imaging revealed significant group differences in both the substantia nigra and anterior olfactory region, with fractional anisotropy of the olfactory region clearly distinguishing the Parkinson's subjects from controls. This study has suggested that there may be value in combining behavioral (olfaction) and MRI testing to identify early Parkinson's disease (Rolheiser et al., 2011; Fulton & Barret, 2008).

Concluding DWI/DTI imaging especially bears several advantages. DWI/DTI imaging may detect diffusion abnormalities in the basal ganglia and infratentorial structures in patients with PD at an early stage of disease. Furthermore, DWI/DTI imaging sequences are widely available on whole body MR scanners and can be acquired within a few minutes.

3.5 Functional Magnetic Resonance Imaging

fMRI is based on the increase in blood flow to the local vasculature that accompanies neural activity in the brain. This results in a corresponding local reduction in deoxyhemoglobin because the increase in blood flow occurs without an increase of similar magnitude in oxygen extraction (Roy & Sherrington, 1890; Fox & Raichle, 1985). Since deoxyhemoglobin is paramagnetic, it alters the T2 weighted magnetic resonance image signal (Ogawa et al, 1990). Thus, deoxyhemoglobin is sometimes referred to as an endogenous contrast enhancing agent, and serves as the source of the signal for fMRI. Using an appropriate imaging sequence, human cortical functions can be observed without the use of exogenous contrast enhancing agents on a clinical strength (1.5 T) scanner (Bandettini et al., 1992, 1993; Kwong, et al, 1992; and Turner, et al, 1993; Schneider et al, 1993). Functional activity of the brain determined from the magnetic resonance signal has confirmed known anatomically distinct processing areas in the visual cortex (Belliveau, et al, 1991; Ogawa, et al, 1992; Schneider, et al, 1993), the motor cortex, and Broca's area of speech and language-related activities (Hinke et al., 1993; Kim et al., 1995). Further, a rapidly emerging body of literature documents corresponding findings between fMRI and conventional electrophysiological techniques to localize specific functions of the human brain (Atlas et al., 1996; Puce, et al, 1995; Burgess, 1995; Detre, et al, 1995; George, et al, 1995; Ives, et al, 1993). Consequently, the number of medical and research centers with fMRI capabilities and investigational programs continues to escalate.

The main advantages to fMRI as a technique to image brain activity related to a specific task or sensory process include:

- the signal does not require injections of radioactive isotopes
- the total scan time required can be very short
- the in-plane resolution of the functional image is generally about 1.5 x 1.5 mm although resolutions less than 1 mm are possible.

The function or dysfunction of the several cortical regions involved in many disease, like PD, can be investigated in vivo by means of functional imaging techniques such as fMRI.

4. Olfactory dysfunction as a early diagnostic marker for Parkinson's Disease

Olfactory dysfunction is a frequent non-motor symptom in PD and may be considered as an early clinical feature of the disease preceding motor symptoms by years (Ansari & Johnson, 1975). More than 96% of patients with PD present with olfactory dysfunction, compared with an established olfactory loss of at least 25% in the normal population over 52 years of age (Haehner et al., 2009). The majority of PD patients are functionally anosmic or severely hyposmic. Several studies have demonstrated an absence of correlation between olfactory loss and both duration of disease (Doty et al., 1988; Hawkes et al., 1997) and the clinical severity of PD (Ramaker et al., 2002), while other studies have found a correlation between the severity of PD and certain measures of olfactory function, such as latencies of olfactory event-related potentials (OERPs) (Hummel, 1999) and results from an odor discrimination task (Tissingh et al., 2001).

The cause of hyposmia in PD is not yet fully understood. It has been proposed that the develop of inclusion bodies, starting from the medulla oblongata and the anterior olfactory nucleus before the involvement of other central nervous structures, constitutes the reason of olfactory impairment before the motor symptoms appearance (Braak et al., 2003).

Moreover olfactory loss in PD is not a primary consequence of damage to the olfactory epithelium but rather result from distinct CNS abnormalities (Hummel et al., 2010). Studies based on biopsies from the olfactory epithelium did not reveal specific changes in the nasal mucosa of PD patients compared to patients who were hyposmic for other reasons (rhinitis, smoking or toxic agents). With regard to volumetrics of the olfactory bulb (OB) results indicated that there is little or no difference between PD patients with anosmia/hyposmia and healthy normosmic controls in terms of OB volume (Huisman et al., 2004; Hummel et al., 2010; Müller et al., 2005). Support for these results has come from a study that found an increase of (inhibitory) dopaminergic neurons in the OB in PD patients (Huisman et al., 2004). These findings have been interpreted within the context of a possible compensatory mechanism in response to the loss of dopaminergic neurons in the basal ganglia.

While cardinal motor symptoms in PD are closely related to a severe loss of dopaminergic cells in the nigro-striatal pathway, early clinical features such as olfactory impairment are more likely to be associated with extranigral pathology. Indeed atrophy in olfactory regions of the limbic and paralimbic cortex in early PD patients was found (Wattendorf et al., 2009). Moreover fMRI in PD patients indicated altered neuronal activity in the amygdaloid complex and hippocampal formation during olfactory stimulation (Takeda et al., 2010; Welge-Lüssen et al., 2009; Westermann et al., 2008). In addition, neuronal activity in components of cortico-striatal loops appears to be up-regulated indicating compensatory processes involving the dopaminergic system (Westermann et al., 2008).

Changes in olfactory function can also be observed using electrophysiological techniques such as recording OERPs (Kobal & Pattig, 1978). OERPs are the result of the sequential activation of numerous brain areas, starting with amygdala and regions of medial temporal lobe followed by the mid-orbito-frontal cortex and insular cortex, along with regions of the temporal lobe (Kettenmann et al., 1997). In PD patients OERPs are typically strongly delayed or even absent (Hawkes et al., 1999).

In a study combining fMRI and OERPs analysis in patients with PD, non-detectable OERPs patients exhibited reduced activity in the anterior cingulate gyrus and portions of the left striatum, while detectable ERP patients exhibited higher activation, especially in the amygdala, parahippocampal cortex, inferior frontal gyrus, insula, cingulate gyrus, striatum, and inferior temporal gyrus. The relationship between the expression of olfactory ERPs and cortical activation patterns seen during olfactory stimulation in fMRI in PD patients supports the idea that OERPs are a sensitive marker of neurodegeneration in olfactory regions, independent of the typically observed nigro-striatal degeneration in PD (Welge-Lüssen et al., 2009).

Olfactory dysfunction is more common in PD compared to atypical parkinsonian syndromes like PSP or MSA (Doty, 1991, 1993; Wenning et al., 1995). In a study including 37 patients with PD (Hoehn and Yahr I to IV) and 13 patients with MSA, CBD or PSP, 86 % of PD patients showed diminished sense of smell, or severe hyposmia, and 14 % were found to have moderate hyposmia, whereas 70 % of the patients with atypical parkinsonian syndromes exhibited moderate to mild hyposmia and 30 % normosmia (Muller et al., 2002).

Olfactory testing may be an additive, helpful and inexpensive diagnostic instrument to support the discrimination of PD from healthy subjects and atypical parkinsonian syndromes, before onset of motor symptoms.

For the clinical assessment of olfactory function, several validated psychophysical tests exist. The best-validated olfactory tests include the University of Pennsylvania Smell Identification Test, the Connecticut Chemosensory Clinical Research Center Test and the Sniffin' Sticks Test (Cain et al., 1988; Doty et al., 1984; Hummel, 1997, 2007; Kobal et al., 2000). The Sniffin' Sticks is based on pen-like odor dispensing devices. It consists of three tests namely for odor threshold, discrimination and identification, the sum of which is defined as "TDI score". This score can give an indication of patient's olfactory performance (normosmia: TDI≥30.5, hyposmia: TDI≤30.5, functional anosmia: TDI≤16.5).

A useful help for the clinical diagnosis of olfactory deficits is represented by system using human electro-physiological methods such as OERPs that requests an adequate methods to produce a selective and controlled stimulation of the olfactory system.

Based on the principles of air-dilution olfactometry, Kobal and Platting introduced a chemosensory stimulation with stimuli having a rectangular shape with rapid onset, precisely controlled in terms of timing, duration, intensity, not simultaneously activating other sensory systems (Kobal & Platting, 1978). This can be achieved by the olfactometer which is a complex instrument for creation of well defined, reproducible smell or pain stimuli in the nose without tactile or thermal stimulation.

In conclusion the detection of early olfactory dysfunction, less frequent in other form of parkinsonism, can be used to assess risk for developing PD in asymptomatic subjects.

5. Conclusions

The defining features of PD are characterized by their insidious onset and inexorable but variable progression. Reliable and well validated early markers for PD to identify individuals "at risk" before motor and non motor symptoms, accurately diagnose individuals at the threshold of clinical PD, and monitor PD progression throughout its course would dramatically improve patient care and accelerate research into both PD cause and therapeutics. During the past two decades, much progress has been made in identifying and assessing PD markers, but as yet, no fully validated marker for PD is available.

Nonetheless, there is increasing evidence that POM evaluation and advanced in vivo brain imaging will provide critical clues to assist in the early diagnosis and medical management of PD patients.

These methods are broadly defined as characteristics that are objectively measured and evaluated as indicators of normal biological processes, pathogenic processes, or pharmacological responses to a therapeutic intervention.

The lack of success of recent disease-modifying therapeutic trials coupled with the huge expense of other methods, such as the nuclear medicine, has highlighted the need for such an ambitious approach to identify and validate early markers of PD progression for future clinical studies of disease-modifying drugs.

6. References

Abe, K.; Terakawa, H.; Takanashi, M.; Watanable, Y.; Tanaka, H. et al. Proton magnetic resonance spectroscopy of patients with parkinsonism. *Brain Research Bulletin,* Vol.52, No.6, (August 2000), pp. 589-595, ISSN 0361-9230

Allen, P.S. In vivo nuclear-magnetic-resonance spectroscopy applied to medicine. *Canadian Association of Radiologists Journal,* Vol.41, No.1, (February 1990), pp. 39-44, ISSN 0008-2902

Ansari, K.A. & Johnson, A. Olfactory function in patients with Parkinson's disease. *Journal of Chronic Diseases,* Vol.28, No.9, (October 1975), pp. 493-497, ISSN 0021-9681

Atlas, S.W.; Howard, II R.S.; Maldijian, J.; Alsop, D.; Detre, J.A. et al. Functional magnetic resonance imaging of regional brain activity in patients with intracerebral gliomas: findings and implications for clinical management. *Neurosurgery,* Vol.38, No2, (February 1996), pp. 329-338, ISSN 0148-396X

Avison, M.J.; Hetherington, H.P. & Shulman R.G. Application of NMR to studies of tissue metabolism. *Annual Review of Biophysics and Biophysical Chemistry,* Vol.15, (June 1986), pp. 377-402, ISSN 0883-9182

Bandettini, P.A.; Jesmanowicz, A.; Wong, E.C. & Hyde, J.S. Processing strategies for time-course data sets in functional MRI of the human brain. *Magnetic Resonance in Medicine,* Vol.30, No2, (August 1993), pp. 161-173, ISSN 07403194

Bares, M.; Bràzdil, M.; Kanovsky, P.; Jurak, P.; Daniel, P.; et al. The effect of apomorphine administration on smooth pursit ocular movements in early Parkinsonian patients. *Parkinsonism & Related Disorders,* Vol. 9, No.3, (January 2003), pp. 139–144, ISSN 1353-8020

Barker, G.J.; Tofts, P.S. & Gass, A. An interleaved sequence for accurate and reproducible clinical measurement of magnetization transfer ratio. *Magnetic Resonance Imaging,* Vol.14, No.4, (1996), pp. 403-411, ISSN 0730-725X

Bonavita, S.; Di Salle, F. & Tedeschi, G. Proton MRS in neurological disorders. *European Journal of Radiology,* Vol.30, No.2, (May 1999), pp. 125-131, ISSN 0720-048X

Bowen, B.C.; Block, R.E.; Sanchez-Ramos, J.; Pattany, P.M.; Lampman, D.A. et al. Proton MR Spectroscopy of the Brain in 14 Patients with Parkinson Disease. *American Journal of Neuroradiology,* Vol.16, No.1, (January 1995), pp. 61-68, ISSN 0195-6108

Braak, H.; Del Tredici, K.; Rüb, U.; De Vos, R.A.I.; Jansen Steur, E.N.H. et al. Staging of brain pathology related to sporadic Parkinson's disease. *Neurobiology of Aging,* Vol.24, No.2, (April 2003), pp. 197-211, ISSN 0197-4580

Brooks, D.J. Morphological and functional imaging studies on the diagnosis and progression of Parkinson's disease. *Journal of Neurololy*, Vol. 247, No2, (April 2000), pp. 11-18, ISSN 0340-5354

Cain, W.S.; Gent, J.F.; Goodspeed, R.B. & Leonard, G. Evaluation of olfactory dysfunction in the Connecticut Chemosensory Clinical Research Center (CCCRC). *Laryngoscope*, Vol.98, No.1, (January 1988), pp. 83-88, ISSN 1531-4995

Clark, J.B. N-acetylaspartate: a marker for neuronal loss or mitochondrial dysfunction. *Developmental Neuroscience*, Vol.20, No.4-5, (July-October 1998), pp. 271-276, ISSN 0378-5866

Clarke, C.E. & Lowry, M. Systematic review of proton magnetic resonance spectroscopy of the striatum in parkinsonian syndromes. *European Journal of Neurology*, Vol.8, No.6, (November 2001), pp. 573-577, ISSN 1351-5101

Davie, C.A.; Wenning, G.K.; Barker, G.J.; Tofts, P.S.; Kendall, B.E. et al. Differentiation of multiple system atrophy from idiopathic Parkinson's disease using proton magnetic resonance spectroscopy. *Annals of Neurology*, Vol.37, No.2, (February 1995), pp. 204-210, ISSN 0364-5134

Dexter. D.T.; Wells, F.R.; Lees, A.J.; Agid, F.; Agid, Y. et al. Increased nigral iron content and alterations in other metal ions occurring in brain in Parkinson's disease. *Journal of Neurochemistry*, Vol.52, No6, (June 1989), pp. 1830-6, ISSN 0022-3042

Di Costanzo, A.; Trojsi, F.; Tosetti, M.; Schirmer, T.; Lechner, S.M. et al. Proton MR spectroscopy of the brain at 3T: an update. *European Radiology*, Vol.17, No.7, (July 2007), pp. 1651-1662, ISSN 0938-7994

Doty, R.L.; Deems, D. & Steller, S. Olfactory dysfunction in Parkinson's disease: a general deficit unrelated to neurologic signs, disease stage, or disease duration. *Neurology*, Vol.38, No.8, (August 1988), pp. 1237-1244, ISSN 0028-3878

Doty, R.L.; Golbe, L.I.; McKeown, D.A.; Stern, M.B.; Lehrach, C.M. et al. Olfactory testing differentiates between progressive supranuclear palsy and idiopathic Parkinson's disease. *Neurology*, Vol.43, No.5, (May 1993), pp. 962-965, ISSN 0028-3878

Doty, R.L.; Perl, D.P.; Steele, J.C.; Chen; K.M.; Pierce, J.D. Jr. et al. Olfactory dysfunction in three neurodegenerative diseases. *Geriatrics*, Vol.46, No.1, (August 1991), pp. 47-51, ISSN 0016-867X

Doty, R.L.; Shaman, P.; Kimmelmann, C.P. & Dann, M.S. University of Pennsylvania Smell identification test: a rapid quantitative olfactory function test for the clinic. *Laryngoscope*, Vol.94, No.2, (February 1984), pp. 176-178, ISSN 1531-4995

Duguid, JR.; De La, P.R. & DeGroot, J. Magnetic resonance imaging of the midbrain in Parkinson's disease. *Annals of Neurology*, Vol.20, No.6, (December 1986), pp. 744-747, ISSN 0364-5134

Eckert, T.; Sailer, M.; Kaufmann, J.; Schrader, C.; Peschel, T. et al. Differentiation of idiopathic Parkinson's disease, multiple system atrophy, progressive supranuclear palsy, and healthy controls using magnetization transfer imaging. *Neuroimage*, Vol.21, No.1, (January 2004), pp. 229-235, ISSN 1053-8119

Edelman, R.R.; Ahn, S.S.; Chien, D.; Li, W.; Goldmann, A. et al. Improved time-of-flight MR angiography of the brain with magnetization transfer contrast. *Radiology*, Vol.184, No.2, (August 1992), pp. 395-399, ISSN 0033-8419

Federico, F.; Simone, I.L.; Lucivero, V.; Iliceto, G.; De Mari, M. et al. Proton magnetic resonance spectroscopy in Parkinson's disease and atypical parkinsonian disorders. *Movement Disorders*, Vol.12, No.6, (November 1997), pp. 903-909, ISSN 0885-3185

Federico, F.; Simone, I.L.; Lucivero, V.; Mezzapesa, D.M.; De Mari, M. et al. Usefulness of proton magnetic resonance spectroscopy in differentiating parkinsonian syndromes. *Italian Journal of Neurological Sciences*, Vol.20, No.4, (August 1999), pp. 223-229, ISSN 0392-0461

Firbank, M.J.; Harrison, R.M. & O'Brien, J.T. A comprehensive review of proton magnetic resonance spectroscopy studies in dementia and Parkinson's disease. *Dementia And Geriatric Cognitive Disorders*, Vol.14, No.2, (July 2002), pp. 64-76, ISSN 1420-8008

Fox, P.T. & Raichle, M.E. Stimulus rate determines regional brain blood flow in striate cortex. *Annals of Neurology*, Vol.17, No3, (March 1985), pp.303-305, ISSN 0364-5134

Fulton, HG. & Barrett, SP. A demonstration of intravenous nicotine self-administration in humans? *Neuropsychopharmacology*, Vol.33, No8, (Jule 2008), pp. 2042-2043, ISSN 0893-133X

George, JS.; Aine, CJ.; Mosher, JC.; Schmidt, MD.; Ranken, DM. et al., Mapping function in the human brain with magneto encephalography, anatomical magnetic resonance imaging, and functional magnetic resonance imaging. *Journal of Clinical Neurophysiology*, Vol.12, No5, (September 1995), pp. 406-429 ISSN 1676-2649

Gupta, A.; Dawson, V.L. & Dawson, T.M. What causes cell death in Parkinson's disease? *Annals of Neurology*, Vol.64, No6, (December 2008), pp. S3-S15, ISSN 0364-5134

Haehner, A.; Boesveldt, S.; Berendse, H.W.; Mackay-Sim, A. Fleischmann, J. et al. Prevalence of smell loss in Parkinson's Disease - a multicenter study. *Parkinsonism & Related Disorders*, Vol.15, No.7, (August 2009), pp. 490-494, ISSN 1353-8020

Hagmann, P.; Jonasson, L.; Maeder, P.; Thiran, J.P.; Wedeen, V.J. et al. Understanding diffusion MR imaging techniques: from scalar diffusion-weighted imaging to diffusion tensor imaging and beyond. *Radiographics*, Vol.26, Sp. Iss, (October 2006), pp. S205-U219, ISSN 0271-5333

Hattingen, E.; Magerkurth, J.; Pilatus, U.; Morez, A.; Seifried, C. et al. Phosphorus and proton magnetic resonance spectroscopy demonstrates mitochondrial dysfunction in early and advanced Parkinson's disease. *Brain*, Vol.132, No.12, (December 2009), pp. 3285-3297, ISSN 0006-8950

Hawkes, C.H.; Shephard, B.C. & Daniel, S.E. Olfactory disfunction in Parkinson's disease. *Journal of Neurology Neurosurgery and Psychiatry*, Vol.62, No.5, (May 1997), pp. 436-446, ISSN 0022-3050

Hawkes, C.H.; Shephardm, B.C. & Daniel, S.E. Is Parkinson's disease a primary olfactory disorder? *Qjm-An International Journal of Medicine*, Vol.92, No.8, (August 1999), pp. 473-480, ISSN 1460-2725

Hinke, R.M.; Hu, X.; Stillman, A.E.; Kim, S.G.; Merkle, H. et al. Functional magnetic resonance imaging of Broca's area during internal speech. *NeuroReport*, Vol.4, No6, (June 1993) pp. 675-678 ISSN 0959-4965

Hirsch, E.C. & Hunot S. Neuroinflammation in Parkinson's disease: a target for neuroprotection? *Lancet Neurology*, Vol.8, No.4, (April 2009), pp. 382-397, ISSN: 1474-4422

Holshouser, B.A.; Komu, M.; Moller, H.E.; Zijlmans, J.; Kolem, H. et al. Localized proton NMR spectroscopy in the striatum of patients with idiopathic Parkinson's disease: a multicenter pilot study. *Magnetic Resonance in Medicine*, Vol.33, No.5, (May 1995), pp. 589-594, ISSN 0740-3194

Horsfield, M.A. Magnetization transfer imaging in multiple sclerosis. *Journal of Neuroimaging*, Vol.15, No.4, (2005), pp. 58-67, ISSN 1051-2284

Huisman, E.; Uylings, H.B. & Hoogland, P.V. A 100% increase of dopaminergic cells in the olfactory bulb may explain hyposmia in Parkinson's Disease. *Movement Disorders*, Vol.19, No.6, (June 2004), pp. 687-692, ISSN 0885-3185

Hummel, T. (1999). Olfactory evoked potentials as a tool to measure progression of Parkinson's disease. In: *Focus medicine – New development in the drug therapy of Parkinson's Disease*, T. Chase & P. Bedard, (Eds.), 47-53, ISBN 0-632-05174-4, Blackwell Science, Oxford, UK

Hummel, T.; Kobal, G.; Gudziol, H. & Mackay-Sim, A. Normative data for the "Sniffin'Sticks" including tests of odor identification, odor discrimination, and olfactory thresholds:an upgrade based on a group of more than 3.000 subjects. *European Archives of Oto-Rhino-Laryngology*, Vol.264, No.3, (March 2007), pp. 237-243, ISSN 0937-4477

Hummel, T.; Sekinger, B.; Wolf, S.; Pauli, E. & Kobal G. "Sniffin' Sticks": olfactory performance assessed by the combined testing of odor identification, odor discrimination and olfactory threshold. *Chemical Senses*, Vol.22, No.1, (February 1997), pp. 39-52, ISSN 0379-864X

Hummel, T.; Witt, M.; Reichmann, H.; Welge-Luessen, A & Haehner A. Immunohistochemical, volumetric, and functional neuroimaging studies in patients with idiopathic Parkinson's disease. *Journal of the Neurological Sciences*, Vol.298, No.1-2, (February 2010), pp. 119-122, ISSN 0022-510X

Inglese, M.; Horsfield, M.A. & Filippi, M. Scan-rescan variation of measures derived from brain magnetization transfer ratio histograms obtained in healthy volunteers by use of a semi-interleaved magnetization transfer sequence. *American Journal of Neuroradiology*, Vol.22, No.4, (April 2001), pp. 681-684, ISSN 0195-6108

Karagulle Kendi, A.T.; Lehericy, S.; Luciana, M.; Ugurbil, K. & Tuite, P. Altered diffusion in the frontal lobe in Parkinson disease. *AJNR American Journal of Neuroradiology*, Vol.38, No3, (March 2008), pp. 501-5, ISSN 1936-959X

Kettenmann, B.; Hummel, C.; Stefan, H. & Kobal, G. Multiple olfactory activity in the human neocortex identified by magnetic source imaging. *Chemical Senses*, Vol.22, No.5, (October 1997), pp. 493-502, ISSN 0379-864X

Kim, K.; Hirsch, J.; DeLaPaz, R.L.; Relkin, N. & Lee, K.M. Comparison of cortical areas activated by primary and secondary languages in human brain using functional magnetic resonance imaging (fMRI). *Abstracts: Society of Neuroscience*, Vol.21, No3, (1993), pp.1763, ISSN 0270-6474

Kobal, G. & Plattig, K.H. Objective olfactometry: methodological annotations for recording olfactory EEG-responses from the awake human. *EEG EMG Z Elektroenzephalogr Elektromyogr Verwandte Geb.*, Vol.9, No.3, (September 1978), pp. 135-145, ISSN 0012-7590

Kobal, G.; Klimek, L.; Wolfensberger, M.; Gudziol, H.; Temmel, A. et al. Multicenter investigation of 1.036 subjects using a standardized method for the assessment of olfactory function combining tests of odor identification, odor discrimination, and olfactory thresholds. *European Archives of Oto-Rhino-Laryngology*, Vol.257, No.4, (April 2000), pp. 205-211, ISSN 0937-4477

Le Bihan, D. Looking into the functional architecture of the brain with diffusion MRI. *Nature Reviews Neuroscience*, Vol.4, No.6, (June 2003), pp. 469-480, ISSN 1471-0048

Lekwuwa, G.U.; Barnes, G.R.; Collins, C.J.S.; Limousin, P. Progressive bradykinesia and hypokinesia of ocular pursuit in Parkinson's disease. *Journal of Neurology Neurosurgery and Psychiatry*, Vol.66, No.6, (June 1999), pp. 746–753, ISSN 0022-3050

Lin, A.; Ross, B.D.; Harris, K. & Wong, W. Efficacy of proton magnetic resonance spectroscopy inneurological diagnosis and neurotherapic decision making. *NeuroRx: the journal of the American Society for Experimental NeuroTherapeutics*, Vol.2, No.2, (April 2005), pp. 197-214, ISSN 1545-5343

Marino, S.; Sessa, E.; Di Lorenzo, G.; Lanzafame, P.; Scullica, G.; et al. Quantitative analysis of pursuit ocular movements in Parkinson's disease by using a video-based eye tracking system. *European Neurology*, Vol. 58, No. 4, (September 2007), pp. 193-7, ISSN 0014-3022

Marino, S.; Lanzafame, P.; Sessa, E.; Bramanti, A.; Bramanti, P. The effect of L-Dopa administration on pursuit ocular movements in suspected Parkinson's disease. *Neurological Sciences*, Vol. 31,No. 3 (June 2010), pp. 381-385, ISSN 0022-510X

Muller, A.; Reichmann, H.; Livermore, A. & Hummel T. Olfactory function in idiopathic Parkinson's disease (IPD): results from cross-sectional studies in IPD patients and long-term follow-up of de-novo IPD patients. *Journal of Neural Transmission*, Vol.109, No.5-6, (May 2002), pp. 805-811, ISSN 0300-9564

Ogawa, S.; Lee, T.M.; Nayak, A. S.; & Glynn, P. Oxygenation-sensitive contrast in magnetic resonance image of rodent brain at high magnetic fields. *Magnetic Resonance in Medicine*, Vol.14, No1, (April 1990) pp.68-78, ISSN 07403194

Pike, G.B.; Hu, B.S.; Glover, G.H. & Enzmann, D.R. Magnetization transfer time-of-flight magnetic resonance angiography. *Magnetic Resonance in Medicine*, Vol.25, No.2, (June 1992), pp. 372-379, ISSN 0740-3194

Ramaker, C.; Marinus, J.; Stiggelbout, A.M. & Van Hilten, B.J. Systematic evaluation of rating scales for impairment and disability in Parkinson's disease. *Movement Disorders*, Vol.17, No.5, (September 2002), pp. 867-876, ISSN 0885-3185

Rolheiser, T.M.; Fulton, H.G.; Good, K.P.; Fisk, J.D.; McKelvey, J.R. et al. Diffusion tensor imaging and olfactory identification testing in early-stage Parkinson's disease. *Journal of Neurology*, (February 2011), ISSN 0340-5354

Ross, B. & Bluml, S. Magnetic resonace spectroscopy of the human brain. *The Anatomical Record*, Vol.265, No.2, (April 2001), pp. 54-84, ISSN 0003-276X

Roy, C. & Sherrington, C. On the regulation of the blood-supply of the brain. *The Journal of Physiology*, Vol.11, No1-2, (January 1890), pp.85-108, ISSN 1469-7793

Rutledge, J.N.; Hilal, S.K.; Silver, A.J.; Defendini, R. & Fahn S. Study of movement disorders and brain iron by MR. *AJR American Journal of Roentgenology*, Vol.149, No2, (August 1987), pp.365-379, ISSN 0361-803X

Savoiardo, M.; Girotti, F.; Strada, L. & Ciceri, E. Magnetic resonance imaging in progressive supranuclear palsy and other parkinsonian disorders. *Journal of Neural Transmission*, Vol.42, (1994), pp. 93-110, ISSN 0303-6995

Schneider, W.; Noll, D.C. & Cohen, J. D. Functional topographic mapping of the cortical ribbon in human vision with conventional MRI scanners. *Nature*, Vol365, No6442, (September 1993), pp. 150-152, ISSN 0028-0836

Schocke, M.F.; Seppi, K.; Esterhammer, R.; Kremser, C.; Mair, K.J. et al. Trace of diffusion tensor differentiates the Parkinson variant of multiple system atrophy and Parkinson's disease. *Neuroimage*, Vol.19, Suppl.9, (2004), pp. S53-S53, ISSN 08853185

Sofic, E.; Riederer, P.; Heinsen, H.; Beckmann, H.; Reynolds, G.P. et al. Increased iron (III) and total iron content in post mortem substantia nigra of parkinsonian brain. *Journal of Neural Transmission*, Vol.74, No3, (August 1988), pp.199-205, ISSN 0300-9564

Srinivasan, R.; Vigneron, D.; Sailasuta, N.; Hurd, R. & Nelson, S. A comparative study of myo-inositol quantification using LCmodel at 1.5 T and 3.0 T with 3D 1H proton spectroscopic imaging of the human brain. *Magnetic Resonance Imaging*, Vol.22, No.4, (May 2004), pp. 523-528, ISSN 0730-725X

Takeda, A.; Saito, N.; Baba, T.; Kikuchi, A.; Sugeno, N. et al. Functional imaging studies of hyposmia in Parkinson's disease. *Journal of the Neurological Sciences*, Vol.298, No.1-2, (February 2010), pp. 36-39, ISSN 0022-510X

Tambasco, N.; Pelliccioli, G.P.; Chiarini, P.; Montanari, G.E.; Leone, F. et al. Magnetization Transfer changes of gray and white matter in Parkinson 's disease. *Neuroradiology*, Vol.45, No.4, (April 2003), pp. 224-230, ISSN 0028-3940

Tedeschi, G.; Litvan, I.; Bonavita, S.; Bertolino, A.; Lundbom, N. et al. Proton magnetic resonance spectroscopic imaging in progressive supranuclear palsy, Parkinson's disease and corticobasal degeneration. *Brain*, Vol.120, No.9, (September 1997), pp. 1541-1552, ISSN 0006-8950

Tessa, C.; Giannelli, M.; Della Nave, R.; Lucetti, C.; Berti, C.A. et al. A whole-brain analysis in de novo Parkinson disease. *AJNR American Journal of Neuroradiology*, Vol.29, No4, (April 2008), pp. 674-680, ISSN 01956108

Tissingh, G.; Berendse, H.W.; Bergmans, P.; DeWaard, R.; Drukarch, B. et al. Loss of olfaction in de novo and treated Parkinson's disease: possible implications for early diagnosis. *Movement Disorders*, Vol.16, No.1, (January 2001), pp. 41-46, ISSN 0885-3185

Watanabe, H.; Fukatsu, H.; Katsuno, M.; Sugiura, M.; Hamada, K. et al. Multiple regional 1H-MR spectroscopy in multiple system atrophy: NAA/Cr reduction in pontine base as a valuable diagnostic marker. *Journal of Neurology, Neurosurgery, and Psychiatry*, Vol.75, No.1, (January 2004), pp. 103-109, ISSN 0022-3050

Wattendorf, E.; Welge-Lüssen, A.; Fiedler K.; Bilecen, D.; Wolfensberger, M. et al. Olfactory Impairment Predicts Brain Atrophy in Parkinson's Disease. *The Journal of Neuroscience*, Vol.29, No.49, (December 2009), pp. 15410-15413, ISSN 0270-6474

Welge-Lüssen, A.; Wattendorf, E.; Schwerdtfeger, U.; Fuhr, P.; Bilecen, D. et al. Olfactory induced brain activity in Parkinson's disease relates to the expression of event-related potentials—an fMRI study. *Neuroscience*, Vol.162, No.2, (August 2009), pp. 537-543, ISSN 0306-4522

Wenning, G.K.; Shephard, B.; Hawkes, C.; Petruckevitch, A.; Lees, A. et al. Olfactory function in atypical parkinsonian syndromes. *Acta Neurologica Scandinavica*, Vol.91, No.4, (April 1995), pp. 247-250, ISSN 0001-6314

Westermann, B.; Wattendorf, E.; Schwerdtfeger, U.; Husner, A.; Fuhr, P. et al. Functional imaging of the cerebral olfactory system in patients with Parkinson's disease. *Journal of Neurology, Neurosurgery, and Psychiatry,* Vol.79, No.1, (January 2008), pp. 19-24, ISSN 0022-3050

Wilms, H.; Zecca, L.; Rosenstiel, P.; Sievers, J.; Deuschl, G. et al. Inflammation in Parkinson's diseases and other neurodegenerative diseases: cause and therapeutic implications. *Current Pharmaceutical Design,* Vol.13, No18, (June 2007), pp. 1925-1928, ISSN: 1381-6128

Wolff, S.D. & Balaban, R.S. Magnetization transfer contrast (MTC) and tissue water proton relaxation in vivo. *Magnetic Resonance in Medicine,* Vol.10, No.1, (April 1989), pp. 135-144, ISSN 0740-3194

Wolff, S.D.; Eng, J. & Balaban, R.S. Magnetization transfer contrast: method for improving contrast in gradient-recalled-echo images. *Radiology,* Vol.179, No.1, (April 1991), pp. 133-137, ISSN 0033-8419

Yonca, A.; Pervin, I.; Ali, D.; Sezer, K. & Naighan, I. Magnetization Transfer Ratio in Early Period of Parkinson Disease. *Academic Radiology,* Vol.14, No.2, (February 2007), pp. 189-192, ISSN 1076-6332

Youdim, M.B.H.; Ben-Schachar, D.; Yehuda, S. & Riederer, P. The role of iron in the basal ganglia. *Advances in Neurology,* Vol.53, (1990) pp.155-162, ISSN: 0091-3952

3

Brain Event - Related Oscillations in Parkinsonian Patients During Discrimination Task Conditions

Juliana Dushanova

Institute of Neurobiology, Bulgarian Academy of Sciences

Bulgaria

1. Introduction

Parkinson's disease (PD) is caused by a disruption of dopaminergic neurotransmission in the basal ganglia, which serve as an integrative centre for the sensory and cognitive processing of information and as a mutual link between this processing and disturbed motor performance. The basal ganglia and the cerebellum transmit information via the thalamus to the cerebral cortex in order to regulate movement. The neurotransmitter changes affect the output of the striatum into the globus pallidus as well as into the thalamus and cerebral cortex beyond. The disease is a common and disabling disorder of movement characterized by poverty, slowness and impaired scaling of voluntary movements (akinesia and bradykinesia), muscle rigidity, and tremor of the limbs at rest. Alterations of the basal ganglia with proven neuronal degenerative disorders of dopaminergic neurons and a reduction in activity in frontostriatal neural circuitry have been suggested to play a role in the executive dysfunction of PD (Taylor et al., 1990; Innis et al., 1993; Lewis et al., 2003; Owen, 2004; Leblois et al., 2006; Anik et al., 2007). The slowed information processing, insufficient encoding strategies and planning, and attentional set-shifting are related to memory deficits and cognitive impairment in PD (Daum et al., 1995; Pillon et al., 1997; Knoke et al., 1998; Robertson & Empson, 1999; Sawamoto et al., 2002; Cools, 2006). Neuropsychological studies of PD patients report cognitive deficits even during the early stages of the disease (van Spaendonck et al., 2006). The primary working memory deficit in PD is associated with impaired free recall performances (Higginson et al., 2003).

Many electroencephalographic (EEG) studies on PD have used the event-related potential (ERP) method, where the early modal dependent and obligatory N1 and P2 components permit analysis of sensory events while the later N2 and P3 potentials reflect the cognitive processes involving the assessment of stimuli, decision making, strategy selection and recognition memory. ERP investigations have shown P3 predominantly with prolonged latencies and/or diminished amplitudes for Parkinsonian patients (PP) when compared to healthy subjects (HS) (Evarts et al., 1981; Tachibana et al., 1992; Philipova et al., 1997; Wascher et al., 1997; Minamoto et al., 2001; Antal et al., 2002; Wang et al., 2002). Such results have been interpreted as electrophysiological signs of cognitive slowing with respect to stimulus classification and attentional processing (Robertson & Empson, 1999).

One valuable means of assessing deviations from the normal state in PD is to study oscillatory brain processes. In the ERP method, however, the functional significance of the responses in different frequency bands is lost. More clarification could be expected when attentional processes in PD during a representation of discrimination tasks (Vieregge et al., 1994) are examined using event-related desynchronization/synchronization (ERD/ERS) method. In the early stages, PD also affects cognitive functions (Cools, 2006). Cognitive processes require transient integration between different brain areas. Hence, dynamic links are formed, mediated by the ERS or ERD of neuronal assemblies. ERD is defined as a relative decrease in the power of a certain frequency band during stimulus processing, while ERS is a relative increase in the power of the same frequency (Pfurtscheller & Klimesch, 1991). The ERD/ERS method has been used to study auditory and visual working memory encoding and categorization processes in PP; studies indicate less theta-ERS and upper alpha-ERD reflected disturbance of both the basal ganglia activity as well as activity related to their thalamo-cortical neuronal nets at frontal electrode locations (Schmiedt et al., 2005; Ellfolk et al., 2006). The encoding of auditory stimuli elicits alpha- and theta-ERS, while memory retrieval during the presentation of a target stimulus elicits theta-ERS and alpha-ERD (Karrasch et al., 1998, 2004; Krause et al., 1996, 1999). Oscillations in the beta frequency band are associated with cognitive control of behaviour or "executive functions" (Pfurtscheller & Lopes da Silva, 1999; Engel et al., 2001). By means of an auditory stop-signal task, the differential participation of beta subbands in voluntary motor control can be revealed: ERD in the 20–30 Hz band is related to initiation of movement, while ERS in a low frequency beta band (12–16 Hz) is exclusively linked to the stopping of planned action (Pfurtscheller & Lopes da Silva, 1999; Engel et al., 2001). One proposed hypothesis for these observations is that lower-frequency beta subbands represent inhibitory components of cognitive control and are more generalized, while higher frequency beta subbands take part in response choice and activation and are more specialized in terms of both function and cortical distribution.

Some recent investigations (Basar, 2001; Ozgoren et al., 2005; Sutoh et al., 2000; Gurtubay et al., 2001) propose that beta and gamma cortical rhythms may serve cognitive processes such as linking perception to action or movement planning (Donoghue et al., 1998). Research both on animals and humans has suggested that gamma-frequency activity also plays an important role in attention as well as working and long-term memory (Herrmann et al., 2004). Current investigations using intracranial and high-density electro- and magnetoencephalographic recordings explore the involvement of gamma-band synchronization in various cognitive paradigms in humans (Engel et al., 2001; Basar et al., 2001; Herrmann et al., 2004; Pantev, 1995; Tallon-Baudry et al., 1996; Farmer, 1998; Fries et al., 2001). Other works associate the changes in EEG spectral power in the gamma frequency band to interactions between the cortex and basal ganglia (Gatev & Wichmann, 2008). Additionally, akinesia in PP has been related in some studies to abnormally increased beta (15–30 Hz) and decreased gamma (35–80 Hz) synchronous oscillatory activity in the basal ganglia (Weinberger et al., 2006). Other results suggest that resting tremor in PD is associated with an altered balance between beta and gamma oscillations in the motor circuits of the subthalamic nucleus (STN) and is exhibited as increased oscillatory activity in the low gamma frequency range (35–55 Hz) during periods with stronger tremor (Weinberger et al., 2008). Therapeutic doses of dopaminergic medication in PP attenuate the beta band power in the STN, giving rise to the hypothesis that the beta prominence is pathological in PD (Cassidy et al, 2002; Kühn et al., 2006; Levy et al., 2001; 2002; Priori et al., 2002). Treatment of PP with dopaminergic therapy leads to increased gamma band activity in the basal ganglia and thus to improvement in motor performance (Brown et al., 2001), hence the suggestion that synchronization of the activity of populations of basal ganglia neurons in the gamma band may facilitate motor processing (Brown, 2003). Investigations based on local field potentials recorded from the STN in PP show increased power in the beta range (13–35 Hz) while the patient is at rest (Cassidy et al., 2002; Levy et al., 2002; Brown et al., 2001; Priori et al., 2004). This suggests that there is excessive synchrony in the basal ganglia networks in PD and some of the clinical signs of the disease, it is proposed, stem from this abnormal synchrony between basal ganglia and cortical circuits (Brown, 2003; Marsden et al., 2001).

The aim of the present study was to investigate the functional relationships between oscillatory EEG-dominant components with ERD/ERS method for PP and HS during auditory discrimination tasks within two poststimulus intervals of 0–250 and 250–600 ms. We first focused on time-frequency analysis of delta, theta and alpha rhythms, the appearance of which is well established in PD and is thought to reflect the degree of cortical activation during the information processing. We later shift our focus to the beta and gamma bands, where our aim is to assess the differences between PP and HS in these frequency bands and check an assumption that some PP clinical symptoms stem from excessive synchrony between the basal ganglia and cortical circuits. This investigation of the oscillatory processes and ERD/ERS in HS and PP could contribute to clarification of the disturbances of the neurophysiological mechanisms of this disease.

2. Methods

2.1 Experimental procedure
2.1.1 Subjects
We investigated eleven voluntary patients with a mean age of 61 ± 12.2 years (±s.d.; 7 males, 4 females) with a diagnosis of idiopathic Parkinson's disease for no longer than 2.8 years, assessed by a neurologist at the University Neurological Hospital, with score of I on the Hoehn–Yahr scale of motor function (Hoehn & Yahr, 1967). Patients receiving levodopa (L-dopa) drugs (Sinemet) were included in order to reduce the heterogeneity in the medication. During the experimental session, all patients were in off-phase of the medication. None of the patients had dementia, depression, a presence of atherosclerosis, attendant neurological complications or pronounced tremor. The same number of healthy volunteers was included as aged-matched healthy controls with a mean age of 59.5 ± 9.5 years. Screening confirmed that subjects were free of past or current psychiatric and neurological disorders. All participants were right handed and without deficits in hearing. Handedness was assessed by a questionnaire adapted from the Edinburgh Handedness Inventory (Oldfield, 1971). The study was performed with the approval of the local ethics committee. The subjects were introduced to the nature of the investigation and their informed written consent was obtained according to the declaration of Helsinki.

2.1.2 Stimuli and task
Each subject was comfortably seated in an ergonomically designed chair inside a Faraday cage, monitored by a Canon Video system. The experimental design included a binary sensory-motor reaction task. Each sensory-motor series consisted of 50 computer generated low frequency (LT – 800 Hz) and 50 high frequency (HT – 1000 Hz) acoustic stimuli with an intensity of 60 dB, duration of 50 ms, and an inter-stimulus interval of 2.5–3.5 s presented to the subject in a randomized order. PP and HS were asked to press a key with the index

finger of each hand and make rapid and accurate choice responses with the left hand to the high frequency (HT) or with the right hand to the low frequency (LT) tone. The movement performance from the stimulus presentation to the onset of voluntary force production (onset of reaction time) and from the stimulus presentation to the force peak (force peak latency) were measured by a force transducer. A surface electromyographic activity pattern of the first dorsal interosseus muscles was also registered.

2.1.3 EEG recording

An electroencephalogram (EEG) was recorded from Fz, Cz, Pz, C3' and C4' (10/20, system), using Ag/AgCl Nihon-Kohden electrodes with a reference to both processi mastoidei and a ground electrode, placed on the forehead. An oculogram (EOG) was recorded from m. orbicularis oculi dex. We placed two EOG electrodes next to the eyes to register eye movements. EEG and EOG data were recorded using a Nihon-Kohden EEG-4314F (cut-off frequencies of 0.3–70 Hz) and recorded together with markers of the movement performance as a force profile and a surface electromyographic activity pattern of the first dorsal interosseus muscles (bandpass filtered 0.03–500 Hz). The signals were digitized on-line (10 bit A/D converter, 256 samples/s). The data recordings for the sensorimotor task were synchronized to the marker of the stimulus onset (-0.2 s before and 0.8 s after the stimulus). Only recordings that were artifact-free with respect to event-related potentials were processed. We applied a Chebyshev Type II bandpass filter (1-70 Hz) and second-order notch filter at frequency 50 Hz (AC) component. We defined an independent reference interval in order to quantify the changes in the time-frequency energy density of the signal. We used stimulus-nonrelated subepochs within the resting condition series, distant enough (-1.4 s) from the stimulus onset, not including event-related properties, and exceeding the period of the lowest frequency studied in the signal (1.5 Hz, 0.67 s). We preselected trials by applying a bootstrap estimation within the reference period and a false discovery rate correction for multiple comparisons (0.05) to the available data across the indexes corresponding to time and number of the trial, eliminating the need for a strict assumption of ergodicity (Durka et al., 2004).

2.2 Analysis

The time-frequency analysis (TF) represented the power of a continuous EEG signal as a function of both time and frequency (Matlab®, Mathworks, Inc.). For time amplitude-frequency distributions, the filtered signal was analyzed with a sliding-window fast Fourier transform with length 200 ms and step 10 ms. The amplitude was computed for every time window t and frequency bin f by the real and imaginary Fourier coefficients. The amplitude modulations obtained for each frequency band for each subject in a group were added across trials in order to compare amplitude changes in the post-stimulus intervals with respect to pre-stimulus interval reference amplitudes, i.e. to derive ERD/ERS. This method characterizes the relative amplitude decrement/increment of the given frequency during the post-stimulus period in relation to pre-stimulus amplitude modulation of the same frequency (Pfurtscheller G, Klimesch, 1991). This resulted in ERD/ERS values which could then be presented as percentage changes with respect to the reference interval. Negative values indicate a relative power decrease (ERD), whereas positive values point to a relative power increase (ERS). Relatively, sensory processing takes place during the first post-stimulus interval (T1: 0–250 ms) and cognitive processing during the second post-stimulus interval (T2: 250–600 ms), defined as beginning when a tone ends. The peak amplitude modulations, defined in 10 ms bins, were specified as dominating components. Afterwards, the high amplitudes in each frequency band, respectively, were added over trials and across subjects to compare their amplitude changes in the post-stimulus intervals with those in the reference interval. Thus, we calculated the ERD/ERS of delta ($\delta \sim 1.5$–4 Hz), theta ($\theta \sim 4.1$–7 Hz) and alpha ($\alpha \sim 7.1$–13 Hz) waves as percentage power differences in each frequency band compared to the reference interval for both 0–250 ms and 250–600 ms post-stimulus intervals. We also defined the ERD/ERS of beta ($\beta_1 \sim 13.1$–20 Hz), ($\beta_2 \sim 20.1$–32 Hz) and gamma ($\gamma \sim 32.1$–50 Hz) frequency rhythms during the post-stimulus intervals T1 (0–250 ms) and T2 (250–600 ms).

We employed the detection of the temporally dynamic processes similar to the approach applied by Foffani et al. (Foffani et al., 2005) that describes the behaviour of β_1-, β_2-, γ - ERS rhythms in zones which vary both in amplitude and frequency. Each zone i is characterized by a value $ERSi$ (t) and a frequency value Fi (t), both dependent on time, which separately describe event-related synchronization and corresponding frequency modulations for the beta1, beta2 and gamma rhythms in two post-stimulus time windows. The significance of the observed ERS values was tested for each frequency band and EEG channel using a permutation test, including corrections for multiple comparisons between time points for time course analysis (Mason & Newton, 1990). The latencies of ERS and corresponding frequency (relative to stimulus onset) were measured as the last zero-crossing before a significant modulation, after subtracting the baseline mean ERS value. Although the ERS clearly occurred, the relationship between the ERS peaks and the maximum of the average event-related synchronization (AERS) was not always evident. Since the AERSs of different channels were not identical, an exact coincidence between the peaks times was not observed. The probabilities for the amplitudes and latencies were not uniform and the activity distribution was clearly not Gaussian. We estimated the latency shift between the largest peaks for each pair of channels.

2.2.1 Statistics

We performed statistical analyses of the ERD/ERS for the two post-stimulus intervals and assessed the statistical difference between the groups (PP and HS) for each tone type and interval by means of a bootstrap nonparametric procedure (Mason & Newton, 1990). The characteristics were grouped by tone, interval, patients and healthy controls and analyzed by means of a permutation test for multiple comparisons (Mason & Newton, 1990). The computed random distribution for interval was analyzed with a nonparametric test (Kruskal-Wallis [KW] test, $p < 0.05$) for pairs comparison of the scalp leads between patient and control group. This procedure reduces the influence of random variations in experimental conditions between trials. The ERD/ERS analysis served to identify the most robust differences between groups and was generally done for the two time windows. The parameters of the movement performance (onset of reaction time, force peak latency and error of performance) were processed statistically by Mann–Whitney U test.

3. Experimental results

3.1 Response parameters

Parkinson's patients showed a longer reaction time onset, but the difference between the two groups was not significant: in response to a low tone – 440.5 ± 135.8 ms in HS and 508.4

± 148.5 ms in PP (mean ± S.D., $p > 0.05$), in response to a high tone − 455.7 ± 134.6 ms in HS and 500.4 ± 146.5 ms in PP ($p > 0.05$). Parkinson's patients had significantly longer force peak latency (FPL) in response to the two tone types. The FPLs were 672.8 ± 154.7 ms in HS and 919.96 ± 163.7 ms in PP in response to the low tone (mean ± s.d, $p < 0.02$). In response to the high tone, the FPLs were 690.7 ± 148.7 ms in HS and 934.9 ± 160.2 ms in PP ($p < 0.05$). The mean errors (false and missing responses) were 4.5 and 5.1 in PP, respectively, in response to the low and high tone. The mean errors were 3.5 and 4.4 in HS, respectively, in response to the low and high tone. The differences of errors between the two groups were not significant ($p > 0.05$).

3.2 Frequency components

The grand average ERD/ERS values as a function of time and frequency band at the frontal, central, parietal, left and right motor areas were used for assessment of group means with the standard errors (±SE) for the post-stimulus intervals T1 (0–250 ms) and T2 (250–600 ms). The statistical group comparison for pair channels are shown graphically to illustrate the delta-, theta-, alpha-, beta-, gamma- ERD/ERS following the low frequency tone type (Figs. 1A, 2A) and high frequency tone type (Figs. 1B, 2B) for the early (0–250 ms) and late (250–600 ms) post-stimulus intervals.

3.2.1 Delta

The patterns of δ-ERD/ERS were different between the groups for both intervals in response to both tone types (Dushanova et al., 2009). In the early post-stimulus interval, central δ-ERS amplitude responses were most pronounced in the HS after both tones (Cz, Fig. 1A, B, 1st row, left plots) and in the PP at the frontal side for the high tone (Fig. 1B, left) and parietal area for the low tone (Fig. 1A, left). The least pronounced δ-ERS were those appearing at the frontal side in the HS and in the left motor area in PP following both tones (Fig. 1A, B, left). The comparison by the bootstrap procedure of δ-ERS between the two groups after the low frequency tone determined that the control δ-ERS was significantly higher than that of the PP for all channels (Fz, Pz, $p < 0.05$; Cz, C3′, C4′, $p < 0.001$). Both groups displayed δ-ERS following the high frequency tone (Fig. 1B, left). This was significantly higher for the HS than the PP at centro-parietal, left and right motor areas (Cz, C3′, C4′ $p < 0.001$; Pz, $p < 0.05$). The PD patients' frontal δ-ERS, however, was greater than that of the HS ($p < 0.001$).

The HS maintained δ-ERS at all electrodes during the late post-stimulus interval T2 following the low frequency tone, while in the PP the early post-stimulus δ-ERS was reversed to become δ-ERD in the late post-stimulus interval (Fig. 1A, B, 1st row, right). The highest δ-ERS was located at parietal side for the HS, whereas the PP had a less enhanced parietal δ-ERD. The PP showed the most enhanced δ-ERD at the left motor area (Fig. 1B, right). Following the high frequency tone, δ-ERS was elicited at all electrodes in the HS (Fig. 1B, right). The PP group, in comparison with the HS, showed a less pronounced central δ-ERS (Cz, $p < 0.001$) and specific δ-ERD at parietal and left motor areas ($p < 0.001$).

3.2.2 Theta

In the first post-stimulus interval following both tone types, the θ-ERS responses were most prominent at parietal electrodes for both groups (Fig. 1, A, B, 2nd row, left). Following the low tone, the θ-ERS elicited was significantly higher for HS than for PP at frontal, left and

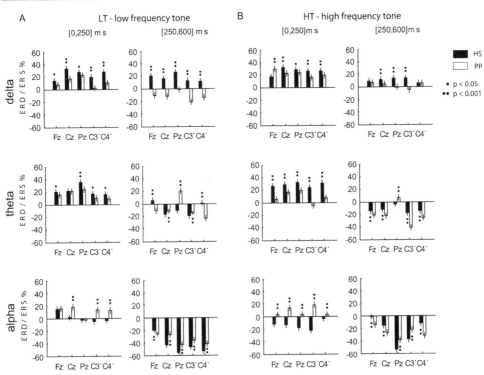

Fig. 1. Group means (±SE) and statistical results of δ-, θ-, α-ERD/ERS over all HS and PP trials after the low tone (A) and high tone type (B) for the early (left) and late time period (right) at all channels.

right motor areas ($p < 0.05$), parietal side ($p < 0.001$), and centrally was non-significantly different (Cz, $p > 0.05$; Fig. 1A, 2nd row, left). Following the high frequency tone, PP produced a significantly lower θ-ERS than the HS at right motor area, fronto-central and parietal sides ($p < 0.001$; Fig. 1B, left). The left motor area showed a pronounced θ-ERS for the HS and a weak θ-ERD in the PP following the high frequency tone.

The comparison of the groups during the late period following the low frequency tone showed θ-ERD in both groups at most electrodes with the following exceptions. PP recorded a large parietal θ-ERS while a less prominent θ-ERS appeared in HS at frontal and right motor areas (Fig. 1A, 2nd row, right). The most pronounced θ-ERDs for HS were at central and left motor areas ($p < 0.001$). The signal at the parietal area was characterized by a very prominent θ-ERS in the patients but by θ-ERD in the control group. In response to the high frequency tone, we found a significant θ-ERD for the PP as compared with the HS at fronto-central, left and right motor areas ($p < 0.001$; Fig. 1B, right). The signal at the parietal area was characterized in a similar manner to that elicited by a low tone, but with a less pronounced θ-ERS in the PP and smaller θ-ERD in the HS.

3.2.3 Alpha

The PP showed fronto-central, left and right motor α-ERS responses following the LT, while the HS had synchronization only at the fronto-central sides but α-ERD at the parietal side, right and left motor areas (Fig. 1A, 3rd row, left). The alpha frequency band in the first interval after the LT showed an enhanced central α-ERS for the PP in comparison with the HS ($p < 0.001$; Fig. 1A, left). The right and left motor areas manifested different reversal alteration as α-ERS for the PP and weakly elicited α-ERD for the HS. Following the high tone, we detected significantly different processes, α-ERS in the PP contrasted with α-ERD in the HS at all electrodes, most prominently at the left motor side (Fig. 1B, left).

Alpha-ERD differences between the groups were observed after low as well as high frequency tones during the late period (Fig. 1A, B, right). After the low tone, the HS α-ERD means were significantly more pronounced than those of the PP at centro-parietal sides, left and right motor areas ($p < 0.001$; Fig. 1A, right). The PP displayed a higher frontal α-ERD than that in the HS ($p < 0.001$). Alpha-ERD differences were observed between the groups following the high tone (Fig. 1B, right). The α-ERD signals of HS at parietal and left motor areas were more pronounced than in the PP ($p < 0.001$). The PP fronto-central and right motor α-ERD signals had greater respective magnitudes than those in HS ($p < 0.001$).

3.2.4 Beta1

During the early post-stimulus interval T1, ERD/ERS β1 patterns appeared in the lower frequency portions of this band for each electrode and group (Dushanova et al., 2010). The maximum synchronized β1 bursts across the channels were localized over fronto-central sides for both groups after LT, but had significantly higher amplitude and shorter durations in PP than HS ($p < 0.001$, bootstrap, KW test; Table 1, **a**). Later β1 ERS bursts were found only in PP over the frontal side and left motor area (Table 1, LT (T1), **b**). Synchronized β1 bursts were centered on right motor side for PP and fronto-central sides for HS, following HT (Table 1, HT (T1), **a**, **b**). In PP, the peaks were of a significantly lower amplitude and peaked later at centro-parietal sides than in HS (Table 1, HT (T1), **a**). During the late post-stimulus interval T2, frontal synchronized β1 peaks at 20 Hz were extracted only in HS after HT and had a prolonged latency of 176 ± 11.5 ms (Table 1, HT (T2), **f**).

3.2.5 Beta2

During T1, ERS β2 bursts were present only in PP after either tone (Table 2, LT(T1), HT(T1)). Their maximum amplitude across the scalp was localized over frontal side for either tone, right and left motor areas respectively for LT and HT (Table 2, **c**). They peaked earlier at the right than at the left motor area, fronto-central leads (Table 2, **c**), and parietal side (Table 2, **d**) for either tone, but in higher β2 frequency range after LT than after HT. During T2, the maximum value of β2 bursts across all recorded areas was centered on right motor area in PP (Table 2, **g**) but on parietal side in HS following LT (Table 2, LT(T2), **j**). More widely distributed, prolonged β2 ERS bursts were pronounced over all locations for PP following HT, but limited to frontal-central and right motor areas for HS (Table 2, HT(T2)). The maximum scalp β2 burst was localized at the right motor area in PP and frontal area in HS after HT (Table 2, **g - j**). At the right motor area, spectral peaks of low β2 exhibited significantly more exaggerated and prolonged bursts in PP than in HS ($p < 0.001$, Table 2, **g - j**). The frontal synchronized high frequency β2 bursts appeared in PP during two subintervals, the first one with a significantly shorter latency than the low frequency β2 bursts in HS ($p < 0.001$, Table 2, **g**). In PP, synchronized bursts of high β2 were generated on the left motor area (Table 2, **g**) earlier than larger synchronized bursts at low β2 (Table 2, **i, j**).

Channels	Fz ERS(%)/ F/ t (±SE) D	Cz ERS(%)/ F/ t (±SE) D	Pz ERS(%)/ F/ t (±SE) D	C3′ ERS(%)/ F/ t (±SE) D	C4′ ERS(%)/F /t (±SE) D
Subjects Tone(period)			HS		
LT (T1)	64.1 (±1.2)/13 Hz 40 (±7.3) ms [8–72] ms (a)	50.1 (±5.8) /13 Hz 36 (±6.9) ms [8–64] ms (a)	18.8 (±0.5)/13 Hz 20 (±5.2) ms [8–32] ms (a)	41 (±3.3)* /13 Hz 36 (±28) ms [8–80] ms (a)	44.9(±5.2)*/13 Hz 32.0 (±6.5)** ms [8–72] ms (a)
HT (T1)	68.6(±10.2)/13.9(±0.3)Hz [13–15] Hz 36 (±6.9) ms [8–64] ms (a)	62.7(±8.5)*/13.7(±0.3)Hz [13–15] Hz 32 (±6.5)** ms [8–56] ms (a)	30.49(±3.3)*/13Hz 28(±6.1)** ms [8–48] ms (a)	54.7(±8.3)*/13.5(±0.3)Hz [13–15] Hz 32(±6.5) ms [8–56] ms (a)	50.4(±6.6)*/13 Hz 32(±6.5) ms [8–56] ms (a)
LT (T2)	-	-	-	-	-
HT (T2)	51 (±3.2)/20 Hz 516 (±11.5) ms [424–600] ms (f)	-	-	-	-
Subjects Tone(period)			PP		
LT (T1)	69.4(±0.9)*/ 13 Hz 12 (±4)** ms [8–80] ms (a)	57.2(±3)*/13 Hz 16 (±4.6)** ms [8–64] ms (a)	-	36.8(±2.8)/13 Hz 12 (±4)** ms [8–16] ms (a)	33.9(±5)/13Hz 48 (±6.5) ms [24–72] ms (a)
	15.8(±0.2)/14(±0.6) Hz 124 (±5.2) ms [112–136] ms (b)	-	-	19.3(±1.3)/18 Hz 148 (±5.2) ms [136–160] ms (b)	-
HT (T1)	-	34.4(±3.8)/13.8(±0.3) Hz 53.6 (±11.2) ms [8–104] ms (a)	21.3(±0.8)/ 13 Hz 46 (±8.7) ms [8–88] ms (a)	35(±1.9)/ 13 Hz 20(±5.2)** ms [8–32] ms (a)	40.2(±2.8)/13 Hz 24 (±5.7) ** ms [8–40] ms (a)
	-	-	-	-	25(±1.1)/16 Hz 92 (±5.2) ms [80–112] ms (b)
LT (T2)	-	-	-	-	-
HT (T2)	-	-	-	-	-

Note: Bold-marked mean ERS β1 bursts (%) (±SE) are maximum across the channels for each condition and subject separately for LT(T1), HT(T1), LT(T2), HT(T2); F (Hz) – mean frequency peaks (±SE) of the maximum ERS β1 bursts across trials; t (ms) – mean times (±SE) of maximum ERS β1 bursts across trials during T1 (or T2) with respect to stimulus onset; D (ms) – time duration of these short–term zones with ERS β1 bursts; [1]* =a significant difference in ERS between the groups HS, PP for each channel and tone separately, marked the higher value (p<0.001, KW test); [2]** =a significant difference in t between the groups for each channel and tone separately, marked the shorter value (p<0.001, KW test). Lower case letters in Table 1 marked consecutive sub-intervals with ERS β1 bursts: a, b during T1; f during T2.

Table 1. Mean ERS β1 bursts (%) across the trials with mean frequency peaks F (Hz) for HS and PP after LT and HT presented in short–term zones D (ms) during early T1 and late T2 period.

Channels	Fz ERS(%)/ F/ t (±SE) D	Cz ERS(%)/F/ t (±SE) D	Pz ERS(%)/ F/ t (±SE) D	C3' ERS(%)/ F/ t (±SE) D	C4' ERS(%)/F /t (±SE) D
Subjects tone(period)			HS		
LT (T1)	-	-	-	-	-
HT (T1)	-	-	-	-	-
LT (T2)	-	-	25.8(±1.6)/32Hz 584 (±6.5) ms [560–600] ms (j)	19.6(±1.3)/30.5(±0.2)Hz 588 (±6.1) ms [576–600] ms (j)	-
HT (T2)	43.9(±3.1)/23.1(±0.1)Hz 516 (±11.5) ms [424–600] ms (g–j)	18.1(±0.6)/21Hz 488(±5.7) ms [472–504] ms (h)	-	-	28.2(±2.3)/ 32 Hz 384 (±6.5)** ms [360–408] ms (g)
	-	-	-	-	40.6(±3.1)/23.4(±0.4)Hz 532 (±10.6) ms [456–600] ms (h–j)
Subjects tone(period)			PP		
LT (T1)	61.1 (±1.1)/ 32 Hz 40 (±5.7) ms [24–56] ms (c)	30.6(±4.7)/32Hz 48 (±5.7) ms [32–64] ms (c)	23.2(±1.7)/25.2(±1.6)Hz 64 (±9.2) ms [8–120] ms (c, d)	22.4(±3.7)/29.7(±0.3)Hz 32 (±4.6) ms [24–40] ms (c)	60.3(±1.1)/32Hz 12 (±4) ms [8–16] ms (c)
HT (T1)	41.2(±2)/24.3(±0.5)Hz 60 (±8.8) ms [32–88] ms (c)	29.8(±1.1)/23Hz 64 (±4.6) ms [56–72] ms (c)	28(±2.7)/24.2(±1.1)Hz 121.6 (±9.1) ms [64–160] ms (d)	46(±2.8)/23.9(±0.4) Hz 64 (±6.5) ms [40–88] ms (c)	38.1(±1.2)/22Hz 56 (±4.6) ms [48–72] ms (c)
	-	-	-	19.3(±0.8)/32 Hz 168 (±4.6) ms [160–176] ms (e)	-
LT (T2)	-	15.5(±0.1)/32Hz 392 (±4.6) ms [384–400] ms (g)	17.9(±1)/ 32 Hz 376 (±4.6) ms [368–384] ms (g)	-	30.7(±2.1)/32 Hz 368 (±8.6) ms [320–416] ms (g)
	-	-	24.7(±1.7)/30.9(±0.1)Hz 528 (±10.8) ms [448–600] ms (h)	26(±1.5)/29.3(±0.5)Hz 492 (±9.5) ms [432–552] ms (h)	-
HT (T2)	36.7(±2.9)/ 32Hz 388(±8.9)** ms [336–440] ms (g)	23.8(±1.3)*/32Hz 376 (±7.3)** ms [344–408] ms (g)	25.3(±0.7)/30(±0.03)Hz 452 (±14.8) ms [296–600] ms (g–j)	34.8(±2)/32Hz 352 (±11.8) ms [256–448] ms (g)	60.6(±2)*/22.2(±0.1)Hz 444 (±15.1) ms [280–600] ms (g–j)
	26.1(±1.0)/ 32Hz 548 (±9.5) ms [488–600] ms (i)	-	-	44.8(±2.5)/25Hz 532 (±10.6) ms [456–600] ms (i, j)	-

Note: Lower case letters in Table 2 marked consecutive sub-intervals with ERS β2 bursts: **c, d, e** during T1 and **g, h, i, j** during T2.

Table 2. Mean ERS β2 bursts (%) across the trials with mean frequency peaks **F** (Hz) for HS and PP after LT and HT presented in short–term zones **D** (ms) during early T1 and late T2 period (same format as **Table 1).**

3.2.6 Gamma

The scalp γ burst topography was localized on frontal area for PP following either tone (Table 3, LT(T1), HT(T1), **a**) and for HS – on right motor area after LT and left motor area after HT during T1 (Table 3, **c**). The ERS γ bursts in PP peaked later than in HS at the fronto-central for either tone, and at right and left motor areas after LT (Table 3, **a, b, c**). They were of significantly greater amplitude and more prolonged duration in PP than in HS at the fronto-central and parietal sides after either tone ($p < 0.001$, Table 3). Later γ burst ERS was also found during T1 over right motor and parietal areas in PP after LT (Table 3, **b; c**), and over left motor area in PP, but parietal and right motor sides in HS, after HT (Table 3, **d**). During T2, synchronized frontal γ bursts were extracted from both groups after either tone (Table 3, **f**) and peaked later in PP. The scalp γ bursts were with significantly higher amplitudes in PP than the equivalent responses from HS ($p < 0.001$, Table 3).

In sum, despite the early short-term $\beta1$ synchrony during the two periods, both groups exhibited mean $\beta1$ ERD following either tone type and interval (Fig. 2A, B, 1st row), which was significantly greater for HS in comparison with PP in all channels ($p < 0.001$, bootstrap, KW test), except frontal mean $\beta1$ ERS for the control group following HT during T2 (Fig. 2B, 1st row; Pz, C3', C4', $p < 0.001$; Cz, $p < 0.05$). The prolonged $\beta2$ synchronized bursts for PP during T1 had an effect on the $\beta2$ band behavior during the entire early time period (T1, Fig. 2, 2nd row, left plot). The mean $\beta2$ ERS were prominent only in PP at frontal-parietal and right motor areas after LT and at parietal and left motor areas following HT during T1 (Fig. 2A, B). The comparison of the groups also showed mean $\beta2$ ERD in HS and $\beta2$ ERS in PP during T2 following either tone in all channels except for the frontal area, which showed mean $\beta2$ ERD in both groups after LT, significantly more prominently in HS (LT, $p < 0.05$; Fig. 2A, B). The results for γ closely resembled the $\beta2$-frequency band behaviour. The mean γ ERS were more prominent than those for $\beta2$ in PP. During the sensory processing (T1), PP showed mean γ ERS responses at fronto-parietal and right motor areas after LT, but not after HT (Fig. 2A, B, 3rd row, left). The γ ERD in HS and γ ERS in PP were observed in all channels after either tone during the cognitive processing (T2), except frontal γ ERS after HT, which was more pronounced in HS than in PP ($p < 0.001$, Fig. 2B, right plot).

Channels	Fz ERS(%)/ F/ t (±SE) D	Cz ERS(%)/ F/ t (±SE) D	Pz ERS(%)/ F/ t (±SE) D	C3' ERS(%)/ F/ t (±SE) D	C4' ERS(%)/F /t (±SE) D
Subjects tone(period)			HS		
LT (T1)	22.7(±2)/ 47 Hz (c) 20 (±5.2)** ms [8–32] ms	19.8(±2.8)/ 33 Hz (a) 12 (±4)** ms [8–16] ms	20.4(±1.1)/39.4(±1.3)Hz [35–48] Hz (a, b, c) 86.4 (±9.9) ms [24–144] ms	18.9(±1.4)/41(±5.2) Hz [32,50] Hz (a, c) 28 (±9.5)** ms [8–48] ms	30.7(±1.9)/47.6(±0.4)Hz [46–49] Hz (c) 40 (±7.3)** ms [8–72] ms
HT (T1)	18.4(±1)/42.2(±2.5)Hz [36,37,47,48] Hz (a, b) 28 (±6.1)** ms [8–48] ms –	19.4(±1.4)/36 Hz (a) 20 (±5.2)** ms [8–32] ms –	19.1(±0.5)/40.8(±0.2)Hz 72 (±8.6)** ms (b) [24–120] ms 32.2(±4)/ 42.6(±0.4) Hz 208 (±8.6) ms [160–250] ms (d)	33.8(±2)/43.8(±0.4) Hz 120 (±12.6) ms (c) [8–250] ms – –	30.1(±2.3)*/39.9(±0.5)Hz 44 (±7.7) ms (b) [8–80] ms 32.8(±3.3)/41.5(±0.2) Hz 216(±8) ms [176–250] ms (d)

LT (T2)	16.9(±0.5)/ 38 Hz 260 (±4)** ms [250-264] ms (f)	21.8(±1.2)/40 (±0.5) Hz [38, 42] Hz 548 (±9.5) ms [488-600] ms (i-j)	36.8(±1.6)/38.8(±0.4)Hz [35-41] Hz 464 (±14.2) ms [320-600] ms (g-j)	24.3(±1.6)/34.1(±0.3)Hz [33-35] Hz 552.6 (±9.9) ms [496-600] ms (i-j)	16.6(±1.1)/39Hz 524(±5.2) ms [512-536] ms (h)
	24.6(±2)/ 35 Hz 568 (±6.5) ms [544-592] ms (j)	-	-	-	-
HT (T2)	36.3(±1.4)/43(±0.6)Hz [37,38,40,46,47] Hz 432 (±15.7) ms [250-600] ms (f, g, j)	25.6(±2.2)/45.9(±0.6) Hz [45, 49] Hz 312 (±7.3)** ms [280-344] ms (f)	53.7(±2)/ 43.2(±0.2) Hz 432(±15.7) ms [250-600] ms (f, j)	55(±3)/ 44.1(±0.3) Hz [39-45] Hz 432 (±15.7) ms [250-600] ms (f, g, i, j)	32.4(±1.9)/40.7(±0.4) Hz [39-44] Hz 376 (±13.1)** ms [250-496] ms (f)
	-	39(±3)/ 45 Hz 444 (±7.7) ms [408-488] ms (g)	-	-	46(±5.7)/39.3(±0.6) Hz 568 (±8) ms [528-600] ms (j)
	-	48(±7)/ 38.6 (±0.2) Hz 572 (±7.7) ms [536-600] ms (j)	-	-	-

Subjects tone(period)	PP				
LT (T1)	49(±5.5)*/ 32 Hz (a) 44 (±7.7) ms [8-80] ms	36.4(±4)*/32.3(±0.7)Hz(a) 36 (±6.9) ms [8-64] ms	32.5(±2.1)*/45.5(±1.1)Hz [42-50] Hz (c) 56 (±8.6)** ms [8-104] ms	28.2(±3.4)*/37.5(±1.6)Hz [34,35,43] Hz (a) 36 (±6.9) ms [8-64] ms	32.4(±4.3)/43.2(±2.2) Hz [32,46,48,49,50]Hz (a,d) 56 (±8.6) ms [8-104] ms
	-	-	21.9(±0.8)/47.8(±1.4)Hz [33,49,50] Hz (c) 196 (±9.5) ms [136-250] ms	-	30.1(±2.7)/37.9(±0.1) Hz 192 (±8) ms (b) [152-232] ms
HT (T1)	49.7(±3.5)*/34 Hz (a) 40 (±7.3) ms [8-72] ms	27.6(±2.4)*/34.9(±0.1)Hz 44 (±7) ms (a) [16-72] ms	34.3(±3)*/ 34.1 (±0.1) Hz 112 (±11.8) ms (a) [16-208] ms	29.5(±2.6)/34.4(±0.2) Hz 36 (±7)** ms (a) [8-64] ms	21.1(±2)/41(±3.5)Hz [34,36,47] Hz (a) 20 (±5.2)** ms [8-32] ms
	-	-	-	29.9(±1.5)/33.4(±0.1) Hz - 188 (±10.1) ms (d) [120-250] ms	-
LT (T2)	39(±2.6)*/42.7(±0.9)Hz [34-42] Hz 468 (±14.0) ms [328-600] ms (g-j)	48.8(±4.2)*/44.3(±1.2)Hz [35-50] Hz 468 (±14) ms [328-600] ms (g-j)	68.9(±5.4) */ 45 (±0.7) Hz [35-50] Hz 432 (±15.7) ms [250-600] ms (g-j)	82.1(±5.2) */47(±0.7) Hz [36-50] Hz 468 (±14.0) ms [328-600] ms (g-j)	54.3(±2.9)*/41.6(±0.7)Hz [38-50] Hz 452 (±14.8) ms [296-600] ms (g-j)
HT (T2)	58(±3.5)*/40.3(±1.1)Hz [34,48,49] Hz 444 (±15.1)ms [280-600] ms (f, g, j)	43(±1.5)/44.9(±0.7)Hz, [47,50, 35,38,39] Hz 432 (±15.7) ms [250-600] ms (f, g, i, j)	52(±2.1)/ 37.8(±0.9) Hz [34,35, 41,45,49,50] Hz 436 (±15.5) ms [264-600] ms (g, i, j)	55.5(±3.2)/36.5(±0.9) Hz [33, 50] Hz 432 (±15.7) ms [250-600] ms (f, g, i, j)	41.6(±2.3)/42.4(±1.2)Hz [34-36, 49,50] Hz 448 (±15) ms [288-600] ms (g, h, i, j)

Note: Lower case letters in Table 3 marked consecutive sub-intervals with ERS γ bursts: **a, b, c** during T1 and **f, g, h, i, j** during T2.

Table 3. Mean ERS γ bursts (%) across the trials with mean spectral peaks **F** (Hz) for HS and PP after LT and HT presented in short–term zones **D** (ms) during early T1 and late T2 period (same format as **Table 1**).

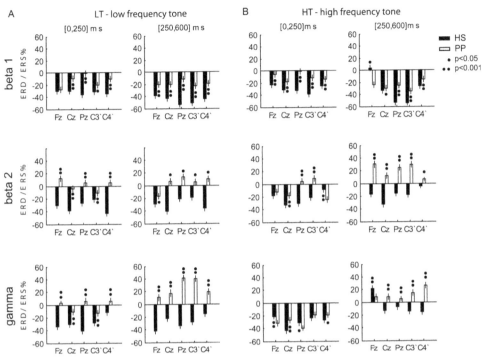

Fig. 2. Beta 1, Beta 2 and gamma band ERD/ERS over T1 and T2. Group means (±SE) are shown graphically to illustrate statistical results of β1-, β2-, γ-ERD/ERS following LT (A) and HT (B) for the early T1 (left) and late T2 (right) time periods. The significant difference in the ERD/ERS of HS and PP are presented for each pair of channels and marked by * (p <0.05) or ** (p <0.001, KW test).

4. Discussion

The data obtained confirmed that event-related oscillatory responses in different frequency bands vary with sensory and cognitive processes. We found functional differences between event-related oscillatory activity for cognitive and sensory-motor information processing, and a clear distinction between PP and HS in both the stimuli encoding (0–250 ms) and cognitive processing (250–600 ms) intervals. Attended stimuli produced theta response synchronizations in both groups, more markedly in HS, in the first period up to 250 ms after stimulation. Enhanced theta waves in the early period (up to 250 ms) of visual and auditory stimuli have also been described by Basar (1980), Schurmann and Basar-Eroglu (1994). Theta frequency rhythms are dominant oscillations within the hippocampal formation, which is of crucial importance for the encoding of new information (Klimesch, 1997; Klimesch et al., 2005). In the late post-stimulus period functionally related to cognitive processing, θ-ERD response was predominant, excluding the parietal θ-ERS in PP in response to both frequency tones and the frontal θ-ERS in HS in response to the low frequency tone.

Prominent differences in the α-ERD/ERS responses between the groups were observed during the first time period of 0–250 ms. A widely distributed fronto-central α-ERS manifested in PP in response to both tone types during the first 250 ms after stimulus was absent in HS. In the second period after stimulus absence, α-ERD was found in both groups in response to both tone types. This was generally more prominent in HS, with the exception of frontal side in response to either a high or low frequency tone. Alpha-ERD was more prominent at central and right motor areas in response to the high frequency tone in PP.

Theta and alpha frequency ERD/ERS were significantly different between subject groups. It is known that the oscillatory alterations to θ-ERS are related to memory encoding (Klimesch et al., 2001; Jensen & Tesche, 2002).

Alpha-ERS most probably demonstrates active working memory or attentional processes (Klimesch, 1997; Jensen et al., 2002), whereas α-ERD is functionally related to mental activity (Basar, 1980) and reflects memory search processes (Klimesch, 1997; Klimesch et al., 2005; Pesonen et al., 2006). The recognition of auditory stimuli elicits widespread α-ERD responses (Krause et al., 1994). It is accepted that alpha oscillations are mainly generated by cortico-cortical and thalamo-cortical neuronal networks (Lopes da Silva et al., 1980; Schmiedt et al., 2005; Ellfolk et al., 2006). This fact, together with the changes in the metabolic patterns of thalamic, premotor and prefrontal cortex, parieto-occipital regions, etc., that occur in PP (Fukuda et al., 2001) could explain the abnormality of early time period α-ERS in the PP compared to the HS. Observed slight activity of the basal ganglia–thalamic and cerebellar–thalamic pathways might be implicated in the development of parkinsonian symptoms (Rolland et al., 2007).

Schmiedt et al. (2005) also found differences between PP and HS in the θ- and α-frequency ERD/ERS responses during working memory encoding but in a visual working memory paradigm. We cannot draw direct parallels between their results and ours in the present study because of the different stimulus modality. The early and late δ post-stimulus activities were enhanced in HS. The late period, related to cognitive information processing, exhibited δ-ERS in HS and δ-ERD in PP at most electrodes in response to a low frequency tone, and at parietal and left motor areas in response to the high frequency tone. Many authors agree that the main power of P300 is in the delta range (Demiralp et al., 1999; Karakas et al., 2000; Klimesch et al., 2000; Klimesch et al., 2006). The lower δ-ERS in PP in the late post-stimulus period, which becomes δ-ERD in some recordings, could explain the lower P3 amplitude observed in PP (Philipova et al., 1997). Our patients were medicated by L-dopa drugs and this medication may have had some effect on the present findings. One of the models (Leblois et al., 2006) supposed that high dopamine depletion could modify the network dynamic state from an imbalance between the feedbacks and lead to synchronous oscillations driven by a hyperdirect loop appearing in basal ganglia after inactivation of the striatum.

A reduction in this α-ERD/ERS abnormality and a consequent improvement in PP performance during working memory tasks have been found as the result of L-dopa (Lewis et al., 2003; Marini et al., 2003; Shohamy et al., 2005; Devos et al., 2004). Nevertheless, we found some differences between the two groups. The memory related and stimulus categorized ERD/ERS responses at all these frequencies reflected different underlying neuropathological and cognitive changes in this neurodegenerative disease. Theta activity is suggested to be mostly engaged in memory operations (Klimesch et al., 1996; Karakas et al., 2000; Jensen et al., 2002b) and this θ pathological synchronized enhancement in PD could explain the cognitive dysfunction commonly occurring even in the early stages of Parkinson's disease (Lewis et al., 2003). We found specific significant differences at left motor area as θ-ERS in the HS and θ-ERD in the PP during sensory-motor processing (early period) following the high frequency tone. We also detected different processes of θ-ERS for the PP and ERD for the HS in the parietal lead during the cognitive information processing (late period) following both tones, which reflects different task-related activation of the associative posterior cortex.

These findings are probably due to the auditory cortex being located in the dorsal and lateral part of the superior temporal gyrus as well as in the inferior parietal lobule (Konig et al., 2005). The absence of α-ERD at the frontal electrode locations in the patients with PD indicated that the PP, compared with HS, used different cognitive strategies for stimulus response processing which are normally implemented by fronto-striatal circuits (Krause, 2006). The late higher fronto-central α-ERD in PP accompanied by a lower P3 component amplitude, especially in the fronto-central sides, reflects a disturbance in the frontal regulation of attentional processes as well a disturbance of the basal ganglia activity and their related thalamo-cortical neuronal nets (Stam et al., 1993; Piccirilli et al., 1989; Schmiedt et al., 2005).

In PP, we found hemispheric lateralization for sensory and cognitive processing concerning θ-ERD/ERS at left and right motor areas as well as a significantly higher α-ERS at left compared to right motor area. This finding corresponds with the results of Magnani et al., 1998, Defebvre et al., 1996. These authors suggested that other cortical areas may be activated both to compensate for a dysfunction of motor preparation and to increase the level of cortical activity necessary for the realization of the movement. Another possible explanation is that this hemispheric lateralization is connected with auditory attention and hemispheric differences in the processing of high and low frequencies (Ivry & Robertson, 1998).

Post-stimulus β1 ERD was elicited from both groups during sensory (T1) and cognitive information (T2) processing, though this was significantly more pronounced in HS in response to both tone types at all electrodes. The greater β1 ERD in HS can be explained by the increased excitability level of the neurons (Pfurtscheller & Lopes da Silva, 1999; Brown & Marsden, 1998). Late post-stimulus frontal β1 ERS (T2) was evident only in HS following HT. This HS ERS, comprising components in the band between 13 and 20 Hz, may represent an inhibited frontal cortical network, at least under certain circumstances (Pfurtscheller & Lopes da Silva, 199; Engel et al., 2001).

A frontal β2 ERD was maintained in both groups during the cognitive information processing (T2) following LT, though this was weaker in PP. β2 ERS was only observed in PP. These were weakly elicited during the sensory stimuli processing (T1) and appeared at fronto-parietal and left motor areas (LT: Fz, C3', Pz; HT: C3', Pz). β2 ERS in PP was more prominent during cognitive processing (T2) after either tone type, but particularly so following HT. The β2 change reversals compared to β1 which we observed for the PD patients support the hypothesis of Marceglia et al. (2009), that two distinct information channels in the cortico-basal ganglia–thalamo-cortical loop, involved in motor and non-motor information processing, are formed in the parkinsonian brain. The frontal β synchronization at 20-30 Hz arises both from communication with, and also from within, the STN (Williams et al., 2003). The β synchrony has been ascribed predominantly to a lack of dopaminergic activity in the striatum which, together with the STN, is the recipient of cortical input to the basal ganglia (Fogelson et al., 2006; Williams et al., 2002). Studies with unmedicated PD patients have revealed prominent oscillations in 'basal ganglia β frequency band' (Weinberger et al., 2006; Kühn et al., 2006; Priori et al., 2004; Fogelson et al., 2006). The engagement of the basal ganglia in β band synchronization is found when there is acute or chronic dopaminergic hypoactivity, and while primarily associated with bradykinesia and rigidity, it has also been associated with impairments to complex movements and motor related cognitive behaviour because of the widespread basal ganglia connectivity with the cerebral cortex (Terman et al., 2002). Further, the pathological β synchrony in the cerebellum might lead to a purer breakdown of simple motor tasks because of more focal cerebellothalamic projections into the cerebral cortex that are concentrated on the primary motor cortex (Leblois et al., 2007). A relative functional division between activities in the β band might be supported by the evidence for different patterns of pharmacological sensitivity (Priori et al., 2004) and cortico-subthalamic coupling (Fogelson et al., 2006). The dopaminergic drug treatment suppressed mainly β1 synchrony, graded by the amount of drug-induced suppression in the STN (Kühn et al., 2006; Wang et al., 2005) and cerebral cortex, correlating with the level of improvement in bradykinesia and rigidity but not in parkinsonian rest tremor (Weinberger et al., 2006; Silberstein et al., 2005), the latter of which probably has an independent pathophysiological substrate (Rivlin-Etzion et al., 2006).

Our group of patients showed a significantly reduced γ–ERD compared with HS over central and left motor areas, and only PP showed γ–ERS over fronto-parietal and right motor areas following LT during the sensory stimuli processing (T1). A widespread γ–ERS appeared during later cognitive processing (T2), and then only in PP, following either tone type, with the exception of a more prominent frontal γ–ERS in HS following HT. In our study, we observed switches between cortical activity in the β2 and γ band oscillations. Hence we concluded that a reduction in β2-band synchronized activity allows higher frequency oscillatory activity in the γ range leading to its synchronization. The observed energy changes in the β2 and γ bands indicate that an increase in one is accompanied by a decrease in the other. These T2 changes in PP were more pronounced in the motor cortex than in the parietal and even frontal cortex data. In the parkinsonian state, there was a tendency towards increased synchronized higher frequency fluctuations, specifically in the motor cortex, where instances of peaks were found after both tone types. Except for the β2 band series of data during cognitive processing (T2) after HT, the difference between magnitude of the peaks in the frontal, parietal and contralateral motor areas did not reach significance. Recent data demonstrate that the disruptions of the beta and gamma range cortical rhythms are based on the disturbed temporal relationship between cortical oscillatory activity and basal ganglia activity in Parkinsonism (Gatev & Wichmann, 2008). This finding is also in agreement with studies of PP following dopaminergic medication, which promoted synchronized oscillatory activity at higher frequencies (γ) predominantly at the level of the frontal cortex and striatum (Levy et al., 2001; 2002; Brown et al., 2001; Williams et al., 2002; Leblois et al., 2007).

In recent MEG investigations of various cognitive and sensory tasks (Kaiser et al., 2003; Lutzenberger et al., 2002) the reported γ band activity over the higher sensory areas has not shown a sustained activation, but rather, a peaking activity. In our sensori-motor study, these transient responses were functionally dissociable between the two groups. We observed stimulus-specific γ band activity components over the fronto-parietal cortex, but this was differently manifest in each group and varied over the time course. The topography was compatible with the notion of an auditory dorsal space processing stream involving the posterior temporal, parietal and superior frontal cortex (Rauschecker, 1998; Arnott et al., 2004). If the cognitive processing (T2) γ band activity components represent similar anticipatory activations both for LT and HT, one might assume that the same cortical networks should underlie the same stimulus representations. However, while all components were mainly localized over fronto-central areas, there was some variation between the conditions, showing significant effects on the parietal γ components for LT, but not for parietal γ activity for HT. This suggests that networks encoding the stimulus features are not fixed, and may vary with task demands.

The assessing EEG stimulus-specific oscillatory activity yielded insights into the temporal dynamics of sound processing in short-term memory. Contrasting oscillatory γ activity between the two stimuli, such as between LT ERS and HT ERD during the sensory processing (T1) in PP, as well as between LT ERD and HT ERS during the cognitive processing (T2) in HS, revealed stimulus-specific γ activity behavior in the 30–50 Hz range over the HS's frontal and PP's fronto-parietal cortex. This suggests that γ band activity reflects the general involvement of cortical networks in particular tasks but may index the specific content of short-term memory in each group.

The pronounced and well-synchronized γ burst in HS was present in the very short-term phases around 25–60 ms after the stimulus onset, with spectral peaks ranging from 30 to 45 Hz (Gurtubay et al., 2001). Despite this short-term high synchrony in HS, the common γ behavior during sensory stimuli processing (T1) was desynchronization. However, the PP processes were with higher short-term energy, which is a prerequisite for all maintenance-related processes, and thus defined a persistent synchronization during sensory stimuli processing, mainly at fronto-parietal and right motor areas following LT. It is clear that there is a difference between groups in the early and well-synchronized response that is basically a sensory phenomenon important to preparing the brain for the subsequent processing. This evidence suggests that γ oscillations may be modulated by attentional processes. Several cognitive paradigms for the auditory system have shown early spectral peak responses in the γ band between 30 and 40 Hz at around 25 ms after stimulus onset that last for about 100 ms (Pantev, 1995; Arnott et al., 2004).

Later peaking activity has been recorded in the 200–400 ms interval following an experimental task. The latency and scalp topography vary according to the type of stimulus, indicating task-dependent local network activation. The significantly varying magnitudes of differentiation demonstrated that the topography of stimulus-specific γ-band activity is also task-dependent within the groups (Tiitinen et al., 1993). We found restricted energy changes over all recorded areas in HS, but not in the frontal area after HT. The significant differences between groups in T2 recorded after both stimuli could be due to memory retrieval processes that are activated during the performance of the paradigms. The lower energy in HS during cognitive processing (T2) could be related to fewer attentional processes required to eventually perform a task. The relative strength of differentiation in the γ–band may suggest that performance depends on the different group's ability to retain a representation in memory of the relevant stimulus feature and thus to be able to neglect the irrelevant stimuli. The acquisition and retention of sound frequency information was accompanied by frontal gamma band activity components (Karakaş & Başar, 1998). The high-frequency stimuli were accompanied by more exaggerated, well–synchronized frontal γ band components in performing the tasks. Memory for low versus high frequency tones selectively enhanced oscillatory activity for the posterior versus the frontal components, thus directly demonstrating differentiation of the group's modulation of cortical activity by task demands.

A mechanism that underlies many of the immediately aforementioned cognitive functions is the match of sensory information with memory contents (Kaiser et al., 2009a; 2009b; Visscher et al., 2007). The 'early' γ-band activity occurring 150 ms after stimulus presentation reflects such a match with memory. The 'late' γ activity, which typically emerges with a latency of more than 150 ms, is a temporal signature of utilization processes such as response selection or context updating. We also found a later (250–400 ms) ERS γ response, following only HT in HS, over the frontal location, where this activity peaked in the 33–45 Hz range. In PP, the specific β2 and γ bursts (30–38 Hz) exhibited maximal scalp projection covering areas to the left and right of the motor areas, and with frontal, central or parietal participation that depended on the stimuli. This oscillatory burst reflects a later stimulus context process, although it has also been associated with the motor responses later in the task (Brown, 2003; Kaiser et al., 2009b). The β2/γ oscillation in the groups points to a direct relation to aspects of post-discrimination processes related to the P300 wave (Haig et al., 2000). This oscillatory burst (letters **g-j** for intervals from 320 to 550 ms) also showed a variable relationship to attention, as it was significantly different during the HT and LT task. The results also showed that EEG activity in the frontal, parietal and motor cortex is significantly different between groups, not only in temporal variations (always with a delay in PP) but also in frequency shifts (β2/γ ERD in HS compared to the ERS in PP). Although these shifts do not follow a simple pattern, they are significantly different from HS, raising the possibility that the interactions between basal ganglia activity and cortical rhythms are functionally relevant. Therefore, the normal higher frequency relationships between cortical and basal ganglia activity are strongly altered in the parkinsonian state (Gatev & Wichmann, 2008). The shifts of β/γ patterns occurring in the groups are probably associated with specific types of basal ganglia events related to transitions between cortical idling and more active states (Williams et al., 2003).

5. Conclusion

Our investigation further demonstrates the close relationship between physiological abnormalities in PD and disturbances in the EEG frequency characteristics. The results of this investigation in PD patients of both sensory and cognitive processing of auditory stimuli suggests that PD should be characterized by multiple impairments in oscillatory networks, which in turn indicates the presence of task-specific disturbances in the temporal and regional integration of all frequency components.

6. References

Anik, Y., Iseri, P., Demirci, A., Komsuoglu, S., Inan, N. (2007) Magnetization transfer ratio in early period of Parkinson disease. *Acad Radiol* 14(2), (2007 Feb), pp. 189–192, ISSN 1076-6332

Antal, A., Kéri, S., Dibó, G., Benedek, G., Janka, Z., Vécsei, L., Bodis-Wollner, I. (2002) Electrophysiological correlates of visual categorization, pp. evidence for cognitive dysfunctions in early Parkinson's disease. *Brain Res Cogn Brain Res* 13(2), (2002 Apr) ,pp. 153–158, ISSN 0926-6410

Arnott, S. R., Binns, M. A., Grady, C. L., Alain, C. (2004) Assessing the auditory dualpathway model in humans. *NeuroImage* 22(1), (2004 May), pp. 401-408, ISSN 1053-8119

Basar, E. (1980) EEG brain dynamics. Relations between EEG and brain evoked potentials. Elsevier, Amsterdam

Başar, E., Basar-Eroglu, C., Karakas, S., Schurmann, M. (2001) Gamma, alpha, delta, and theta oscillations govern cognitive processes. *Int J Psychophysiol* 39(2-3), (2001 Jan) pp. 241-248, ISSN 0167-8760

Brown, P. & Marsden, C. D. (1998) What do the basal ganglia do? Lancet 351(9118), (1998 Jun 13), pp. 1801-1804, ISSN 0140-6736

Brown, P., Oliviero, A., Mazzone, P., Insola, A., Tonali, P. & Di Lazzaro, V. (2001) Dopamine dependency of oscillations between subthalamic nucleus and pallidum in Parkinson's disease. *J Neurosci* 21 (3), (2001 Feb 1) pp. 1033-1038, ISSN 0270-6474

Brown, P. (2003) Oscillatory nature of human basal ganglia activity: relationship to the pathophysiology of Parkinson's disease. *Mov Disord* 18(4), (2003 Apr), pp. 357-363, ISSN 0885-3185

Cassidy, M., Mazzone, P., Oliviero, A., Insola, A., Tonali, P., Di Lazzaro, V., Brown, P. (2002) Movement-related changes in synchronization in the human basal ganglia. Brain 125(Pt 6), (2002 Jun), pp. 1235-1246, ISSN 0006-8950

Cools R (2006) Dopaminergic modulation of cognitive functionimplications for L-DOPA treatment in Parkinson's disease. *Neurosci Biobehav Rev* 30(1), (2005 Jun 1), pp. 1–23, ISSN 0149-7634

Gurtubay, I. G., Alegre, M., Labarga, A., Malanda, A., Iriarte, J., Artieda, J. (2001) Gamma band activity in an auditory oddball paradigm studied with the wavelet transform. *Clin Neurophysiol* 112(7), (2001 Jul), pp. 1219-1228, ISSN 1388-2457

Daum, I., Schugens, M. M., Spieker, S., Poser, U., Schönle, P. W., Birbaumer, N. (1995) Memory and skill acquisition in Parkinson's disease and frontal lobe dysfunction. *Cortex* 31(3), (1995 Sep), pp. 413–432, ISSN 0010-9452

Defebvre, L, Bouniez, JL, Destke, A, Guieu, JD (1996) Movement related ERD pattern preceding voluntary movement in untreated Parkinson's disease. *J Neurol Neurosurg Psychiatry* 60(3), (1996 Mar), pp. 307–312, ISSN 0022-3050

Demiralp, T., Ademoglu, A., Schürmann, M., Bas,ar-Eroglu, C., Başar, E. (1999) Detection of P300 waves in single trials by the wavelet transform (WT). *Brain Lang* 66(1), (1999 Jan), pp. 108–128, ISSN 0093-934X

Devos, D., Labyt, E., Derambure, P., Bourriez, J. L., Cassim, F., Reyns, N., Blond, S., Guieu, J. D., Destée, A., Defebvre, L. (2004) Subthalamic nucleus stimulation modulates motor cortex oscillatory activity in Parkinson's disease. *Brain* 127(2), (2004 Feb), pp. 408–419, ISSN 0006-8950

Donoghue, J. P., Sanes, J. N., Hatsopoulos, N. G., Gaal, G. (1998) Neural discharge and local field potential oscillations in primate motor cortex during voluntary movements. *J Neurophysiol* 79(1), (1998 Jan), pp. 159-173, ISSN 0022-3077

Durka, P. J., Zygierewicz, J., Klekowicz, H., Ginter, J., Blinowska, K. J. (2004) On the statistical significance of event-related EEG desynchronization and synchronization in the time-frequency plane. *IEEE Trans Biomed Eng* 51(7), (2004 Jul), pp. 1167–1175, ISSN 0018-9294

Dushanova, J., Philipova, D., Nikolova., G. (2009) Event-related synchronization/ desynchronization during discrimination task conditions in patients with

Parkinson's disease. *Cell Mol Neurobiol* 29(6-7), (2009 Sep), pp. 971-980, ISSN 0272-4340

Dushanova, J., Philipova, D., Nikolova, G. (2010) Beta and gamma frequency-range abnormalities in parkinsonian patients under cognitive sensorimotor task. *Journal of the Neurological Sciences* 293(1-2), (2010 Jun 15), pp. 51-58, ISSN 0022-510X

Ellfolk, U., Karrasch, M., Laune, M., Pesonen, M., Krause, K. (2006) Event related desynchronisation/ERS during an auditory-verbal memory task in mild Parkinson's disease. *Clin Neurophysiol* 117(8), (2006 Aug), pp. 1737-1745, ISSN 1388-2457

Engel, A. K., Fries, P., & Singer, W. (2001) Dynamic predictions: oscillations and synchrony in top-down processing. *Nat Rev Neurosci* 2(10), (2001 Oct), pp. 704-716, ISSN 1471-003X

Evarts, E. V., Teräväinen, H., & Calne, D. B. (1981) Reaction time in Parkinson's disease. *Brain* 104(1), (1981 Mar), pp. 167-186, ISSN 0006-8950

Farmer, S. F. (1998) Rhythmicity, synchronization and binding in human and primate motor systems. *J Physiol* 509(1), (1998 May 15), pp. 3-14, ISSN 0022-3751

Fries, P., Reynolds, J. H., Rorie, A. E., Desimone, R. (2001) Modulation of oscillatory neuronal synchronization by selective visual attention. *Science* 291(5508), (2001 Feb 23), pp. 1560-1563, ISSN 0036-8075

Foffani, G., Bianchi ,A. M., Baselli, G., Priori, A. (2005) Movement-related frequency modulation of beta oscillatory activity in the human subthalamic nucleus, *J Physiol* 568(2), (2005 Oct 15), pp 699-711, ISSN 0022-3751

Fogelson, N., Williams, D., Tijssen, M., van Bruggen, G., Speelman, H., Brown, P. (2006) Different functional loops between cerebral cortex and the subthalmic area in Parkinson's disease. *Cereb Cortex* 16(1), (2006 Jan), pp. 64-75, ISSN 1047-3211

Fukuda, M., Edward, C., Eidelberg, D. (2001) Functional brain networks in Parkinson's disease. *Parkinsonism Relat Disord* 8(2), (2001 Oct), pp. 91–94, ISSN 1353-8020

Gatev, P., & Wichmann, T. (2008) Interactions between Cortical Rhythms and Spiking Activity of Single Basal Ganglia Neurons in the Normal and Parkinsonian State. *Cereb Cortex* 19(6), (2009 Jun), pp. 1330-44, ISSN 1047-3211

Haig, A. R., Gordon, E., Pascalis, V. D., Meares, R. A., Bahramali, H., Harris, A. (2000) Gamma activity in schizophrenia: evidence of impaired network binding? *Clin Neurophysiol* 111(8), (2000 Aug), pp. 1461–1468, ISSN 1388-2457

Herrmann, C. S., Munk, M. H. J., Engel, A. K. (2004) Cognitive functions of gamma-band activity: memory match and utilization. *Trends Cogn Sci* 8(8), (2004 Aug), pp. 347-355, ISSN 1364-6613

Higginson, C. I., King, D. S., Levine, D., Wheelock , V. L., Khamphay, N. O., Sigvardt, K. A. (2003) The relationship between executive function and verbal memory in Parkinson's disease. *Brain Cogn* 52(3), (2003 Aug), pp. 343–352, ISSN 0278-2626

Hoehn, M. M., Yahr, M. D. (1967) Parkinsonism: onset progression and mortality. *Neurology* 17(5), (1967 May), pp. 427-442, ISSN 0028-3878

Innis, R. B., Seibyl, J. P., Scanley, B. E., Laruelle, M., Abi-Dargham, A., Wallace, E., Baldwin, R. M., Zea-Ponce, Y., Zoghbi, S., Wang, S. (1993) Single photon emission computed tomographic imaging demonstrates loss of striatal dopamine transporters in

Parkinson disease. *Proc Natl Acad Sci USA* 90(24), (1993 Dec 15), pp. 11965–11969, ISSN 0027-8424

Ivry, R. B., Robertson, L. C. (1998) The two sides of perception. MIT Press, Cambridge, MA, ISBN 0-262-09034-1

Jensen, O., Tesche, C. D. (2002) Frontal theta activity in humans increases with memory load in a working memory task. *Eur J Neurosci* 15(8), (2002 Apr), pp. 1395–1399, ISSN 0953-816X

Jensen, O., Gelfand, J., Kounios, J., Lisman, J. E. (2002) Oscillations in the alpha band (9–12 Hz) increase with memory load during retention in a short-term memory task. *Cereb Cortex* 12(8), (2002 Aug), pp. 877– 882, ISSN 1047-3211

Kaiser, J., Ripper, B., Birbaumer, N., Lutzenberger, W. (2003) Dynamics of gamma-band activity in human magnetoencephalogram during auditory pattern working memory. *NeuroImage* 20(2), (2003 Oct), pp. 816-827, ISSN 1053-8119

Kaiser, J., Rahm, B., Lutzenberger, W. (2009a) Temporal dynamics of stimulus-specific gamma-band activity components during auditory short-term memory. *Neuroimage* 44(1), (2009 Jan 1), pp. 257-264, ISSN 1053-8119

Kaiser, J., Lutzenberge, W., Decker, C., Wibral, M., Rahm, B. (2009b) Task- and performance-related modulation of domain-specific auditory short-term memory representations in the gamma band. *Neuroimage* 46(4), (2009 Jul 15), pp. 1127-36, ISSN 1053-8119

Karakaş ,S., & Başar, E. (1998) Early gamma response is sensory in origin: a conclusion based on cross-comparison of results from multiple experimental paradigms. *Int J Psychophysiol* 31(1), (1998 Dec), pp. 13-31, ISSN 0167-8760

Karakas, S., Erzengin, O. U., & Başar, E. (2000) A new strategy involving multiple cognitive paradigms demonstrates that ERP components are determined by the superposition of oscillatory signals. *Clin Neurophysiol* 111(10), (2000 Oct), pp. 1719–1732, ISSN 1388-2457

Karrasch, M., Krause, C. M., Laine, M., Lang, H. A., Lehto, M. (1998) Eventrelated ERD and ERS during an auditory lexical matching task. *Electroencephalogr Clin Neurophysiol* 107(2), (1998 Aug), pp. 112–121, ISSN 0013-4694

Karrasch, M., Laine, M., Rapinoja, P., Krause, C. M. (2004) Effects of normal ageing on event-related ERD/ERS during a memory task in humans. *Neurosci Lett* 366(1), (2004 Aug 5), pp. 18–23, ISSN 0304-3940

Klimesch, W. (1997) EEG a-rhythms and memory processes. *Int J Psychophysiol* 26(1-3), (1997 Jun), pp. 319–340, ISSN 0167-8760

Klimesch, W., Doppelmay, M., Russegger, H., Pachinger, T. (1996) Theta band power in the human scalp EEG and the encoding of new information. *Neuroreport* 7(7), (1996 May 17), pp. 1235–1240, ISSN 0959-4965

Klimesch, W., Doppelmayr, M., Schwaiger, J., Winkler, T., Gruber W. (2000) Theta oscillations and the ERP old/new effect: independent phenomena? *Clin Neurophysiol* 111(5), (2000 May), pp. 781–793, ISSN 1388-2457

Klimesch, W., Doppelmayr, M., Stadler, W., Pollhuber, D., Sauseng, P., Rohm, D. (2001) Episodic retrieval is reflected by a process specific increase in human electroencephalographic h activity. *Neurosci Lett* 302(1), (2001 Apr 13), pp. 49–52, ISSN 0304-3940

Klimesch, W., Schnack, B., Sauseng, P. (2005) The functional significance of h and upper a-oscillations. *Exp Psychol* 52(2), pp. 99–108, ISSN 1618-3169

Klimesch, W., Hanslmayr, S., Sauseng, P., Gruber, W., Brozinsky, C. J., Kroll, N. E., Yonelinas, A. P., Doppelmayr, M. (2006) Oscillatory EEG correlates of episodic trace decay. *Cereb Cortex* 16(2), (2006 Feb), pp. 280–290, ISSN 1047-3211

Konig, R., Heil, P., Budinger, E., Scheich, H. (2005) The auditory cortex: a synthesis of human and animal research. Lawrence Erlbaum Associates, NJ. ISBN 0-8058-4938-6

Krause, C. M. (2006) Cognition- and memory-related ERD/ERS responses in the auditory stimulus modality. *Prog Brain Res* 159, pp. 197–207, ISSN 0079-6123

Krause, C. M., Lang, H. A., Laine, M., Helle, S. I., Kuusisto, M. J., Pörn, B. (1994) Event-related desynchronization evoked by auditory stimuli. *Brain Topogr* 7(2), (1994 Winter), pp. 107–112, ISSN 0896-0267

Krause, C. M., Lang, A. H., Laine, M., Kuusisto, M., Pörn, B. (1996) Eventrelated EEG desynchronization and synchronization during an auditory memory task. *Electroencephalogr Clin Neurophysiol* 98(4), (1996 Apr), pp. 319–326, ISSN 0013-4694

Krause, C. M., Aström, T., Karrasch, M., Laine, M., Sillanmäki, L. (1999) Cortical activation related to auditory semantic matching of concrete versus abstract words. *Clin Neurophysiol* 110(8), (1999 Aug), pp. 1371– 1377, ISSN 1388-2457

Knoke, D., Taylor, A. E., Saint-Cyr, J. A. (1998) The differential defects of ceing on recall in Parkinson's Disease and normal subjects. *Brain Cogn* 38(2), (1998 Nov), pp. 261–274, ISSN 0278-2626

Kühn, A. A., Kupsch, A., Schneider, G. H., Brown, P. (2006) Reduction in subthalamic 8–35 Hz oscillatory activity correlat with clinical improvement in PD. *Eur J Neurosci* 23(7), (2006 Apr), pp. 1956-1960, ISSN 0953-816X

Leblois, A., Boraud, T., Meissner, W., Bergman, H., Hansel, D. (2006) Competition between feedback loops underlies normal and pathological dynamics in the basal ganglia. *J Neurosci* 26(13), (2006 Mar 29), pp. 3567– 3583, ISSN 0270-6474

Leblois, A., Meissner, W., Bioulac, B., Gross, C. E., Hansel, D., Boraud, T. (2007) Late emergence of synchronized oscillatory activity in the pallidum during progressive parkinsonism. *Eur J Neurosci* 26(6), (2007 Sep), pp. 1701-1713, ISSN 0953-816X

Lewis, S. J., Dove, A., Robbins, T. W., Barker, R. A., Owen, A. M. (2003) Cognitive impairments in early Parkinson's disease are accompanied by reductions in activity in frontostriatal neural circuitry. *J Neurosci* 23(15), (2003 Jul 16), pp. 6351–6356, ISSN 0270-6474

Levy, R., Dostrovsky, J. O., Lang, A. E., Sime, E., Hutchison, W. D., Lozano, A. M. (2001) Effects of apomorphine on subtalamic nucleus and globus pallidus internus neurons in patients with Parkinson's disease. *J Neurophysiology* 86(1), (2001 Jul), pp. 249-260, ISSN 0022-3077

Levy, R., Hutchison, W. D., Lozano, A. M., Dostrovsky, J. O. (2002) Synchronized neuronal discharge in the basal ganglia of parkinsonian patients is limited to oscillatory activity. *J Neuroscience* 22(7), (2002 Apr 1), pp. 2855-2861, ISSN 0270-6474

Lopes da Silva, F. H., Vos, J. E., Mooibroek, J., Van Rotterdam, A. (1980) Relative contributions of intracortical and thalamo-cortical processes in the generation of a-rhythms, revealed by partial coherence analysis. *Electroencephalogr Clin Neurophysiol* 50(5-6), (1980 Dec), pp. 449–456, ISSN 0013-4694

Lutzenberger, W., Ripper, B., Busse, L., Birbaumer, N., Kaiser, J. (2002) Dynamics of gamma-band activity during an audiospatial working memory task in humans. J Neurosci 22(13), (2002 Jul 1), pp. 5630-5638, ISSN 0270-6474

Magnani, G., Cursi, M., Leocani, L., Volonté, M. A., Locatelli, T., Elia, A., Comi, G. (1998) Event-related ERD to contingent negative variation and self-paced movement paradigms in Parkinson's disease. *Mov Disord* 13(4), (1998 Jul), pp. 653–660, ISSN 0885-3185

Marsden, J. F., Limousin-Dowsey, P., Ashby, P., Pollak, P. & Brown, P. (2001) Subthalamic nucleus, sensorimotor cortex and muscle interrelationships on Parkinson's disease. *Brain* 124(2), (2001 Feb), pp. 378-388, ISSN 0006-8950

Mason, M., & Newton, M. (1990) A rank statistics approach to the consistency of the general bootstrap, *Ann. Statist* 20, pp. 1611–1624, ISSN 0090-5364

Marceglia, S., Fiorio, M., Foffani, G., Mrakic-Sposta, S., Tiriticco, M., Locatelli, M., Caputo, E., Tinazzi M., Priori, A. (2009) Modulation of beta oscillations in the subthalamic area during action observation in Parkinson's disease. *Neuroscience* 161(4), (2009 Jul 21), pp. 1027-1036, ISSN 0306-4522

Minamoto, H., Tachibana, H., Sugita, M., Okita, T. (2001) Recognition memory in normal ageing and Parkinson's disease: behavioural and electrophysiological measures. *Brain Res Cogn Brain Res* 11(1), (2001 Mar), pp. 23–32, ISSN 0926-6410

Oldfield, R. C. (1971) The assessment and analysis of handedness: the Edinburgh inventory. *Neuropsychologia* 9(1), (1971 Mar), pp. 97-113, ISSN 0028-3932

Owen, A. M. (2004) Cognitive dysfunction in Parkinson's disease: the role of frontostriatal circuitry. *Neuroscientist* 10(6), (2004 Dec), pp. 525–537, ISSN 1073-8584

Ozgoren, M., Basar-Eroglu, C., Basar, E. (2005) Beta oscillations in face recognition. *Int J Psychophysiol* 55(1), (2005 Jan), pp. 51-59, ISSN 0167-8760

Pantev, C. (1995) Evoked and induced gamma-band activity of the human cortex. *Brain Topogr* 7(4), (1995 Summer), pp. 321-330, ISSN 0896-0267

Pesonen, M., Björnberg, C. H., Hämäläinen, H., Krause, C. M. (2006) Brain oscillatory 1–30 Hz EEG ERD/ERS responses during the different stages of an auditory memory search task. *Neurosci Lett* 399(1–2), (2006 May 15), pp. 45–50, ISSN 0304-3940

Philipova, D., Gatchev, G., Vladova, T., Georgiev, D (1997) Event related potentials under auditory discrimination tasks. *Int J Psychophysiol* 27(1), (1997 Jul), pp. 69–78, ISSN 0167-8760

Piccirilli M., D'Alessandro P., Finali G., Piccinin G. L., Agostini L. (1989) Frontal lobe dysfunction in Parkinson's disease: prognostic value for dementia? *Eur Neurol* 29(2), pp. 71–76, ISSN 0014-3022

Pillon, B., Ertle, S., Deweer, B., Bonnet, A., Vidailhet, M., Dubois, B. (1997) Memory for spatial location in 'de novo' parkinsonian patients. *Neuropsychologia* 35(3), (1997 Mar), pp. 221–228, ISSN 0028-3932

Priori, A., Foffani, G., Pesenti, A., Bianchi, A., Chiesa, V., Baselli, G. (2002) Movement-related modulation of neural activity in human basal ganglia and its l-DOPA dependency: recordings from deep brain stimulation electrodes in patients with

Parkinson's disease. *Neurol Sci* 23(Suppl. 2), (2002 Sep), pp. S101-S102, ISSN 1590-1874

Priori ,A., Foffani, G., Pesenti, A., Tamma, F., Bianchi, A. M., Pellegrini, M., Locatelli, M., Moxon, K. A., Villani, R. M. (2004) Rhythm-specific pharmacological modulation of subthalamic activity in Parkinson's disease. *Exp Neurol* 189(2), (2004 Oct), pp. 369-379, ISSN 0014-4886

Pfurtscheller, G., & Klimesch, W. (1991) Event-related ERD during motor behaviour and visual information processing. *Electroencephalogr Clin Neurophysiol Suppl* 42, pp. 58-65, ISSN 0424-8155

Pfurtscheller, G., & Lopes da Silva, F. H. (1999) Event-related desynchronization Handbook of Electroencephalography and Clinical Neurophysiulogy. Revised Series, Vol. 6, ISBN 0-444-82999-7

Rauschecker J. P. (1998) Cortical processing of complex sounds. *Curr Opin Neurobiol* 8(4), (1998 Aug), pp. 516-521, ISSN 0959-4388

Rivlin-Etzion, M., Marmor, O., Heimer, G., Raz, A., Nini, A., Bergman, H. (2006) Basal ganglia oscillations and pathophysiology of movement disorders. *Curr Opin Neurobiol* 16(6), (2006 Dec), pp. 629-637, ISSN 0959-4388

Robertson, C., Empson, J. (1999) Slowed cognitive processing and high workload in Parkinson's disease. *J Neurol Sci* 162(1), (1999 Jan 1), pp. 27-33, ISSN 0022-510X

Rolland, A.-S., Herrero, M.-T., Garcia-Martinez, V., Ruberg, M., Hirsch, E. C., Francois, C. (2007) Metabolic activity of cerebellar and basal ganglia-thalamic neurons is reduced in parkinsonism. *Brain* 130(1), (2007 Jan), pp. 265-275, ISSN 0006-8950

Sawamoto, N., Honda, M., Hanakawa, T., Fukuyama, H., Shibasaki, H. (2002) Cognitive slowing in Parkinson's disease: a behavioural evaluation independent of motor slowing. *J Neurosci* 22(12), (2002 Jun 15), pp. 5198-5203, ISSN 0270-6474

Schmiedt, C., Meistrowitz, A., Schwendemann, G., Herrmann, M., Basar-Eroglu, C. (2005) Theta and alpha oscillations reflect differences in memory strategy and visual discrimination performance in patients with Parkinson's disease. *Neurosci Lett* 388(3), (2005 Nov 18), pp. 138-143, ISSN 0304-3940

Schurmann, M., Basar-Eroglu, E. (1994) Topography of alpha and theta oscillatory responses upon auditory and visual stimuli in humans. *Biol Cybern* 72(2), pp. 161-174, ISSN 0340-1200

Shohamy, D., Myers, C. E., Grossman, S., Sage, J., Gluck, M. A. (2005) The role of dopamine in cognitive sequence learning: evidence from Parkinson's disease. *Behav Brain Res* 156(2), (2005 Jan 30), pp. 191-199, ISSN 0166-4328

Silberstein, P., Pogosyan, A., Kühn, A. A., Hotton, G., Tisch, S., Kupsch, A., Dowsey-Limousin, P., Hariz, M. I., Brown, P. (2005) Cortico-cortical coupling in Parkinson's disease and its modulation by therapy. *Brain* 128(6), (2005 Jun), pp. 1277-1291, ISSN 0006-8950

Stam, C. J., Visser, S. L., Op de Coul, A. A., De Sonneville, L. M., Schellens, R. L., Brunia, C. H., de Smet. J. S., Gielen, G. (1993) Disturbed frontal regulation of attention in Parkinson's disease. *Brain* 116(5), (1993 Oct), pp. 1139-1158, ISSN 0006-8950

Sutoh T., Yabe H., Sato Y., Hiruma T., Kaneko S. (2000) Event-related desynchronization during an auditory oddball task. *Clin Neurophysiol* 111(5), (2000 May), pp. 858-862, ISSN 1388-2457

Tachibana, H., Toda, K., Sugita, M. (1992) Actively and passively evoked P3 latency of event-related potentials in Parkinson's disease. *J Neurol Sci* 111(2), (1992 Sep), pp. 134–142, ISSN 0022-510X

Taylor, A. E., Saint-Cyr, J. A., Lang, A. E. (1990) Memory and learning in early Parkinson's disease: evidence for a "frontal lobe syndrome". *Brain Cogn* 13(2), (1990 Jul), pp. 211–232, ISSN 0278-2626

Tallon-Baudry, C., Bertrand, O., Delpuech, C., Pernier, J. (1996) Stimulus specificity of phase-locked and non-phase-locked 40 Hz visual responses in human. *J Neurosci* 16(13), (1996 Jul 1), pp. 4240-4249, ISSN 0270-6474

Terman, D., Rubin, J. E., Yew, A. C., Wilson, C. J. (2002) Activity patterns in a model for the subthalamopallidal network of the basal ganglia. *J Neurosci* 22(7), (2002 Apr 1), pp. 2963-2976, ISSN 0270-6474

Tiitinen, H., Sinkkonen, J., Reinikainen, K., Alho, K., Lavikainen, J., Näätänen, R. (1993) Selective attention enhances the auditory 40-Hz transient response in humans. *Nature* 364(6432), (1993 Jul 1), pp. 59-60, ISSN 0028-0836

van Spaendonck, K. P., Berger, H. J., Horstink, M. W., Cools, A. R. (1998) Cognitive deficits in Parkinson's disease. *Tijdschr Gerontol Geriatr* 29(4), (1998 Aug), pp. 189-195, ISSN 0167-9228

Vieregge, P., Verleger, R., Wascher, E., Stüven, F., Kömpf, D. (1994) Auditory selective attention is impaired in Parkinson's disease event-related evidence from EEG potentials. *Brain Res Cogn Brain Res* 2(2), (1994 Sep), pp. 117–129, ISSN 0926-6410

Visscher, K. M., Kaplan, E., Kahana, M. J., Sekuler, R. (2007) Auditory short-term memory behaves like visual short-term memory. *PLoS Biol* 5(3), (2007 Mar) e56, ISSN 1544-9173

Wang, H., Wang, Y., Wang, D., Cui L., Tian, S., Zhang, Y. (2002) Cognitive impairment in Parkinson's disease revealed by event-related potential N270. *J Neurol Sci* 194(1), (2002 Feb 15), pp. 49–53, ISSN 0022-510X

Wang, S. Y., Aziz, T. Z., Stein, J. F. & Liu, X. (2005) Time-frequency analysis of transient neuromuscular events: dynamic changes in activity of the subthalamic nucleus and forearm muscles related to the intermittent resting tremor. *J Neurosci Methods* 145(1-2), (2005 Jun 30), pp. 151-158, ISSN 0165-0270

Wascher, E., Verleger, R., Vieregge, P., Jaskowski ,P., Koch, S., Kömpf, D. (1997) Responses to cued signals in Parkinson's disease. Distinguishing between disorders of cognition and of activation. *Brain* 120(8), (1997 Aug), pp. 1355–1375, ISSN 0006-8950

Weinberger, M., Mahant, N., Hutchison, W. D., Lozano, A. M., Moro, E., Hodaie, M., Lang, A E., Dostrovsky, J. O. (2006) Beta oscillatory activity in the subthalamic nucleus and its relation to dopaminergic response in Parkinson's disease. *J Neurophysiol* 96(6), (2006 Dec), pp. 3248-3256, ISSN 0022-3077

Weinberger, M., Hutchison, W. D., Lozano, A. M., Hodaie, M., Dostrovsky, J. O. (2008) Increased gamma oscillatory activity in the subthalamic nucleus during tremor in Parkinson's disease patients. *J Neurophysiol* 101(2), (2009 Feb), pp. 789-802, ISSN 0022-3077

Williams, D., Kühn, A., Kupsch, A., Tijssen, M., van Bruggen, G., Speelman, H., Hotton, G., Yarrow, K. & Brown, P. (2003) Behavioural cues are associated with modulations of synchronous oscillations in the human subthalamic nucleus. *Brain* 126(9), (2003 Sep), pp. 1975-1985, ISSN 0006-8950

Williams, D., Tijssen, M., van Bruggen, G., Bosch, A., Insola, A., Di Lazzaro, V., Mazzone, P., Oliviero, A., Quartarone, A., Speelman, H., & Brown, P (2002) Dopamine dependent changes in the functional connectivity between basal ganglia and cerebral cortex in the human. *Brain* 125(7), (2002 Jul), pp. 1558-1569, ISSN 0006-8950

4

Developing an MRI-Based Biomarker for Early Diagnosis of Parkinson's Disease

Jorge E. Quintero[1], Xiaomin Wang[3] and Zhiming Zhang[1,2,*]
*[1]Department of Anatomy and Neurobiology, Morris K. Udall Parkinson's Disease
Research Center of Excellence,
[2]Magnetic Resonance Imaging and Spectroscopy Center, University of Kentucky Chandler
Medical Center, Lexington,
[3]Department of Physiology, Key Laboratory for Neurodegenerative Disorders of the
Ministry Education, Capital Medical University, Beijing
[1,2]USA
[3]PR of China*

1. Introduction

Parkinson's disease (PD) is a relentlessly progressive disorder causing disability in most individuals and cannot be controlled with available medication. PD is currently considered a systemic disease with complex motor disorders and non-motor deficits which appear before or in parallel with motor deficits and then worsen with disease progression (Chaudhuri *et al.*, 2006; Ferrer *et al.*, 2010). In a recent survey, the projected number of individuals with PD will dramatically increase in 20 years especially in the most populated countries like China, India, Brazil and the United States (Dorsey *et al.*, 2007). Current causative theories for PD include complex interactions between genetic susceptibility and environmental factors. These and possibly other mechanisms lead to a progressive and variable degree of dopamine (DA) neuron loss in the substantia nigra compacta (SNc) resulting in DA depletion in the striatum (Hornykiewicz & Kish, 1987; Marsden & Obeso, 1994) that then leads to the clinical manifestation of PD. Studies have demonstrated that PD is characterized by a presymptomatic phase, likely lasting years, or even decades, during which neuronal degeneration is occurring but before clinical symptoms appear (Hubble, 2000; DeKosky & Marek, 2003; Katzenschlager & Lees, 2004). In addition, studies have demonstrated that most patients when diagnosed with PD have already lost a significant amount of SNc DA neurons in the range of 50% cell loss. Based on detailed pathological studies, Fearnley and Lees (1991) have proposed the notion that the loss of nigral neurons would occur exponentially, with greater loss occurring within the first decade in the disease process, and then reaching over 90% loss at the time of death.

While our understanding of PD has grown over the course of the last two centuries and PD is one of the best understood neurodegenerative diseases, our ability to treat PD remains limited. Given the progressive nature of the disease, the question becomes is it possible to divert or change the rate of the progression? Inherent to this question is our ability to identify where an individual is along the path of this disease. Thus it would behoove us to be able to establish indicators of the disease stage while intervention remains a possibility. Here we describe the development of using non-invasive functional imaging as a biomarker for the early diagnosis of PD.

1.1 Difficulty of early detection of PD

The diagnosis and treatment of PD is fraught with problems: 1) so far, no objective measures are available for the diagnosis of PD (Wu et al., 2011); 2) it is unknown whether a linear relationship exists between a worsening in the Unified Parkinson's Disease Rating Scale (UPDRS), or other clinical scales, and the progressive degeneration of the nigrostriatal system; 3) no objective measures are available for testing responsiveness of therapy. Therefore, biomarkers of disease progression before the appearance of symptoms would be of onsiderable value; thus, neuroimaging techniques may be good candidates for meeting the challenges. In the past decade, radiotracer imaging of the nigrostriatal dopaminergic system has been extensively explored with positron emission tomography (PET) and single photon emission computed tomography (SPECT) imaging protocols and has become a prominent biomarker in PD although these techniques are still controversial in some aspects such as the interpretation of imaging data and disconnection with clinical outcomes (Brooks et al., 2003; Ravina et al., 2005). However, the spatial resolution of these techniques is relatively poor, thus reducing their utility in mapping subtle changes in neuroanatomy and neurochemistry with PD progression (Snow et al., 2000). Furthermore, PET imaging is not widely available and is expensive (~US$3,000-$6,000) because of the need to generate and use radioactive nucleotides onsite. Clearly there is a need for imaging techniques that do not require radioactive isotopes but ones that would still be sensitive enough to usefully and longitudinally monitor the development, progression, and treatment of PD. The ideal technique would 1) permit high-resolution imaging of brain sites affected by PD processes, 2) provide valid assessment of the underlying neuroanatomical state, and 3) be safe to allow repeated tests. A hypothesis for PD is that the disease severity corresponds to the magnitude and pattern of histological and neuroimaging abnormalities (DeKosky & Marek, 2003; Eckert & Eidelberg, 2004; Seibyl et al., 2005). Based on our own previous studies, and those of others in rodents, nonhuman primates, and humans, pharmacological MRI (phMRI; or functional MRI with specific pharmacological stimulation) would be a good candidate because of its high resolution, sensitivity, reproducibility, wide availability, and low cost (Nguyen et al., 2000; Tracey, 2001; Honey & Bullmore, 2004; Jenkins et al., 2004; Chin et al., 2008; Thiel, 2009; Rasmussen Jr, 2010).

1.2 Why is a new imaging protocol needed for PD?

In the past decade, PET and SPECT have become the most widely used and accepted imaging methods for PD research (de la Fuente-Fernandez & Stoessl, 2002; Eckert & Eidelberg, 2004). Worsening motor disability along with ^{18}F-dopa uptake decreases in the putamen (Brooks et al., 1990) correlate with the storage of DA within vesicles (Hoshi et al., 1993) and with the number of functioning DA terminals in the striatum (Snow et al., 1993). Currently, in vivo measurements can be conducted using SPECT with ligands for the DA transporter (DAT) such as [(123)I]N-omega-fluoropropyl-2beta-carbomethoxy-3beta-{4-iodophenyl}nortropane (FP-CIT) that provide a measure of DA terminal integrity (DeKosky & Marek, 2003; Andringa et al., 2005). Although the aforementioned studies have shown that these neuroimaging techniques are capable of mapping changes in dopaminergic function in the basal ganglia, much controversy still exists. Recent problems have been encountered in clinical trials that have used radioligand imaging to quantify medication response. For example, there appears to be a discrepancy between current imaging protocols and clinical outcomes. In National Institutes of Health (NIH) sponsored randomized double-blind studies on PD patients receiving either fetal tissue transplants or sham surgery, a 40% increase in ^{18}F-dopa uptake in the putamen contrasted with a modest (non-significant) 18% improvement in the mean UPDRS in one study involving 40 patients (Freed et al., 2001). In the second study involving 34 patients, a 20-30% increase of ^{18}F-dopa uptake was seen in the striatum, but clinical changes failed to reach statistical significance (Brooks, 2004). Most recently, a significant increase was found in ^{18}F-dopa uptake in the putamen of PD patients receiving trophic therapy, while clinical improvements did not differ significantly from the control group (Lang et al., 2006).

1.3 What are imaging biomarkers for PD?

In general, biomarkers must be biologically and clinically relevant, analytically sound, operationally practical, timely, interpretable and cost effective. On the other hand, biomarkers must be objectively measured indicators of biological and pathobiological process or pharmacologic responses to treatment. The biomarkers should be used to substitute for a clinical endpoint (predict benefit or harm) based on epidemiologic, therapeutic, pathophysiologic or other scientific evidence (Biomarkers definition working group, 2001). Specifically for PD, the biomarkers must be indicators of biological processes that change with the progression of the nigrostriatal system. The biomarkers should 1) correlate to some extents with severity of PD assessed by behavior and with pathophysiological changes such as the number of surviving neurons in the SNc; 2) reflect true disease status or predict clinical outcomes; 3) be used to assess efficacy and/or responsiveness of treatment, and 4) be used as surrogate endpoints.

1.4 What is BOLD-phMRI?

Our preliminary studies have shown evidence that blood-oxygenation-level-dependent (BOLD)-phMRI can be used as a non-invasive imaging modality to detect functional changes of the dopamine system in parkinsonian monkeys. More importantly, the studies were conducted in a conventional clinical MRI scanner without the injection of contrast agents. Using this imaging method, a significant correlation was found between the amphetamine-evoked BOLD response and the number of surviving dopamine neurons in the substantia nigra, which was also significantly correlated with bradykinesia scores on the nonhuman primate parkinsonian rating scale (Ovadia et al., 1995), suggesting that phMRI may be used as a biomarker to assess dopamine neuronal loss in PD. Recently, fMRI has become a popular tool for imaging of functionally active brain regions in healthy and diseased brains. The use of fMRI is promoting the emergence of a new area of research, one that is complementary to more invasive techniques for measuring neural activity in animal models while better understanding the function and dysfunction of the human brain. The most common method of fMRI is the BOLD imaging technique. fMRI takes advantage of the coupling between neural activity and hemodynamics (the local control of blood flow and oxygenation) in the brain to allow the non-invasive localization and measurement of brain activity (Fig. 1).

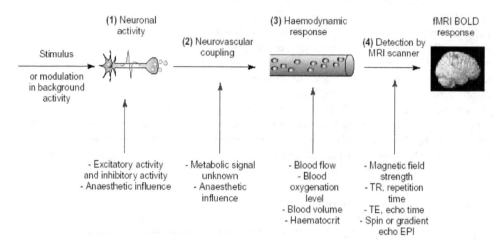

Fig. 1. fMRI provides an insight into neural activity. The BOLD signal has several constituents: (1) the neuronal response to a stimulus or background modulation; (2) the complex relationship between neuronal activity and triggering a haemodynamic response (termed neurovascular coupling); (3) the haemodynamic response itself; and (4) the detection of the response by an MRI scanner (from Arthurs & Boniface, 2002).

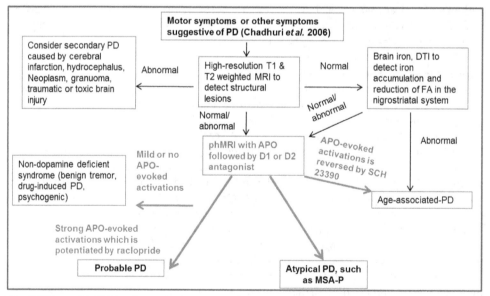

Fig. 2. Using phMRI for the early diagnosis of PD. As part of a multi-factor approach, phMRI provides a possible means of screening for the underlying neurological changes in parkinsonism or PD.

We hypothesize that the BOLD-fMRI response to a specific DA stimulation could serve as a potential biomarker for PD because of its unique features which are different from other neuroimaging technologies as follows: 1) High sensitivity and reproducibility, and relatively high specificity, 2) Minimal invasiveness or patient discomfort ("subject friendly"), 3) Low per-usage cost (this is especially important if widespread screening is contemplated), and 4) wide availability.

2. phMRI detects dopamine deficiency in parkinsonian monkeys

2.1 An animal model of dopamine deficiency in rhesus monkeys

A reliable and reproducible model of dopamine deficiency/a model simulating human PD is developed by unilateral administration of neurotoxin 1-methyl-4-phenyl-1,2,3,6-etrahydropyridine (MPTP) through the carotid artery. The specific neurotoxic actions of MPTP are produced when it is metabolized by monoamine oxidase B into 1-methyl-4-phenylpyridinium (MPP +), a complex I mitochondrial neurotoxin with relative specificity for dopamine neurons in the substantia nigra (Langston & Ballard, 1983; Nicklas et al., 1987; Richardson et al., 2007). Ding and colleagues (2008) described the key features modeled by MPTP toxicity including 1) all animals show parkinsonian features often seen in idiopathic PD such as bradykinesia, rigidity, postural, and balance instability, 2) these PD features can be partially normalized by levodopa treatment, which is the most efficacious drug to treat PD motor symptoms and is widely considered the "gold standard" treatment for the disease, 3) massive neuronal loss of dopaminergic neurons in the SNc and dopaminergic fibers in the striatum, and 4) remarkable declines in DA and DA metabolites.

2.2 phMRI procedures

1) Mapping of MPTP-induced functional changes with d-amphetamine stimulations (from a pre-synaptic perspective) and 2) Mapping of MPTP-induced functional changes with APO challenge (from a post-synaptic perspective). In early studies, the scans were conducted on a Siemens VISION 1.5 T MRI scanner using the body coil to transmit radio frequency and an 8 cm diameter surface coil placed above the monkey's head for RF signal reception. The anatomical structures of interest were visualized using a 3D FLASH sequence with 1 mm isotropic resolution (TR/TE=21/6 ms, flip angle = 30°, image matrix size = 128x128x90, field of view = 128 mm). The functional MR images from pharmacological challenges were acquired continuously using a FLASH 2D multiple gradient-recalled-echo (MGRE) navigator sequence (Chen et al., 1996). The ROI dimensions were 3x3x3 mm, each representing a 27 mm³ volume. ROIs were manually selected in both hemispheres of MPTP-lesioned and normal control animals based on the co-registered 3D anatomical images acquired from the FLASH sequence. Because of variability in the inherent noise level due to differences in positioning animals for each scan and the movements during scanning, the replicate scans were treated as independent observations in the analysis. For later studies, images were acquired on a Siemens 3T Trio clinical MRI system using a dedicated receive-only coil for reception, which was designed and developed by our group. The BOLD-effect weighted MR images used to measure the phMRI response were acquired in an anatomically coronal plane. The image planes of the acquisition were arranged to cover the motor cortex and the basal ganglia. A segmented gradient-echo EPI sequence with TE=28 ms and a turbo factor of 7 was used to reduce echo train length and minimize magnetic susceptibility-related artifacts. The EPI sequence acquisition parameters are FOV=112x98 mm and image matrix 64x56 for an in-plane resolution of 1.75 mm. A total of 15 contiguous

slices, each 2 mm-thick, were acquired at a rate of 15 s per EPI volume. The overall scan duration was 80 minutes with 128 volumes acquired prior to apomorphine (APO) administration as a baseline and 192 after APO to track the response. Images were motion corrected and spatially smoothed using a Gaussian kernel of width 3.5 mm. phMRI response was calculated as the fractional signal change in % of the average of the post-APO image data relative to the pre-APO baseline. A co-registered high-resolution (0.67×0.67×1 mm) T1-weighted anatomical MRI scan was acquired in each session for spatial localization of the activation response. Prior to the administration of d-amphetamine (2.0mg/kg) or APO (0.1 mg/kg), a total of 40 image frames were collected over 20 min to determine the baseline state. Following injection of d-amphetamine or APO, an additional 40 frames were collected to track the dynamic response (Zhang *et al.*, 2001; Andersen *et al.*, 2002). The change in R_2^*, i.e. ΔR_2^* which represents the phMRI activation response to drug, was determined as the difference between the mean R_2^* across 20 images post drug administration during the period of peak response (5-15 min) and the mean R_2^* within the 40 baseline images. A reduction ("negative" change) in R_2^* associated with a local decrease of paramagnetic deoxyhemoglobin is an indicator of BOLD-effect activation (Chen *et al.*, 1996).

2.3 phMRI-responses correlate with severity of PD

Six out of six animals responded positively to APO treatment represented by 44% improvements in parkinsonian symptoms. The same dose of APO also evoked phMRI responses by increasing the phMRI signal intensity. The typical phMRI (BOLD effect) responses to APO were gradually increased after APO administration only in the structure on the ipsilateral side receiving MPTP administration. Interestingly, but not surprising, APO-induced behavioral changes (PD features) were significantly correlated with APO-induced phMRI responses in the putamen, premotor cortex, and cingulate gyrus. When compared with standard but objective measures, there was a significant negative correlation between the phMRI responses in the putamen and distance travelled and movement speed. Similar relationships were also seen between phMRI responses in the motor cortex and daytime home-cage activity and between phMRI responses in the caudate nucleus and movement speed.

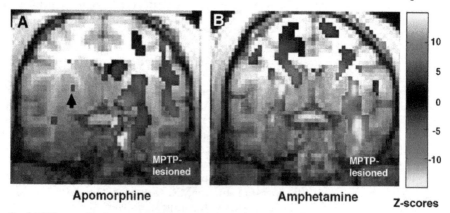

Fig. 3. phMRI reveals nigrostriatal system responsiveness to dopamine stimulation. Coronal MRI scans depicting areas of activation and deactivation (represented by the pseudocolor) in the brain after an APO or amphetamine challenge in unitalteral MPTP-lesioned nonhuman primates (from Zhang *et al.*, 2006).

2.4 phMRI-response and MPTP-induced dopamine deficiency
2.4.1 phMRI responses in MPTP-lesioned structures

Apomorphine administration strongly activated the MPTP-denervated putamen (Figs. 3A and 4C) and substantia nigra (Fig.4D). An opposite response (a positive ΔR_2^* value) was evident in the contralateral putamen (Fig. 4G) and substantia nigra (Fig. 4H). The differences between the intact and lesioned substantia nigra and between the intact and lesioned putamen were highly significant, P < 0.01(t-test), in both cases. In contrast, ΔR_2^* responses in the caudate nucleus and in the corpus callosum were not significant, nor were there significant hemispheric differences in activation or deactivation with the contralateral caudate or with a comparable region in the contralateral callosum (Figs. 4A and 4E).

The phMRI responses to amphetamine treatment in the putamen (Figs. 3B and 4G) and substantia nigra (Fig. 4H) were the inverse of those seen with apomorphine. Amphetamine-induced decreases (positive $\Delta R2^*$ values) in the lesioned putamen and substantia nigra suggested diminished neuronal activity in both sites. In contrast, amphetamine induced the opposite $\Delta R2^*$ response in the intact left side, tending to increase activation in the putamen and substantia nigra. The responses in the intact putamen and intact substantia nigra were significantly different from their lesioned counterparts. Again, the corpus callosum and the caudate nucleus displayed only small, insignificant changes in response to amphetamine stimulation (Figs. 4E and 4F).

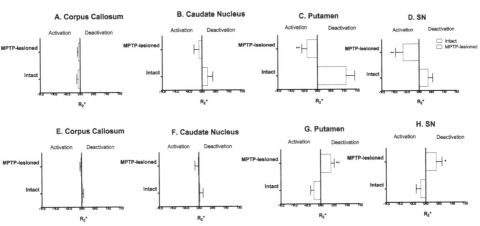

Fig. 4. phMRI responses in the nigrostriatal system. Depending on the means of stimulation, phMRI reveals a differential activations and deactivations in the nigrostriatal system. After APO stimulation (A-D) or d-amphetamine stimulation (E-H). **P<0.01; *P<0.05; unpaired t-test (from Zhang et al., 2006).

2.4.2 phMRI-responses and loss of DA neurons in the SN

In a later study, post-mortem histopathological evaluation revealed that the unilateral MPTP administration (received 5 years before the analysis) produced a massive (85%) loss of the rate-limiting enzyme for DA formation, tyrosine hydroxylase, (TH$^+$) cells in the midbrain on the ipsilateral side receiving the infusion of the neurotoxin. TH$^+$ cell numbers were significantly higher on the un-lesioned side compared to the MPTP-lesioned side. More importantly, the number of TH$^+$ cells was strongly correlated with the phMRI responses in the caudate nucleus and in the cingulate gyrus. When comparing d-amphetamine-induced DA release in the putamen and DA neuron counts in the SNc, a significant correlation was also seen. In an earlier study (Zhang *et al.*, 2006), amphetamine administration evoked a BOLD response in the SN that correlated with the number of TH+ dopamine neurons in the same structure. These data support that there is a strong relationship between BOLD-responses to dopaminergic challenge and the number of dopaminergic neurons in the midbrain.

2.4.3 phMRI-responses and loss of DA fibers in the striatum

Similar to the effect on dopaminergic neurons, the MPTP administration also produced a remarkable reduction of TH+ fibers on the ipsilateral side of the lesion. A comparison of the fiber density in the putamen on the MPTP-lesioned side with other elements of the cortico-basal ganglia-cortical circuit (Braak & Del Tredici, 2008) such as ipsilateral phMRI responses in the motor cortex (Fig. 5A) and caudate nucleus (Fig. 5B) showed strong correlations. In addition, the fiber density in the MPTP-lesioned caudate nucleus was strongly correlated with phMRI responses in the premotor cortex, caudate nucleus, and cingulate gyrus. Those changes in TH+ fiber density were also correlated with behavior and DA levels in the striatum and with the number of DA neurons in the SNc.

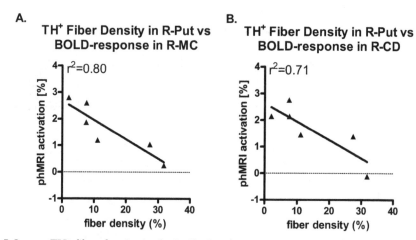

Fig. 5. Lower TH+ fiber density in the ipsilesional putamen corresponds with higher phMRI activation. TH+ fiber density in the right putamen (R-Put) is inversely correlated with phMRI activation in A) the right motor cortex (R-MC) and B) the right caudate nucleus (R-CD).

2.4.4 phMRI-responses correlate with dopamine overflow

The microdialysis experiments were conducted months after the parkinsonian symptoms had been fully developed and stabilized. First, the single administration of MPTP produced significant reduction in both potassium- and d-amphetamine-evoked overflow of DA in the putamen (Fig. 6A) and SNc (Fig.6B) on the ipsilateral side of the lesion. Second, there were several important correlations between DA levels in the putamen and SNc and the phMRI responses. For example, both potassium- and d-amphetamine-evoked overflow of DA in

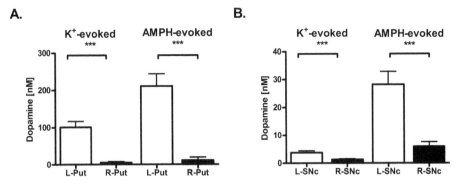

Fig. 6. Hemiparkinsonian nonhuman primates have markedly dimished dopaminergic function. K+ (100 mM)- and amphetamine (250 μM)-evoked DA release was significantly attenuated in the ipsilesional A) putamen (Put) and B) SNc; ***: P < 0.0001 (paired *t*-test).

the putamen (each measured for a single time point, 30 minutes after stimulus administration) had significant correlations with phMRI responses in the putamen. DA levels in the putamen were also significantly correlated with phMRI responses in the premotor cortex and cingulate gyrus, as well as in the caudate nucleus. Finally, d-amphetamine-evoked DA release in the SNc was found to have a significant, but negatively correlated relationship with the motor cortex (Fig. 7).

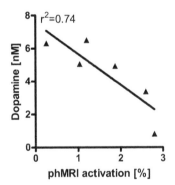

Fig. 7. DA levels in the right SNc correlate with the BOLD responses in the right motor cortex. In animals with lower DA levels in the right SNc, less activation was observed in the right motor cortex

3. Using phMRI to monitor therapeutic effects in parkinsonian monkeys

There is a great need for the development of noninvasive, highly sensitive, and widely available imaging methods which can potentially be used to longitudinally monitor treatment of PD. We reported the monitoring of glial-cell-line-derived neurotrophic factor (GDNF) induced functional changes of the basal ganglia in hemiparkinsonian monkeys via phMRI measuring the BOLD response to a direct dopamine agonist, APO, (Luan *et al.*, 2008). The effectiveness of GDNF to protect and restore the nigrostriatal dopaminergic system in rodent and nonhuman primate models of PD has been extensively documented (Beck *et al.*,

1995; Tomac *et al.*, 1995; Gash *et al.*, 1996; Kordower *et al.*, 2000; Grondin *et al.*, 2002). This trophic factor has also shown promise in Phase I clinical trials for the treatment of PD (Gill *et al.*, 2003; Slevin *et al.*, 2005). Ample evidence supports the idea that GDNF can protect and promote survival of pre-synaptic dopaminergic neurons in the SNc and axons in the striatum (Gash *et al.*, 1996). After testing BOLD responses to APO in their normal state, additional scans were taken with the same dose of APO stimulation after MPTP-induced hemiparkinsonism. Then, the animals were chronically treated with GDNF for 18 weeks by a programmable pump and catheter system. The catheter was surgically implanted into the right putamen and connected to the pump via flexible polyurethane tubing. phMRI scans were taken at both 6 and 18 weeks while they received 22.5μg of GDNF per day (Fig. 8). In addition, behavioral changes were monitored throughout the entire study. The primary finding of this study was that APO-evoked activations in the DA denervated putamen were attenuated by the chronic intraputamenal infusion of GDNF accompanied by improvements of parkinsonian features, movement speed and APO-induced rotation compared to data collected before the chronic GDNF treatment. The results suggest that phMRI methods in combination with administration of a selective DA agonist may be useful for monitoring neurorestorative therapies in PD patients in the future.

A. Pre-GDNF   B. Post-GDNF

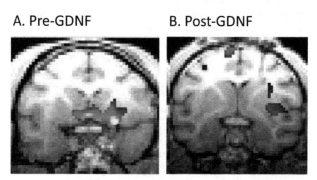

Fig. 8. phMRI (BOLD)-responses to APO can be used to monitor GDNF-induced neurorestorative therapeutic effects in rhesus monkeys with MPTP-induced hemiparkinsonisms. phMRI activation reveals differences in dopaminergic activity after GDNF treatment (from Luan *et al.*, 2008).

4. Brain iron and motor deficits in rhesus monkeys

Schuff (2009) notes in a recent review, perhaps the most consistently reported MRI findings in PD have been the detection of signal changes related to excessive iron, most likely related to ferritin, the main iron-storage protein within the brain. Under normal condition, iron is essential for normal metabolism and used in production of DA. Brain iron may also play an essential role in learning and memory (Fretham *et al.*, 2011). Several years ago, we reported a correlation of R_2 with total iron concentration in the brains of rhesus monkeys (Hardy *et al.*, 2005). The results show that the transverse relaxation rate $R_2 = 1/T_2$ is highly correlated to and varies linearly with iron content. In the study, Hardy and colleagues demonstrated that R_2 was highly correlated with the total iron concentration and that the relationship between R_2 and tissue iron concentration appeared to depend upon the iron concentration. In another multidiscipline study of brain iron in a large group of rhesus monkeys ranging in age from 4 to 32 years old, Cass and colleagues (2006) found significant decreases in motor performance, decreases in striatal DA release, and increases in striatal iron levels in rhesus monkeys as they aged from young adulthood. A comprehensive statistical analysis relating age, motor performance, DA release, and iron content indicated that the best predictor of decreases in motor ability, above and beyond levels of performance that could be explained by age alone, was iron accumulation in the striatum. Compared to the young animals, the relaxation rate $1/T_2^*$ used as an indicator of iron content was elevated by 38-43% in all three regions in the middle-aged monkeys (Fig. 9). In the aged animals, iron content was increased by 55%, 61%, and 79% in the caudate, putamen, and nigra, respectively, compared to the young animals (Fig. 9). Iron content in the nigra of the aged animals was also 30% higher than in the middle-aged animals. ROI data for $1/T_2$ measures are not shown but exhibited a similar dependence on age. Regression analysis extended the group statistics and further confirmed the strong age-associated increase of the MRI relaxation rate $1/T_2^*$ (equivalent to a T_2^*-shortening) in each of the three regions of interest (n = 24; p<0.0001). The intercept and rate of increase were 16.537+ 0.598 sec^{-1}/year, 15.728+0.734 sec^{-1}/year, and 19.047+0.791 sec^{-1}/year for the caudate, putamen, and substantia nigra, respectively. This suggests that striatal iron levels may be a biomarker of motor dysfunction in aging; and as such, can be monitored non-invasively by longitudinal brain MRI scans.

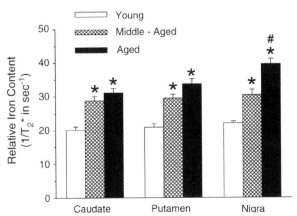

Fig. 9. Using MR imaging of iron content to identify alterations in the aging brain. The use of MR imaging to identify the relative iron content in particular brain structures illustrates the potential usefulness for a non-invasive means of assessing changes in the nigrostriatal system with aging. *: P <0.05; #: P <0.01 (one-way ANOVA). (from Cass *et al.*, 2006)

5. Diffusion Tensor Image (DTI) and dopamine deficiency in rhesus monkeys

Diffusion tensor imaging (DTI) has been increasingly used in PD related research (Schuff, 2009). DTI can be used to noninvasively investigate and identify white matter (WM) changes associated with PD. DTI is able to obtain quantitative information about fractional anisotropy (FA) and mean diffusivity (MD). A diminished FA is thought to reflect axonal loss and demyelination. A recent DTI study was conducted by our group in normal (n=9) and hemiparkinsonian (n=8) monkeys to explore the MPTP-effects on WM using the DTI parameters of FA and MD. Under general anesthesia, DTI data was obtained on a 3T Siemens

Trio MRI scanner with a custom-built, single channel, receive-only coil, built on a fiberglass frame and used to enhance the received signal. Imaging consisted of single shot (SS), double pulsed gradient spin echo (double-PGSE), diffusion weighted, echo planar imaging (EPI) with a spatial resolution of $1.23 \times 1.23 \times 2.0$ mm^3. Images were processed and analyzed by using the publicly available image processing software FSL (http://www.fmrib.ox.ac.uk/fsl) (Smith et al., 2004; Smith et al., 2006). All of the processing tools referred to by their FSL acronyms are available for download at the website. First, we observed a WM tract in the vicinity of the basal ganglia (BG) with FA greater (P<0.01, t-test) in the aged-matched control animals than MPTP-treated animals in the same structure. Second, we observed multiple WM tracts in the sensory cortex, with FA greater (P<0.05, t-test) in the MPTP-treated than untreated side in the same animals. The result from the pilot study supports the idea that high resolution DTI has the potential to distinguish animals with a MPTP-lesioned nigrostriatal system from normal age-matched, healthy controls on an animal-by-animal basis.

6. Conclusion and perspectives

Since a diagnosis of PD still solely depends on the judgment of the clinician, there is an urgent demand for the development of reliable and applicable test systems or biomarkers to provide a level of certainty to the diagnosis. Objective biomarkers of PD are pivotal to tracking the disease progression and confirm the therapeutic effects. Non- or minimally-invasive imaging techniques provide a unique, real-time opportunity to assess the changes that occur with neurodegenerative diseases. In addition, with the rapidly expanding use of fMRI to provide a dramatically greater understanding of brain function, imaging techniques such as phMRI are only bound to benefit from this new wealth of knowledge.

The advantage of MRI is that MRIs are far more widely available than other imaging modalities and are most commonly used in clinical practice to differentiate idiopathic PD from secondary cause of parkinsonism (Pavese & Brooks, 2009). Recent advancement in high field MRI technology offers even better opportunities for noninvasively, longitudinally, and objectively assessing brain alterations in PD. For example functional and pharmacological MRI has been increasingly employed for preclinical and clinical research of the disease. Ample evidence supports that MRI signals have the potential to be developed as a noninvasive state biomarker in PD. For example, several MRI methodologies such as structural MRI, imaging of brain iron, DTI, functional MRI and pharmacological MRI have provided meaningful insight of brain alteration in PD. That said, we note that while we have gained greater understanding of the changes that occur in disorders of dopaminergic dysfunction with the use of phMRI in the rhesus model of PD, nevertheless the studies are works in progress and ones that still require cautious interpretation because conditions in patients with PD are more complex than in the animal model used in these studies.

In our hands, MRI studies conducted at the University of Kentucky have demonstrated that phMRI-responses to dopaminergic challenges in MPTP-treated monkeys are highly correlated with 1) the severity of parkinsonism, 2) the loss of dopamine neurons and terminals, 3) the decline of dopamine overflow and 4) the functional recovery from GDNF treatment. In addition, results from imaging brain iron suggest that striatal iron levels may constitute a biomarker for motor dysfunction in aged animals with parkinsonism. As shown in Fig. 10, combining various MRI methodologies may be used to screen populations at high risk, to differentiate idiopathic PD from second causes of parkinsonisms, and to monitor progression of the disease and the therapeutic effects.

Developing an MRI-based diagnostic kit for early detection of Parkinson's disease

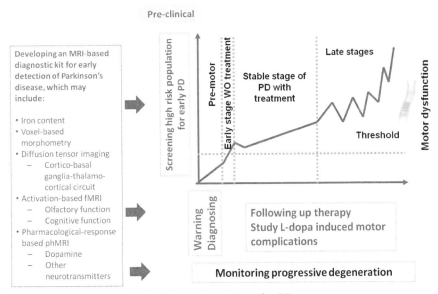

Fig. 10. Employing MRI methodologies in the clinic for PD.

7. Acknowledgment

We thank Drs. Anders Andersen, Peter Hardy, and Richard Grondin for their technical help in data analysis, behavioral evaluation, and discussions. Support provided by USPHS NIH grants NS50242, NS39787, and AG13494.

8. References

Andersen, A.H., Zhang, Z., Barber, T., Rayens, W.S., Zhang, J., Grondin, R., Hardy, P., Gerhardt, G.A. & Gash, D.M. (2002) Functional MRI studies in awake rhesus monkeys: methodological and analytical strategies. *J Neurosci Methods*, 118, 141-152.

Andringa, G., Drukarch, B., Bol, J.G., de Bruin, K., Sorman, K., Habraken, J.B. & Booij, J. (2005) Pinhole SPECT imaging of dopamine transporters correlates with dopamine transporter immunohistochemical analysis in the MPTP mouse model of Parkinson's disease. *Neuroimage*, 26, 1150-1158.

Arthurs, O.J. & Boniface, S. (2002) How well do we understand the neural origins of the fMRI BOLD signal? *Trends Neurosci*, 25, 27-31.

Beck, K.D., Valverde, J., Alexi, T., Poulsen, K., Moffat, B., Vandlen, R.A., Rosenthal, A. & Hefti, F. (1995) Mesencephalic dopaminergic neurons protected by GDNF from axotomy-induced degeneration in the adult brain. *Nature*, 373, 339-341.

Braak, H. & Del Tredici, K. (2008) Cortico-basal ganglia-cortical circuitry in Parkinson's disease reconsidered. *Exp Neurol*, 212, 226-229.

Brooks, D.J. (2004) Neuroimaging in Parkinson's disease. *NeuroRx*, 1, 243-254.

Brooks, D.J., Frey, K.A., Marek, K.L., Oakes, D., Paty, D., Prentice, R., Shults, C.W. & Stoessl, A.J. (2003) Assessment of neuroimaging techniques as biomarkers of the progression of Parkinson's disease. *Exp Neurol*, 184 Suppl 1, S68-79.

Brooks, D.J., Ibanez, V., Sawle, G.V., Quinn, N., Lees, A.J., Mathias, C.J., Bannister, R., Marsden, C.D. & Frackowiak, R.S. (1990) Differing patterns of striatal 18F-dopa uptake in Parkinson's disease, multiple system atrophy, and progressive supranuclear palsy. *Ann Neurol*, 28, 547-555.

Cass, W.A., Grondin, R., Andersen, A.H., Zhang, Z., Hardy, P.A., Hussey-Andersen, L.K., Rayens, W.S., Gerhardt, G.A. & Gash, D.M. (2006) Iron accumulation in the striatum predicts aging-related decline in motor function in rhesus monkeys. *Neurobiol.Aging*.

Chaudhuri, K.R., Healy, D.G. & Schapira, A.H.V. (2006) Non-motor symptoms of Parkinson's disease: diagnosis and management. *The Lancet Neurology*, 5, 235-245.

Chen, Q., Andersen, A.H., Zhang, Z., Ovadia, A., Gash, D.M. & Avison, M.J. (1996) Mapping drug-induced changes in cerebral R2* by Multiple Gradient Recalled Echo functional MRI. *Magn Reson Imaging*, 14, 469-476.

Chin, C.L., Tovcimak, A.E., Hradil, V.P., Seifert, T.R., Hollingsworth, P.R., Chandran, P., Zhu, C.Z., Gauvin, D., Pai, M., Wetter, J., Hsieh, G.C., Honore, P., Frost, J.M., Dart, M.J., Meyer, M.D., Yao, B.B., Cox, B.F. & Fox, G.B. (2008) Differential effects of cannabinoid receptor agonists on regional brain activity using pharmacological MRI. *British Journal of Pharmacology*, 153, 367-379.

de la Fuente-Fernandez, R. & Stoessl, A.J. (2002) Parkinson's disease: imaging update. *Curr Opin Neurol*, 15, 477-482.

DeKosky, S.T. & Marek, K. (2003) Looking backward to move forward: early detection of neurodegenerative disorders. *Science*, 302, 830-834.

Ding, F., Luan, L., Ai, Y., Walton, A., Gerhardt, G.A., Gash, D.M., Grondin, R. & Zhang, Z. (2008) Development of a stable, early stage unilateral model of Parkinson's disease in middle-aged rhesus monkeys. *Exp Neurol*, 212, 431-439.

Dorsey, E.R., Constantinescu, R., Thompson, J.P., Biglan, K.M., Holloway, R.G., Kieburtz, K., Marshall, F.J., Ravina, B.M., Schifitto, G., Siderowf, A. & Tanner, C.M. (2007) Projected number of people with Parkinson disease in the most populous nations, 2005 through 2030. *Neurology*, 68, 384-386.

Eckert, T. & Eidelberg, D. (2004) The role of functional neuroimaging in the differential diagnosis of idiopathic Parkinson's disease and multiple system atrophy. *Clin Auton Res*, 14, 84-91.

Fearnley, J.M. & Lees, A.J. (1991) Ageing and Parkinson's disease: substantia nigra regional selectivity. *Brain*, 114 (Pt 5), 2283-2301.

Ferrer, I., Martinez, A., Blanco, R., Dalfó, E. & Carmona, M. (2010) Neuropathology of sporadic Parkinson disease before the appearance of parkinsonism: preclinical Parkinson disease. *Journal of Neural Transmission*, 1-19.

Freed, C.R., Greene, P.E., Breeze, R.E., Tsai, W.Y., DuMouchel, W., Kao, R., Dillon, S., Winfield, H., Culver, S., Trojanowski, J.Q., Eidelberg, D. & Fahn, S. (2001) Transplantation of embryonic dopamine neurons for severe Parkinson's disease. *N Engl J Med*, 344, 710-719.

Fretham, S.J.B., Carlson, E.S. & Georgieff, M.K. (2011) The Role of Iron in Learning and Memory. *Advances in Nutrition: An International Review Journal*, 2, 112-121.

Gash, D.M., Zhang, Z., Ovadia, A., Cass, W.A., Yi, A., Simmerman, L., Russell, D., Martin, D., Lapchak, P.A., Collins, F., Hoffer, B.J. & Gerhardt, G.A. (1996) Functional recovery in parkinsonian monkeys treated with GDNF. *Nature*, 380, 252-255.

Gill, S.S., Patel, N.K., Hotton, G.R., O'Sullivan, K., McCarter, R., Bunnage, M., Brooks, D.J., Svendsen, C.N. & Heywood, P. (2003) Direct brain infusion of glial cell line-derived neurotrophic factor in Parkinson disease. *Nat Med*, 9, 589-595.

Grondin, R., Zhang, Z., Yi, A., Cass, W.A., Maswood, N., Andersen, A.H., Elsberry, D.D., Klein, M.C., Gerhardt, G.A. & Gash, D.M. (2002) Chronic, controlled GDNF infusion promotes structural and functional recovery in advanced parkinsonian monkeys. *Brain*, 125, 2191-2201.

Group, B.D.W. (2001) Biomarkers and surrogate endpoints: Preferred definitions and conceptual framework*. *Clin Pharmacol Ther*, 69, 89-95.

Hardy, P.A., Gash, D., Yokel, R., Andersen, A., Ai, Y. & Zhang, Z. (2005) Correlation of R2 with total iron concentration in the brains of rhesus monkeys. *J Magn Reson Imaging*, 21, 118-127.

Honey, G. & Bullmore, E. (2004) Human pharmacological MRI. *Trends Pharmacol Sci*, 25, 366-374.

Hornykiewicz, O. & Kish, S.J. (1987) Biochemical pathophysiology of Parkinson's disease. *Adv Neurol*, 45, 19-34.

Hoshi, H., Kuwabara, H., Leger, G., Cumming, P., Guttman, M. & Gjedde, A. (1993) 6-[18F]fluoro-L-dopa metabolism in living human brain: a comparison of six analytical methods. *J Cereb Blood Flow Metab*, 13, 57-69.

Hubble, J.P. (2000) Pre-clinical studies of pramipexole: clinical relevance. *Eur J Neurol*, 7 Suppl 1, 15-20.

Jenkins, B.G., Sanchez-Pernaute, R., Brownell, A.L., Chen, Y.C. & Isacson, O. (2004) Mapping dopamine function in primates using pharmacologic magnetic resonance imaging. *J Neurosci*, 24, 9553-9560.

Katzenschlager, R. & Lees, A.J. (2004) Olfaction and Parkinson's syndromes: its role in differential diagnosis. *Curr Opin Neurol*, 17, 417-423.

Kordower, J.H., Emborg, M.E., Bloch, J., Ma, S.Y., Chu, Y., Leventhal, L., McBride, J., Chen, E.Y., Palfi, S., Roitberg, B.Z., Brown, W.D., Holden, J.E., Pyzalski, R., Taylor, M.D., Carvey, P., Ling, Z., Trono, D., Hantraye, P., Deglon, N. & Aebischer, P. (2000) Neurodegeneration prevented by lentiviral vector delivery of GDNF in primate models of Parkinson's disease. *Science*, 290, 767-773.

Lang, A.E., Gill, S., Patel, N.K., Lozano, A., Nutt, J.G., Penn, R., Brooks, D.J., Hotton, G., Moro, E., Heywood, P., Brodsky, M.A., Burchiel, K., Kelly, P., Dalvi, A., Scott, B., Stacy, M., Turner, D., Wooten, V.G., Elias, W.J., Laws, E.R., Dhawan, V., Stoessl, A.J., Matcham, J., Coffey, R.J. & Traub, M. (2006) Randomized controlled trial of intraputamenal glial cell line-derived neurotrophic factor infusion in Parkinson disease. *Ann Neurol*, 59, 459-466.

Langston, J.W. & Ballard, P.A., Jr. (1983) Parkinson's disease in a chemist working with 1-methyl-4-phenyl-1,2,5,6-tetrahydropyridine. *N Engl J Med*, 309, 310.

Luan, L., Ding, F., Ai, Y., Andersen, A., Hardy, P., Forman, E., Gerhardt, G.A., Gash, D.M., Grondin, R. & Zhang, Z. (2008) Pharmacological MRI (phMRI) monitoring of treatment in hemiparkinsonian rhesus monkeys. *Cell Transplant*, 17, 417-425.

Marsden, C.D. & Obeso, J.A. (1994) The functions of the basal ganglia and the paradox of stereotaxic surgery in Parkinson's disease. *Brain*, 117 (Pt 4), 877-897.

Nguyen, T.V., Brownell, A.L., Iris Chen, Y.C., Livni, E., Coyle, J.T., Rosen, B.R., Cavagna, F. & Jenkins, B.G. (2000) Detection of the effects of dopamine receptor supersensitivity using pharmacological MRI and correlations with PET. *Synapse*, 36, 57-65.

Nicklas, W.J., Youngster, S.K., Kindt, M.V. & Heikkila, R.E. (1987) MPTP, MPP+ and mitochondrial function. *Life Sci*, 40, 721-729.

Ovadia, A., Zhang, Z. & Gash, D.M. (1995) Increased susceptibility to MPTP toxicity in middle-aged rhesus monkeys. *Neurobiol Aging*, 16, 931-937.

Pavese, N. & Brooks, D.J. (2009) Imaging neurodegeneration in Parkinson's disease. *Biochim Biophys Acta*, 1792, 722-729.

Rasmussen Jr, I. (2010) Psychopharmacological MRI. *Acta Neuropsychiatrica*, 22, 38-39.

Ravina, B., Eidelberg, D., Ahlskog, J.E., Albin, R.L., Brooks, D.J., Carbon, M., Dhawan, V., Feigin, A., Fahn, S., Guttman, M., Gwinn-Hardy, K., McFarland, H., Innis, R., Katz, R.G., Kieburtz, K., Kish, S.J., Lange, N., Langston, J.W., Marek, K., Morin, L., Moy, C., Murphy, D., Oertel, W.H., Oliver, G., Palesch, Y., Powers, W., Seibyl, J., Sethi, K.D., Shults, C.W., Sheehy, P., Stoessl, A.J. & Holloway, R. (2005) The role of radiotracer imaging in Parkinson disease. *Neurology*, 64, 208-215.

Richardson, J.R., Caudle, W.M., Guillot, T.S., Watson, J.L., Nakamaru-Ogiso, E., Seo, B.B., Sherer, T.B., Greenamyre, J.T., Yagi, T., Matsuno-Yagi, A. & Miller, G.W. (2007) Obligatory role for complex I inhibition in the dopaminergic neurotoxicity of 1-methyl-4-phenyl-1,2,3,6-tetrahydropyridine (MPTP). *Toxicol Sci*, 95, 196-204.

Schuff, N. (2009) Potential role of high-field MRI for studies in Parkinson's disease. *Mov Disord*, 24 Suppl 2, S684-690.

Seibyl, J., Jennings, D., Tabamo, R. & Marek, K. (2005) The role of neuroimaging in the early diagnosis and evaluation of Parkinson's disease. *Minerva Med*, 96, 353-364.

Slevin, J.T., Gerhardt, G.A., Smith, C.D., Gash, D.M., Kryscio, R. & Young, B. (2005) Improvement of bilateral motor functions in patients with Parkinson disease through the unilateral intraputaminal infusion of glial cell line-derived neurotrophic factor. *J Neurosurg.*, 102, 216-222.

Smith, S.M., Jenkinson, M., Johansen-Berg, H., Rueckert, D., Nichols, T.E., Mackay, C.E., Watkins, K.E., Ciccarelli, O., Cader, M.Z., Matthews, P.M. & Behrens, T.E. (2006) Tract-based spatial statistics: voxelwise analysis of multi-subject diffusion data. *Neuroimage*, 31, 1487-1505.

Smith, S.M., Jenkinson, M., Woolrich, M.W., Beckmann, C.F., Behrens, T.E., Johansen-Berg, H., Bannister, P.R., De Luca, M., Drobnjak, I., Flitney, D.E., Niazy, R.K., Saunders, J., Vickers, J., Zhang, Y., De Stefano, N., Brady, J.M. & Matthews, P.M. (2004) Advances in functional and structural MR image analysis and implementation as FSL. *Neuroimage*, 23 Suppl 1, S208-219.

Snow, B.J., Tooyama, I., McGeer, E.G., Yamada, T., Calne, D.B., Takahashi, H. & Kimura, H. (1993) Human positron emission tomographic [18F]fluorodopa studies correlate with dopamine cell counts and levels. *Ann Neurol*, 34, 324-330.

Snow, B.J., Vingerhoets, F.J., Langston, J.W., Tetrud, J.W., Sossi, V. & Calne, D.B. (2000) Pattern of dopaminergic loss in the striatum of humans with MPTP induced parkinsonism. *J Neurol Neurosurg Psychiatry*, 68, 313-316.

Thiel, C.M. (2009) Neuropharmacological fMRI. *Neuropharmakologisches fMRT*, 40, 233-238.

Tomac, A., Lindqvist, E., Lin, L.F., Ogren, S.O., Young, D., Hoffer, B.J. & Olson, L. (1995) Protection and repair of the nigrostriatal dopaminergic system by GDNF in vivo. *Nature*, 373, 335-339.

Tracey, I. (2001) Prospects for human pharmacological functional magnetic resonance imaging (phMRI). *J Clin Pharmacol*, Suppl, 21S-28S.

Wu, Y., Le, W. & Jankovic, J. (2011) Preclinical Biomarkers of Parkinson Disease. *Arch Neurol*, 68, 22-30.

Zhang, Z., Andersen, A., Grondin, R., Barber, T., Avison, R., Gerhardt, G. & Gash, D. (2001) Pharmacological MRI mapping of age-associated changes in basal ganglia circuitry of awake rhesus monkeys. *Neuroimage*, 14, 1159-1167.

Zhang, Z., Andersen, A.H., Ai, Y., Loveland, A., Hardy, P.A., Gerhardt, G.A. & Gash, D.M. (2006) Assessing nigrostriatal dysfunctions by pharmacological MRI in parkinsonian rhesus macaques. *Neuroimage*, 33, 636-643.

5

Neuroimaging in Manganese-Induced Parkinsonism

Yangho Kim

Department of Occupational and Environmental Medicine,
Ulsan University Hospital, University of Ulsan College of Medicine,
Ulsan,
Korea

1. Introduction

Over the last 20 years, the impact of imaging on the clinical sciences has been immense. Tremendous progress has been made in medical imaging of the human body since the invention of computed tomography (CT) and magnetic resonance imaging (MRI). Neuroimaging of patients with metal neurotoxicity can be divided into two types: morphological neuroimaging (anatomy-based imaging) including CT and MRI; and functional neuroimaging (physiology-based imaging) such as magnetic resonance spectroscopy (MRS), single-photon emission computed tomography (SPECT), positron emission tomography (PET), diffusion tensor imaging (DTI), and functional MRI (fMRI). Neuroimaging is undergoing a shift from morphological to functional imaging as new technologies are introduced and technical problems associated with the local production of radioisotopes are solved (Lang, 2000; Walker et al., 2004). MRI, PET, and SPECT have been used for 10 years or more to evaluate workers exposed to manganese (Mn), and to examine the neurological consequences of such exposure. Very recently, functional neuroimaging modalities such as fMRI, MRS, and DTI have been applied to this end.
The objectives of this chapter are (1) to review the use of neuroimaging in Mn-induced parkinsonism, and (2) to discuss recent developments in the functional neuroimaging in Mn-induced parkinsonism.

2. The pallidal MRI T1-signal reflects the target organ dose of Mn exposure

The Mn ion (Mn^{2+}) has five unpaired electrons in the 3d orbital, which results in a large magnetic moment, resulting in the shortening of proton T1-relaxation time and an increased signal intensity on T1-weighted MRI. Because of this paramagnetic quality of Mn^{2+}, a bilateral symmetrical increase in signal intensity, mainly confined to the globus pallidus and midbrain, can be observed on T1-weighted MRI, but with no concomitant alteration on the T2-weighted image (Kim et al., 1999a) (Fig. 1).
However, Mn-induced high signals on T1-weighted MRI do not correspond to any abnormal findings on brain CT (Park et al., 2003). The characteristic high signal caused by Mn can be differentiated from signals that increase in intensity for other reasons. Thus, high signals from fat, hemoglobin breakdown products, melanomas, neurofibromatosis, and

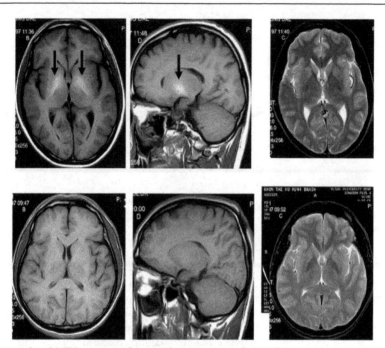

Fig. 1. T1-weighted MRI scans with or without increased signal intensities. Axial and sagittal sections show increase in signal intensities mainly confined to the globus pallidus, but with no concomitant alteration on T2-weighted image in workers exposed to manganese (Mn) in the upper row. In the lower row, worker without Mn exposure does not show increased signal intensities (Arrow indicates high signal. Left and middle column: T1-weighted image; right column: T2-weighted image.

calcification, can be seen on T1-weighted images. High signals from hemoglobin breakdown products, melanomas, and neurofibromatosis can be differentiated from Mn-induced high signals on the basis of signal site and symmetry. Iron deposits cause a greater shortening of the T2-relaxation time than the T1-relaxation time, resulting in low signal intensity upon T2-weighted imaging, distinct from that of an Mn deposit. Calcification can be easily identified by CT (Ahn et al., 2003). Krieger et al. (1995) coined the term "pallidus index" (PI) to quantify Mn accumulation in the globus pallidus, defined as the ratio of the signal intensity in the globus pallidus to that in the subcortical frontal white matter (WM) in axial T1-weighted MRI planes, multiplied by 100. An increase in signal upon T1-weighted imaging was observed during experimental Mn poisoning of non-human primates (Erikson et al., 1992; Newland et al., 1989). Nelson et al. (1993) were the first to report increased signal intensities in a patient with occupational Mn neurointoxication. A similar MRI pattern has also been observed in patients receiving total parenteral nutrition (TPN) by direct intravenous administration (Ejima et al., 1992; Mirowitz et al., 1991) and in patients with portal systemic shunts such as individuals with liver cirrhosis, leading to an inability to clear Mn via biliary excretion (Butterworth et al., 1995; Hauser et al., 1994, 1996; Krieger et al., 1995; Park et al., 2003; Spahr et al., 1996). A high pallidal signal is very frequently observed in patients with established liver cirrhosis, but who lack exposure to Mn (Park et al., 2003). Mn-induced high signals can occasionally be observed in patients with severe iron-deficiency anemia (Kim et al., 2005). Kim et al. (1999a) showed, for the first time, that the characteristic high T1 signals were also frequently observed in asymptomatic workers exposed to Mn. The cited authors found a high prevalence (41.6%) of increased MRI signals in Mn-exposed workers, and, interestingly, 73.5% of welders showed increased signal intensities compared to none of the non-exposed clerical workers in the same factories. The cited authors found that the increased signal intensities resolved significantly approximately 1 year after Mn exposure ceased (Kim et al., 1999b). The disappearance of high signal abnormalities on MRI following withdrawal of the Mn source has been shown after the cessation of occupational exposure (Nelson et al., 1993), after discontinuation of TPN (Mirowitz et al., 1991), and after liver transplantation in patients with hepatic failure (Choi et al., 2005; Pujol et al., 1993). These findings suggest that increased signal intensities on a T1-weighted image reflect exposure to Mn, but do not necessarily indicate the presence of manganism. This is very important when the similarities and differences between idiopathic Parkinson's disease (IPD) and manganism are considered. Many reports have shown that blood Mn concentration is highly correlated with PI in liver cirrhotics (Hauser et al., 1996; Krieger et al., 1995; Spahr et al., 1996). In Mn-exposed workers, blood Mn concentration was also found to correlate with PI (Chang et al., 2009a; Dietz et al., 1999; Jiang et al., 2007; Kim et al., 1999a).

A recent study showed that PI was significantly associated with digit symbol test results, digit span backward ratings, scores on the Stroop Word and Stroop Error indices, and Grooved Pegboard (dominant hand) data (Chang et al., 2009a). This means that PI is a good predictor of neurobehavioral performance in welders without clinical manganism. In particular, PI was a better predictor of neurobehavioral performance than was blood Mn levels in such welders.

Taken together, the data suggest that PI on MRI may reflect a target organ dose of occupational Mn exposure (Kim, 2006). In addition, Mn in brain has a longer half-life than in blood (Lucchini and Kim, 2009). Thus, PI reflects the cumulative dose better than does blood Mn level. However, the level of signal intensity indicating progression to manganism from Mn exposure remains to be determined. The development of an animal model of manganism would assist in this regard, but the fact that the routes of exposure in humans differ, and that data on non-human species may not be transferable to human situations, are limiting factors. Hence, a prospective study correlating increases in T1 signal intensities with clinical and neuropsychological findings in Mn-exposed workers is needed.

3. PET/SPECT as an index of the integrity of the dopaminergic nigrostriatal pathway

The dopaminergic nigrostriatal pathway is the primary focus of neurodegeneration in IPD (Brooks et al., 1990; Morrish et al., 1995, 1996). In IPD, dopamine uptake is reduced in the striatum, particularly the posterior putamen. This finding is in accord with the 40-60% loss of dopaminergic cells seen in the nigrostriatal pathway of patients with IPD. In non-human primates and humans intoxicated with Mn, [18F]-dopa (fluorodopa) PET scans are normal (Erikson et al., 1992; Kim et al., 1998; Shinotoh et al., 1995, 1997; Wolters et al., 1989). This supports the view that, in instances of Mn intoxication, the nigrostriatal pathway is relatively well preserved, consistent with many pathological observations showing that Mn-induced damage occurs primarily in pathways postsynaptic to the nigrostriatal system. Dopamine transporter (DAT) imaging using (1r)-2b-carboxymethoxy-3b-(4-iodophenyl)tropane (β-CIT), employed as a SPECT ligand, reveals the density of DAT, and therefore explores the integrity of the nigrostriatal dopaminergic system. DAT is a protein located in the presynaptic nerve terminals of this system. β-CIT binds to DAT with high affinity and a low level of nonspecificity (Laruelle et al., 1993). In IPD, [123I]-β-CIT SPECT reveals that specific striatal β-CIT uptake is reduced (Seibyl et al., 1995). Earlier data showed that this method can distinguish IPD patients from normal controls (Jeon et al., 1998a, 1998b). Further, striatal DAT uptake is nearly normal in patients with Mn-induced parkinsonism, but is markedly reduced in IPD patients (Huang et al., 2003). Various ligands that bind to DAT, such as [123I]-β-CIT, [123I]-fluoropropyl-CIT, and [99mTc]-TRODAT-1 have been used in SPECT studies (Huang et al., 2003; Kim et al., 2002). DAT SPECT is more easily accessible and less expensive than is fluorodopa PET. Fluorodopa and DAT uptake values are (nearly) normal in patients with manganism (Huang et al., 2003; Kim et al., 1998; Shinotoh et al., 1997; Wolters et al., 1989), whereas uptake is markedly reduced in IPD patients. However, Guilarte et al. (2008) reported that, in the non-human primate brain, chronic Mn exposure inhibited dopaminergic transmission, leading to motor deficits, in the absence of changes to presynaptic dopaminergic nerve terminals.

Racette et al. (2005) found relatively symmetrical and severely reduced fluorodopa uptake on PET in the posterior putamen of a patient with manganism secondary to liver failure, together with T1 hyperintensities in the basal ganglia on MRI. This is the only reported case of secondary manganism accompanied by abnormal fluorodopa PET findings. However, SPECT data from our secondary manganism patients (Kim et al., 2010) revealed two different patterns of clinical and neuroradiological features. Four of five patients showed atypical parkinsonism, with normal DAT density, which could be clearly differentiated from PD, whereas one patient showed levodopa-responsive parkinsonism with reduced DAT density (classical PD). These findings are remarkably different from those of Racette et al. (2005). PET/SPECT findings in patients with manganism caused by liver failure should be further studied, with respect to both clinical and pathological features. Further, the pathogenesis, clinical characteristics, and neuroimaging might differ between patients with primary and secondary manganism. Liver cirrhosis might confound the symptoms and accelerate the signs of parkinsonism. It is unclear whether secondary manganism caused by liver cirrhosis, for example, differs (from a neuroimaging standpoint) from manganism associated with occupational or environmental exposure to Mn.

Some welders showed clinical features and PET/SPECT findings typical of IPD, with concurrent Mn exposure (Kim et al., 1999b, 2002; Racette et al., 2001). Initially, Kim et al. (1999b) reported that one welder showed IPD with incidental exposure to Mn. However, they subsequently developed the hypothesis that Mn might have been a risk factor for development of IPD, although they could not exclude the possibility that the patient simply suffered from IPD, with coincidental exposure to Mn (Kim et al., 2002). Racette et al. (2001) suggested that welding might be a possible risk factor for development of early-onset IPD. However, it remains unclear whether Mn causes or accelerates IPD. The link between Mn exposure and an increased risk of IPD should be further examined in clinical, pathological, and epidemiological studies focusing on PET/SPECT findings.

Neuroimaging modalities such as MRI and PET/SPECT may be useful for the differential diagnosis of parkinsonism (Calne et al., 1994; Kim, 2006) (Fig. 2).

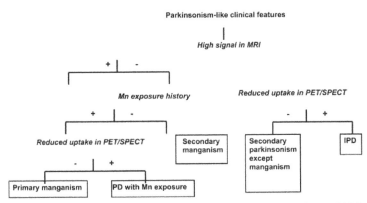

Fig. 2. Differential diagnosis of manganism from parkinson's disease (Kim, 2006)

When a patient exhibits parkinsonian features, MRI is recommended. Observation of bilateral symmetrical increases in signal intensities, mainly confined to the globus pallidus on T1-weighted MRI, in a patient confirms recent CNS exposure to Mn. It should be noted that a negative MRI signal can occur when worker exposure to Mn ceased more than 6–12 months prior to testing. When a patient with a high T1 signal and an Mn exposure history also shows normal uptake by PET/SPECT, primary manganism should be highly suspected. If a patient who has a high T1 signal and an Mn exposure history also shows reduced uptake upon PET/SPECT, the patient should be categorized as suffering from IPD with coincidental Mn exposure. When a patient yielding a high T1 signal upon MRI does not have an Mn exposure history, but shows normal uptake upon PET/SPECT, he/she may be diagnosed with secondary manganism attributable to liver cirrhosis or TPN. If a patient without a high T1 signal shows reduced uptake on PET/SPECT, he/she could possibly have IPD. When a patient without a high T1 signal on MRI shows normal uptake on PET/SPECT, he/she would be under suspicion of a form of secondary parkinsonism other than manganism (Kim 2006). However, neuroimaging should be combined with clinical evaluation for the differential diagnosis of parkinsonism (Ravina et al., 2005).

4. Recent developments in functional neuroimaging in Mn-induced parkinsonism

4.1 MRS

In vivo proton magnetic resonance spectroscopy ([1H]-MRS) is an image-guided, noninvasive method for monitoring of neurochemical metabolites in the brain (Rosen and Lenkinski, 2007). Currently, [1H]-MRS is the biomedical technique that is most commonly employed to obtain metabolic information to aid in the diagnosis of many neurological diseases, and also allows disease progression to be followed and response to treatment to be evaluated (Ross et al., 2006). Although MRS permits noninvasive, in vivo measurement of brain metabolites, only a few MRS investigations have been performed to date in efforts to assess the neurological effects of heavy metals in the environmental or occupational health. Recently, a few reports have analyzed the impact of lead exposure on brain metabolism in vivo in adults and children (Meng et al., 2005; Trope et al., 2001; Weisskopf, 2007; Weisskopf et al., 2007). However, little is known about the effects of chronic Mn exposure on brain metabolites in vivo. Two reports employed MRS to investigate the potential neurotoxic effects of chronic Mn exposure on the brain (Guilarte et al., 2006; Kim et al., 2007). Guilarte et al. (2006) assessed the toxic effects of chronic Mn exposure on the levels of brain metabolites in non-human primates. This [¹H]-MRS study found a decrease in the N-acetylaspartate/creatine (NAA/Cr) ratio in the parietal cortex and frontal WM at the end of the period of exposure to Mn, relative to baseline, indicating ongoing neuronal degeneration or dysfunction. NAA is known to serve as a neuronal marker (Birken and Oldendorf, 1989). A reduction in NAA levels in the brain can be interpreted as indicating neuronal dysfunction or even neuronal loss (Vion-Dury et al., 1994). Kim et al. (2007) investigated the potential neurotoxic effects of chronic Mn exposure in welders. Using point-resolved spectroscopy (PRESS) at 1.5 T, the cited authors measured the NAA/Cr, choline/creatine (Cho/Cr), and NAA/Cho ratios in the basal ganglia, and found no significant differences between welders and control subjects.

In a recent study, Chang et al., (2009b) sought to determine whether metabolic differences existed between 35 welders chronically exposed to Mn and 20 healthy age-matched control individuals, by measuring brain metabolites using [¹H]-MRS. MRI and in vivo single-voxel MRS were performed using the GE 3T MRI system (Signa Excite HD, General Electric Medical Systems, Milwaukee, WI) equipped with an eight-channel RF head coil. The MRS spectra of individual metabolites were analyzed using a Linear Combination Model (Provencher, 1993) running a Linux system. Five brain metabolites—NAA; the Glx complex, including both glutamine (Gln) and glutamate (Glu); total creatine (tCr); total choline (tCho); and myoinositol (mI)—were measured in the anterior cingulate cortex (ACC) and parietal WM. Further, the cited authors investigated correlations between neurochemical changes in the ACC of the brain and neurobehavioral alterations, to assess possible associations between chronic Mn exposure and cognitive deficits (Chang et al., 2009b). The means and standard deviations of blood Mn concentration in welders and controls were found to be 1.53 ± 0.42 and 1.06 ± 0.29 µg/dL, respectively. The mean value of workplace Mn air concentrations was 0.15 mg/m³. The welders had worked for 21.3 ± 7.2 (mean $\pm$ SD) years. All welders were shown to be devoid of clinical manganism, by neurological examination. This study on welders using proton-MRS showed that the NAA/tCr, Glx/tCr, and tCho/tCr ratios in both the ACC and parietal WM did not differ significantly between welders and controls. However, the mI levels in the ACC, but not in the parietal WM, were significantly lower in welders compared with control individuals. Further, in the frontal lobe of the brain, the mI/tCr ratio was significantly correlated with verbal memory scores as well as blood Mn concentrations. Kim et al. (2007) found no statistically significant differences in the levels of brain metabolites (NAA and Cho only were measured) between welders and controls. However, although the cited authors used a PRESS sequence with a short echo time, mI levels was not analyzed, unlike in the study of Chang et al. cited above. The results of the latter work agree with those of a previous study (Kim et al., 2007), but a direct comparison of mI levels is not possible. Guilarte et al. (2006) reported a decrease in NAA level in the parietal cortex and frontal WM of the brains of Mn-exposed monkeys. However, when the spectroscopic findings of the work of Chang (2009b) and that of Guilarte et al. (2006) are compared, it is important to consider methodological differences between a human and animal study. MI is known to serve as a cerebral osmoregulator (Strange et al., 1994), and hence may play a role as an intracellular osmolyte. Thus, ml depletion may reflect glial cell swelling associated with long-term exposure to Mn. Previous [¹H]-MRS studies on the brains of cirrhotic patients with overt hepatic encephalopathy (HE) often found a large increase in Glx concentration, and depletion of mI, but no change in

NAA level, in the ACC and basal ganglia; these changes are considered to be typical metabolic abnormalities associated with HE (Geissler et al., 1997; Laubenberger et al., 1997; Weissenborn & Kolbe, 1998). In the early stages of HE, spectral alterations in mI and/or choline levels have been observed, but without corresponding increases in the Glx concentration (Kreis et al., 1992; Laubenberger et al., 1997; Miese et al., 2006; Naegele et al., 2000; Spahr et al., 2000). Compared with HE patients, welders did not show any abnormal change in Glx metabolism in a study by Chang et al. (2009b). The MRS results in welders are compatible with findings in patients in the early stages of HE. The cited study suggested that the depletion of mI in welders may reflect a possible glial cell effect rather than a neuronal effect, associated with long-term exposure to Mn. More recently, Dydak et al. (2011) used MRS to investigate brain metabolites in the globus pallidus, putamen, thalamus, and frontal cortex of 10 Mn-exposed smelters and 10 age- and gender-matched controls. Additionally, they used the MEGA-PRESS sequence to determine GABA levels in the thalamus. In addition to a significant decrease in the NAA/Cr ratio in the frontal cortex of exposed subjects, a significant increase in GABA level was observed in the thalamus, attributable to Mn exposure. The authors recommended that a combination of PI assessment and measurement of GABA level may provide a powerful, non-invasive biomarker of both Mn exposure and pre-symptomatic Mn neurotoxicity. Further studies using MRS are needed to identify brain metabolites in Mn-exposed workers.

4.2 fMRI

The use of fMRI to study neurological diseases has become much more common over the last decade. However, employing fMRI to assess neurotoxicity in humans is a rather novel approach. Chang et al. (2010a) performed the first-ever fMRI experiment, using sequential finger-tapping, to investigate the behavioral significance of additionally recruited brain regions in welders who had experienced chronic Mn exposure. The study population consisted of 42 males, aged 40 years or older, who were current full-time welders, with more than 5 years of welding experience in a factory (Chang et al., 2010a). The control population consisted of 26 age- and gender-matched non-welding production workers from the same factory, who were not exposed to other hazardous materials such as paint. MRI examinations were performed using a 3.0 T whole-body scanner (Signa Excite HD), and blood oxygenation level-dependent (BOLD) contrast data were collected for each participant. T2*-weighted echo planar imaging was used in fMRI acquisition. In the finger-tapping test, each participant was asked to place the thumb on the tip of the index finger, middle finger, ring finger, little finger, ring finger, middle finger, index finger and another finger, in that order, as quickly and precisely as possible. In the cited study, the mean and standard deviation of blood Mn concentrations in welders and control individuals were 1.55 ± 0.45 and 1.15 ± 0.31 µg/dL, respectively. The mean workplace air Mn concentration was 0.14 mg/m³. The welders had an average welding experience of 20.5 years. All welders were shown to be devoid of clinical manganism by neurological examination. Performance on the Grooved Pegboard and finger-tapping tests (right and left hand) were significantly lower among welders than controls. Maximum frequencies, as determined by evaluation of hand pronation/supination, and finger-tapping test results using CAT SYS 2000 (Danish Product Development), were significantly lower among welders than controls. No difference in the results of other rhythmic tests (slow/fast), again using CAT SYS 2000, was evident between the groups.

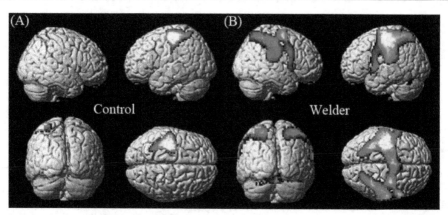

Fig. 3. Statistical parametric maps (SPM) of sequential finger tapping movement with right hand for control (A) and welder group (B) displayed on 3D SPM template brain. All activation voxels are significant at P<0.00001 FDR corrected for multiple comparison across whole brain. Chang et al. (2010a)

During finger-tapping tasks conducted on welders who were chronically exposed to Mn, significant activation foci were noted in the bilateral primary sensorimotor cortex (SM1), the bilateral supplementary motor area (SMA), the bilateral dorsolateral premotor cortex (dPMC), the bilateral superior parietal cortex, and the bilateral dentate nucleus, when data from movement and rest periods were compared. In contrast, control participants exhibited significant activation of the contralateral (left) SM1 (Fig. 3). Activation of the bilateral SM1, bilateral SMA, bilateral dPMC, bilateral superior parietal cortex, and ipsilateral dentate nucleus was higher in the welding group than in the control group. No region showed significantly more activation in controls compared to welders. PI correlated with activation observed in the contralateral SM1, in terms of finger-tapping test data from the left hand. The fMRI variables correlated with motor behavior. Grooved Pegboard performance (right hand) correlated with activation, as seen also in ipsilateral and contralateral SMA data obtained during finger-tapping with the right hand. Left-hand finger-tapping data collected during the first 10 sec of the task significantly correlated with activation of the ipsilateral and contralateral SMA when finger-tapping was evaluated on the left side. Bilateral SM1 hyperactivity may reflect motor re-organization in the brains of Mn-exposed welders, which might compensate for existing subclinical motor deficits. It seems likely that the mechanisms regulating sensorimotor control (i.e., systems operative from the basal ganglial output to the cortical sensorimotor regions, via the thalamus) may compensate for abnormalities in the basal ganglia and thereby prevent the appearance of symptoms in presymptomatic welders. In addition, hyperactivity of the SMA suggests that it is more difficult for welders (compared to controls) to perform a simple sequential finger-tapping task; thus, more SMA activity is recruited via the basal ganglial-thalamo-cortical loop, which allows for successful performance of the sequential finger-tapping task. However, these findings do not agree with those reported for patients with IPD. Functional neuroimaging of participants performing tasks requiring motor selection and initiation showed that the SMA was hypoactivated in patients with IPD, compared to normal participants (Sabatini et al., 2000). In summary, the collective findings suggest that, when relatively simple tasks are set, fMRI may uncover evidence of compromised brain functioning in patients with subclinical manganism. The finding of excessive recruitment of the cortical motor network in chronically Mn-exposed group is in line with the emerging concept of use of adaptive neural mechanisms to compensate for latent dysfunction in the basal ganglia (Buhmann et al., 2005).

Chang et al. (2010b) also performed fMRI, combined with two-back memory tests, to assess the neural correlates of Mn-induced memory impairment in response to subclinical dysfunction in the working memory networks of welders exposed to Mn for extended periods of time. The study population consisted of 23 males, aged 40 years or older, who were current full-time welders with more than 5 years of welding experience in a factory. The control population consisted of 21 age- and gender-matched non-welding production workers from the same factory, who were not exposed to other hazardous materials such as paint. The MRI equipment and the fMRI protocol were identical to those used in the report on fMRI data obtained using the finger-tapping task (this work is summarized above). The working memory paradigm consisted of a two-back memory task combined with a "rest" control task. Stimuli were projected onto a viewing screen, attached within the bore of the scanner, and viewed at a distance of approximately 20 cm from the eyes of the participant, after reflection from two mirrors positioned on top of the head coil. In the cited study, Mn exposure status was similar to that of subjects recruited for the fMRI study that employed the finger-tapping task. All welders were shown to be devoid of clinical manganism, by neurological examination. Welders showed significantly lower performance on cognitive neurobehavioral tests, including the Korean Auditory Verbal Learning Test (K-AVLT) (i.e., delayed recall and recognition), the Korean Complex Figure Test (K-CFT) (i.e., copy,

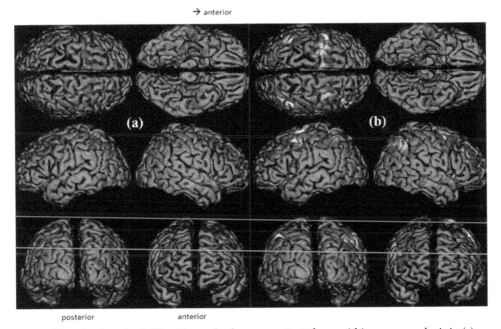

Fig. 4. The activations in fMRI with two-back memory tests from within group analysis in (a) controls and (b) welders (p < 0.05, FDR corrected for multiple comparison). Chang et al. (2010b)

immediate recall, and delayed recall), digit span tests (both forward and backward), and the Stroop tests, compared to controls. Chronic Mn exposure caused increased brain activity in working memory networks during the two-back verbal working memory task.

The cited authors observed activation of the inferior frontal cortex, the basal ganglia (including the putamen), and the bilateral cerebellum, as well as activation of the common memory-related network of frontal and parietal cortical areas including the premotor cortex, the middle frontal cortex, the inferior and superior frontal cortex, the inferior and superior parietal cortex, the precuneus, and the cuneus, in welders exposed to Mn (Fig. 4). Between-group analysis revealed increased brain activity in the left (contralateral) SM1, the right inferior parietal cortex, the anterior and posterior cingulated cortex, the bilateral inferior frontal cortex, and the basal ganglia of welders, compared to controls, during the memory task. No region was significantly more activated in controls compared to welders. After controlling for age and educational level, the percentage change in activation of the parietal cortex was associated with K-AVLT (i.e., delayed recall and recognition). The percentage change in activation of the inferior frontal cortex was significantly associated with scores on the Stroop color and error indices. The percentage change in activation of the ACC was significantly associated with K-AVLT (i.e., recognition) and digit span (i.e., forward) test results.

The basal ganglial-thalamo-cortical circuitry was originally viewed as almost exclusively involved in control of movement. However, these structures are now considered to be essential for non-motor function (DeLong & Wichmann, 2009). Considering that the basal ganglia are the brain regions that receive most Mn deposits, a speculative explanation of the higher basal ganglial activity in welders is that, if performance is to be matched to that of normal subjects, an increased recruitment of basal ganglial cells is required in welders to compensate for a diminished working memory capacity. Together, the fMRI findings indicate that welders might need to recruit more neural resources to the working memory network, to compensate for subtle working memory deficits and alterations in working memory processes, if they are to perform tasks at the same level as is possible by healthy control individuals.

4.3 DTI

DTI is a unique method used to characterize WM micro-integrity, and relies on the principle that water diffusion is highly anisotropic in brain WM structures (Beaulieu, 2002). Thus, DTI reveals the orientation of WM tracts in vivo, and yields indices of microstructural integrity by quantification of the directionality of water diffusion (Le Bihanetal, 2001; Moseley et al., 1990). Although a few previous studies have explored the neurotoxicity associated with exposure to heavy metals such as Hg (Kinoshita et al., 1999) and Mn (McKinney et al., 2004) using diffusion-weighted image (DWI), no report on DTI-detected alteration of microscopic integrity within the WM of subjects experiencing chronic Mn exposure has appeared. Kim et al. (2011) used DTI to investigate whether welders exposed to Mn exhibited differences in WM integrity, compared to control subjects. MRI examinations were performed using a 3.0 T whole body scanner (Signa Excite HD). Fractional anisotropy (FA), mean diffusivity (MD), axial diffusivity (AD), and radial diffusivity (RD) were measured on a voxel-wise basis in 30 male welders exposed to Mn and in 19 age- and gender-matched control subjects (Kim et al., 2011). In the cited study, the means and standard deviations of blood Mn concentration in welders and control individuals were 1.52 ± 0.47 µg/dL and 1.17 ± 0.33 µg/dL, respectively.

The mean workplace Mn air concentration was 0.15 mg/m^3. The welders had an average welding experience of 20.6 years. All welders were shown to be devoid of clinical manganism by neurological examination. Welders showed significantly lower performances in all of the digit symbol, digit span, Stroop, Grooved Pegboard, and finger-tapping tests, compared to controls. Further, the results of the digit symbol, digit span, and Stroop tests were significantly associated with PI and blood Mn level after controlling for age, educational level, smoking status, and alcohol consumption. In addition, relationships between dependent measures and PI were stronger than those seen when blood Mn was used as an independent variable. Direct comparisons between welders and controls using investigator-independent Statistical Parametric Mapping (SPM) voxel-wise analysis of DTI metrics revealed a reduction in FA in the genu, body, and splenium of the corpus callosum (CC), and the frontal WM, in Mn-exposed welders. PI showed a statistically significant correlation with FA in the genu (left), body, and splenium of the CC. Blood Mn levels showed statistically significant correlations with FA in the genu (left) and body of the CC, and in the frontal WM. Further, marked increases in RD, but negligible changes in AD, were evident in the genu, body, and splenium of the CC, and the frontal WM. PI was significantly correlated with RD in the body of the CC. However, the blood Mn level did not show a statistically significant correlation with RD. All of these findings suggested that microstructural changes in the CC and the frontal WM result from a compromised radial directionality of fibers in such areas, primarily caused by demyelination. As the digit span (forward) test is more likely to measure attention and immediate recall, and the digit span (backward) test more specifically explores working memory, the statistically significant positive correlation between FA and digit span performance score (forward) suggests that the reduced FA in the frontal WM is in part responsible for the impaired attention of welders. The Stroop word and color/word tests are often used to measure executive function. Therefore, correlations between FA in the frontal WM, and the Stroop word and color/word test scores, suggest that poor performance on executive functioning, as measured using the Stroop word test (information processing) and the color/word test (executive function), are closely associated with lower FA values in the frontal WM.

In summary, correlation of DTI matrices with motor and cognitive neurobehavioral performance indices suggested that the observed microstructural abnormalities were associated with subtle motor and cognitive differences between welders and controls. This was the first study to use DTI to examine Mn-exposed workers (Kim et al., 2011). However, the functional significance of reduced frontal WM integrity evident in welders with chronic Mn exposure needs to be established in further work.

5. Conclusion

Neuroimaging is undergoing a shift from morphological to functional approaches as new technologies are gradually introduced. For morphological neuroimaging reflecting Mn exposure, PI on T1-weighted MRI data exploring target organ dosages of Mn reflects the cumulative Mn dose better than does assessment of blood Mn. For use in functional neuroimaging exploring Mn exposure, fluorodopa-PET/DAT SPECT serves as an index of the integrity of the dopaminergic nigrostriatal pathway, and is useful to differentiate between manganism and IPD. Recently, proton MRS has been used to identify brain metabolites in Mn-exposed workers. Chang et al. (1999b) suggested that subclinical neurologic effects attributable to long-term Mn exposure are associated with possible glial cell effect rather than neuronal deficits. The use of fMRI, combined with motor tasks, has suggested that cortical hyperactivity may reflect motor re-organization in the brains of Mn-exposed welders, to compensate for subclinical motor deficits. When cognitive tasks are set, fMRI findings indicate that welders might need to recruit more neural resources to the working memory network to compensate for subtle subclinical working memory deficits. Therefore, fMRI is useful to detect subclinical cortical deficits in subjects who have experienced chronic exposure to Mn. DTI revealed microstructural deficits in WM integrity in welders exposed to Mn. Thus, functional neuroimaging can evaluate both subclinical WM integrity and cortical function in those exposed to Mn. Such neuroimaging combined with neurobehavioral performance evaluation shows promise in the elucidation of the pathophysiology of Mn neurotoxicity.

6. References

Ahn, J., Yoo, C-I., Lee, C.R., Lee, J.H., Lee, H., Park, J.K., Sakai, T., Yoon, C.S. & Kim, Y. (2003). Calcification mimicking manganese-induced increased signal intensities in T1-weighted MR images in a patient taking herbal medicine: case report. *Neurotoxicology* Vol.24, No.6, (December 2003), pp. 835-838, ISSN 0161-813X

Beaulieu, C. (2002). The basis of anisotropic diffusion imaging in the nervous system. *NMR Biomed* Vol.15, No.7-8, (November-December 2002), pp. 435–455. ISSN 0952-3480

Birken, D.L., & Oldendorf, W.H. (1989). N-Acetyl-L-aspartic acid: a literature review of a compound prominent in 1H-NMR spectroscopic studies of brain. *Neurosci Biobehav Rev* Vol.13, No.1, (Spring 1989), pp. 23–31, ISSN 0149-7634

Brooks, D.J., Salmon, E.P., Mathias, C.J., Quinn, N., Leenders, K.L., Bannister. R., Marsden, C.D. & Frackowiakm R.S. (1990). The relationship between locomotor disability, autonomic dysfunction, and the integrity of the striatal dopaminergic system in patients with multiple system atrophy, pure autonomic failure and Parkinson's disease, studied with PET. *Brain* Vol.113, No.5, (October 1990), pp. 1539–1552, ISSN 0006-8950

Buhmann, C., Binkofski, F., Klein, C., Büchel, C., van Eimeren, T., Erdmann, C., Hedrich, K., Kasten, M., Hagenah, J., Deuschl, G., Pramstaller, P.P. & Siebner, H.R. (2005) Motor reorganization in asymptomatic carriers of a single mutant Parkin allele: a human model for presymptomatic parkinsonism. *Brain* Vol.128, No.10, (October 2005), pp. 2281-2290, ISSN 0006-8950

Butterworth, R.F., Spahr, L., Fontaine, S. & Layrargues, G.P. (1995) Manganese toxicity, dopaminergic dysfunction and hepatic encephalopathy. *Metab Brain Dis* Vol.10, No.4, (December 1995), pp. 259–267, ISSN 0885-7490

Calne, D.B., Chu, N.S., Huang, C.C., Lu, C.S. & Olanow W. (1994) Manganism and idiopathic parkinsonism: similarities and differences. *Neurology* Vol.44, No.9 (September 1994), pp. 1583–1586, ISSN 0028-3878

Chang, Y., Kim, Y., Woo, S-T., Song, H-J., Kim, S.H., Lee, H., Kwon, Y.J., Ahn, J.H., Park, S-J., Chung, I-S. & Jeong, K.S. (2009) High signal intensity on magnetic resonance imaging is a better predictor of neurobehavioral performances than blood manganese in asymptomatic welders. *Neurotoxicology* Vol.30, No.4 (July 2009), pp. 555-563, ISSN 0161-813X

Chang, Y., Woo, S-T., Lee, J-J., Song, H-J., Lee, H.J., Yoo, D-S., Kim, S.H., Lee, H., Kwon, Y.J., Ahn, H.J., Ahn, J.H., Park, S-J., Weon, Y.C., Chung, I-S., Jeong, K.S. & Kim, Y. (2009)

Neurochemical changes in welders revealed by proton magnetic resonance spectroscopy. *Neurotoxicology* Vol.30, No.6, (November 2009), pp. 950-957, ISSN 0161-813X

Chang, Y., Song, H-J., Lee, J-J., Seo, J.H., Kim, J-H., Lee, H.J., Kim, H.J., Ahn, J-H., Park, S-J., Kwon, J.H., Jeong, K.S., Jung, D-K. & Kim, Y. (2010a) Neuroplastic changes within the brains of manganese-exposed welders: Recruiting additional neural resources for successful motor performance. *Occup Environ Med* Vol.67, No.12, (December 2010), pp. 809-815, ISSN 1351-0711

Chang, Y., Lee, J.J., Seo, J.H., Song, H.J., Kim, J.H., Bae, S.J., Ahn, J.H., Park, S.J., Jeong, K.S., Kwon. Y.J., Kim, S.H. & Kim, Y. (2010b) Altered working memory process in the manganese-exposed brain. *Neuroimage* Vol.53, No.4, (December 2010), pp. 1279-1285, ISSN 1053-8119

Choi, Y., Park, J.K., Park, N.H., Shin, J.W., Yoo, C-I., Lee, C.R., Lee, H., Kim, H.K., Kim, S-R., Jung, T-H., Park, J., Yoon, C.S. & Kim, Y. (2005) Whole blood and red blood cell manganese reflected signal intensities of T1-weighted MRI better than plasma manganese in liver cirrhotics. *J Occup Health* Vol.47, No.1, (January 2005), pp. 68–73, ISSN 1341-9145

DeLong, M. & Wichmann, T. (2009) Update on models of basal ganglia function and dysfunction. *Parkinsonism Relat Disord* Suppliment 3., pp. 237–240, ISSN 1353-8020

Dietz, M.C., Ihrig, A., Bader, M., Wradzillo, W. & Triebig, G. (1999) Effects on the nervous system of manganese exposed workers in a dry cell battery factory. In: Proceedings of the seventh international symposium on neurobehavioral methods and effects in occupational and environmental health.

Dydak, U., Jiang, Y.M., Long, L.L., Zhu, H.,Chen, J., Li, W.M., Edden, R.A., Hu, S., Fu, X., Long, Z., Mo, X.A., Meier, D., Harezlak, J., Aschner, M., Murdoch, J.B. & Zheng, W. (2011) In vivo measurement of brain GABA concentrations by magnetic resonance spectroscopy in smelters occupationally exposed to manganese. *Environ Health Perspect* Vol.119, No.2, (February 2011), pp. 219–224,, ISSN 0091-6765

Ejima, A., Imamur, T., Nakamura, S., Saito, H., Matsumoto, K. & Momono, S. (1992) Manganese intoxication during total parental nutrition. *Lancet* Vol.339, No.8790, (February 1992), pp. 426, ISSN 0140-6736

Erikson, H., Tedroff, J., Thuomas, K.A., Aquilonius, S.M., Hartvig, P., Fasth, K.J., Bjurling, P., Långström, B., Hedström, K.G. & Heilbronn, E. (1992) Manganese induced brain lesions in Macaca fasciulularis as revealed by positron emission tomography and magnetic resonance imaging. *Arch Toxicol* Vol.66, No.6. (June 1992), pp. 403–407, ISSN 0340-5761

Geissler, A., Lock, G., Frund, R., Held, P., Hollerbach, S., Andus, T., Schölmerich, J., Feuerbach, S. & Holstege, A. (1997) Cerebral abnormalities in patients with cirrhosis detected by proton magnetic resonance spectroscopy and magnetic resonance imaging. *Hepatology* Vol.25, No.1, (January 1997), pp. 48–54, ISSN 0270-9139

Guilarte, T.R., McGlothan, J.L., Degaonkar, M., Chen, M.K., Barker, P.B., Syversen, T. & Schneider, J,S. (2006) Evidence for cortical dysfunction and widespread manganese accumulation in the nonhuman primate brain following chronic manganese exposure: a 1H-MRS and MRI study. *Toxicol Sci* Vol.94, No.2 (December 2006):351–358, ISSN 1096-6080

Guilarte, T.R., Burton, N.C., McGlothan, J.L., Vernia, T., Zhou, Y., Alexander, M., Pham, L., Griswold, M., Wong, D.F., Syversen, T. & Schneider, J.S. (2008) Impairment of nigrostriatal dopamine neurotransmission by manganese is mediated by presynaptic mechanism(s): implications to manganese-induced parkinsonism. *J Neurochem* Vol.107, No.5, (December 2008), pp. 1236–1247, ISSN 0022-3042

Hauser, R.A., Zesiewicz, T.A., Rosemurgy, A.S., Martinez, C. & Olanow, C.W. (1994) Manganese intoxication and chronic liver failure. *Ann Neurol* Vol.36, No.6 (December 1994), pp. 871–875, ISSN 0364-5134

Hauser, R.A., Zesiewicz, T.A., Martinez, C., Rosemurgy, A.S. & Olanow, C.W. (1996) Blood manganese correlates with brain magnetic resonance imaging changes in patients with liver disease. *Can J Neurol Sci* Vol.23, No.2, (May 1996), pp. 95–98, ISSN 0317-1671

Huang, C.C., Weng, Y.H., Lu, C.S., Chu, N.S. & Yen, T.C. (2003) Dopamine transporter binding in chronic manganese intoxication. *J Neurol* Vol.250, No.11. (November 2003), pp. 1335–1339, ISSN 0340-5354

Jeon, B., Jeong, J.M., Park, S.S., Kim, J.M., Chang, Y.S., Song, H.C., Kim, K.M., Yoon, K.Y., Lee, M.C. & Lee, S.B. (1998a) Dopamine transporter density measured by [123I]beta-CIT single-photon emission computed tomography is normal in dopa-responsive dystonia. *Ann Neurol* Vol.43, No.6, (June 1998), pp. 792–800, ISSN 0364-5134

Jeon, B., Kim, J.M., Jeong, J.M., Kim, K.M., Chang, Y.S., Lee, D.S. & Lee. M.C. (1998b) Dopamine transporter imaging with [123I]beta-CIT demonstrates presynaptic nigrostriatal dopaminergic damage in Wilson's disease. *J Neurol Neurosurg Psychiatry* Vol.65, No.1, (July 1998), pp. 60–64, ISSN 0022-3050

Jiang, Y.M., Zheng, W., Long, L.L, Zhao, W.J., Li, X.R., Mo, X.A., Lu, J., Fu, X., Li, W., Liu, S., Long, Q., Huang. J. & Pira, E. (2007) Brain magnetic resonance imaging and manganese concentrations in red blood cells of smelting workers: search for biomarkers of manganese exposure. *Neurotoxicology* Vol.28, No.1, (January 2007). pp. 126–135, ISSN 0161-813X

Kim, E.A., Cheong, H.K., Choi, D.S., Sakong, J., Ryoo, J.W., Park, I. & Kang. D.M. (2007) Effect of occupational manganese exposure on the central nervous system of welders: 1H magnetic resonance spectroscopy and MRI findings. *Neurotoxicology* Vol.28, No.2, (March 2007), pp. 276–283, ISSN 0161-813X

Kim, Y. (2006) Neuroimaging in manganism. *Neurotoxicology* Vol.27, No.3, (May 2006), pp. 369–372, ISSN 0161-813X

Kim, J.M., Kim, J.S., Jeong, S.H., Kim, Y.K., Kim, S.E., Kim, S.H. & Kim, Y. (2010) Dopaminergic neuronal integrity in parkinsonism associated with liver cirrhosis. *Neurotoxicology.* Vol.31, No.4, (August 2010), pp. 351-355, ISSN 0161-813X

Kim, J.W., Kim, Y., Cheong, H.K. & Ito, K. (1998) Manganese induced parkinsonism: a case report. *J Korean Med Sci* Vol.13, No.4, (August 1998), pp. 437–439, ISSN 1011-8934

Kim, Y., Kim, K.S., Yang, J.S., Park, I.J., Kim, E., Jin, Y., Kwon, K.R., Chang, K.H., Kim, J.W., Park, S,H,, Lim,. H.S., Cheong, H.K., Shin, Y.C., Park, J. & Moon, Y. (1999a) Increase in signal intensities on T1-weighted magnetic resonance images in asymptomatic manganese-exposed workers. *Neurotoxicology* Vol.20, No.6, (December 1999), pp. 901–907, ISSN 0161-813X

Kim, Y., Kim, J., Ito, K., Lim, H-S., Cheong, H-K., Kim, J.Y., Shin, Y.C., Kim, K.S. & Moon, Y (1999b) Idiopathic parkinsonism with superimposed manganese exposure: utility of positron emission tomography. *Neurotoxicology* Vol.20, No.2-3, (April 1999), pp. 249–252, ISSN 0161-813X

Kim, Y., Kim, J.M., Kim, J., Yoo, C., Lee, C.R., Lee, J.H., Kim, H.K., Yang, S.O., Park, J., Chung, H.K., Lee, D.S. & Jeon, B. (2002) Dopamine transporter density is decreased in parkinsonian patients with a history of manganese exposure; what does it mean? *Mov Disord* Vol.17, No.3, (May 2002) pp. 568–575, ISSN 0885-3185

Kim, Y., Park, J.K., Choi, Y., Yoo, C-I., Lee, C.R., Lee, H., Lee, J-H., Kim, S-R., Jung, T-H., Yoon, C.S. & Park J-H. (2005) Blood manganese concentration is elevated in iron deficiency anemia patients, whereas globus pallidus signal intensity is minimally affected. *Neurotoxicology* Vol.26, No.1, (January 2005), pp. 107-111, ISSN 0161-813X

Kim, Y., Jeong, K.S., Song, H-J., Lee, J-J., Seo, J-H., Kim, G-C., Lee, H.J., Kim, H.J., Ahn, J-H., Park, S-J., Kim, S.H., Kwon, Y.J. & Chang, Y. (2011) Altered white matter microstructural integrity revealed by voxel-wise analysis of diffusion tensor imaging in welders with manganese exposure. *Neurotoxicology* Vol.32, No.1, (January 2011), pp. 100-109, ISSN 0161-813X

Kinoshita, Y., Ohnishi, A., Kohshi, K. & Yokota, A. (1999) Apparent diffusion coefficient on rat brain and nerves intoxicated with methylmercury. *Environ Res* Vol.80, No.4, (May 1999) pp. 348–354, ISSN 0013-9351

Kreis, R., Ross, B.D., Farrow, N.A. & Ackerman, Z. (1992) Metabolic disorders of the brain in chronic hepatic encephalopathy detected with H-1 MR spectroscopy. *Radiology* Vol.182, No.1, (January 1992), pp. 19–27, ISSN 0033-8419

Krieger, D., Krieger, S., Jansen, O., Gass, P., Theilmann, L. & Lichtnecker, H. (1995) Manganese and chronic hepatic encephalopathy. *Lancet* Vol.346, No.8970, (July 1995) pp. 270–274, ISSN 0140-6736

Lang, C.J. (2000) The use of neuroimaging techniques for clinical detection of neurotoxicity: a review. *Neurotoxicology* Vol.21, No.5, (October 2000), pp. 847-855, ISSN 0161-813X

Laubenberger, J., Haussinger, D., Bayer, S., Gufler, H., Hennig, J. & Langer, M. (1997) Proton magnetic resonance spectroscopy of the brain in symptomatic and asymptomatic patients with liver cirrhosis. *Gastroenterology* Vol.112, No.5, (May 1997), pp. 1610–1616 ISSN 0016-5085

Laruelle, M., Baldwin, R.M., Malison, R.T., Zea-Ponce, Y., Zoghbi, S.S., al-Tikriti, M., Sybirska, E.H., Zimmermann, R.C., Wisniewski, G. & Neumeyer, J.L. (1993) SPECT imaging of dopamine and serotonin transporters with [123I]beta-CIT SPECT: pharmacological characterization of brain uptake in nonhuman primates. *Synapse* Vol.13, No.4, (April 1993), pp. 295–309, ISSN 0887-4476

Le Bihan, D., Mangin, J.F., Poupon, C., Clark, C.A., Pappata, S., Molko, N. & Chabriat, H. (2001) Diffusion tensor imaging: concepts and applications. J Magn Reson Vol.13, No.4, (April 2001), pp. 534–546, ISSN 1090-7807

Lucchini, R. & Kim, Y. (2009) Manganese, Health Effects. In Vojtisek, M and Prakash, R Eds. Metals and Neurotoxicity. Society for Science and Environment. 81-92, India.

McKinney, A.M., Filice, R.W., Teksam, M., Casey, S., Truwit, C., Clark, H.B., Woon, C. & Liu, H.Y. (2004) Diffusion abnormalities of the globi pallidi in manganese neurotoxicity. *Neuroradiology* Vol.46, No.4 (April 2004), pp. 291–295, ISSN 0028-3940

Meng, X.M., Zhu, D.M., Ruan, D.Y., She, J.Q. & Luo, L. (2005) Effects of chronic lead exposure on 1H MRS of hippocampus and frontal lobes in children. *Neurology* Vol.64, No.9, (May 2005), pp. 1644–1647, ISSN 0028-3878

Miese, F., Kircheis, G., Wittsack, H.J., Wenserski, F., Hemker, J., Mödder, U., Häussinger, D. & Cohnen, M. (2006) 1H-MR spectroscopy, magnetization transfer, and diffusion-weighted imaging in alcoholic and nonalcoholic patients with cirrhosis with hepatic encephalopathy. *AJNR Am J Neuroradiol* Vol.27, No.5, (May 2006):1019–1026, ISSN 0195-6108

Mirowitz, S.A., Westrich, T.J. & Hirsch, J.D. (1991) Hyperintense basal ganglia on T1-weighted MR images in patients receiving parenteral nutrition. *Radiology* Vol.181, No.1, (October, 1991), pp. 117–120, ISSN 0033-8419

Morrish, P.K., Sawle, G.V. & Brooks, D.J. (1995) Clinical and [18F]dopa PET findings in early Parkinson's disease. *J Neurol Neurosurg Psychiatry* Vol.59, No.6, (December 1995), pp. 597–600, ISSN 0364-5134

Morrish, P.K., Sawle, G.V. & Brooks, D.J. (1996) An [18F]dopa-PET and clinical study of the rate of progression in Parkinson's disease. *Brain* Vol.119, No.2 (April 1996), pp. 585–591, ISSN 0006-8950

Moseley, M.E., Cohen, Y. & Kucharczyk, J. (1990) Diffusion-weighted MR imaging of anisotropic water diffusion in cat central nervous system. *Radiology* Vol.176, No.2, (August 1990), pp.439–446, ISSN 0033-8419

Naegele, T., Grodd, W., Viebahn, R., Seeger, U., Klose, U., Seitz, D., Kaiser, S., Mader, I., Mayer, J., Lauchart, W., Gregor, M. & Voigt, K. (2000) MR imaging and (1)H spectroscopy of brain metabolites in hepatic encephalopathy: time-course of renormalization after liver transplantation. *Radiology* Vol.216, No.3, (September 2000), pp. 683–691, ISSN 0033-8419

Nelson, K., Golnick, J., Korn, T. & Angle, C. (1993) Manganese encephalopathy: utility of early magnetic resonance imaging. *Br J Ind Med* Vol.50, No.6, (June 1993), pp. 510–513, ISSN 0007-1072

Newland, M.C., Ceckler, T.L., Kordower, J.H. & Weiss, B. (1989) Visualizing manganese in the primate basal ganglia with magnetic resonance imaging. *Exp Neurol* Vol.106, No.3, (December 1989), pp. 251–258, ISSN 0014-4886

Park, N.H., Park, J.K., Choi, Y., Yoo, C-I., Lee, C.R., Lee, H., Kim, H.K., Kim, S-R., Jung, T.H., Park, J., Yoon, C.S. & Kim, Y (2003) Whole blood manganese correlates with high signal intensities on T1-weighted MRI in patients with liver cirrhosis. *Neurotoxicology* Vol.24, No.6, (December 2003), pp. 909–915, ISSN 0161-813X

Pujol, A., Pujol, J., Graus, F., Rimola, A., Peri, J., Mercader, J.M., García-Pagan, J.C., Bosch, J., Rodés, J. & Tolosa, E. (1993) Hyperintense globus pallidus on T1-weighted MRI in cirrhotic patients is associated with severity of liver failure. *Neurology* Vol.43, No.1, (January 1993), pp. 65–69, ISSN 0028-3878

Racette, B.A., McGee-Minnich, L., Moerlein, S.M., Mink, J.W., Videen, T.O. & Perlmutter, J.S. (2001) Welding-related parkinsonism: clinical features, treatment, and pathophysiology. *Neurology* Vol.56, No.1, (January 2001), pp. 8–13, ISSN 0028-3878

Racette, B.A., Antenor, J.A., McGee-Minnich, L., Moerlein, S.M., Videen, T.O., Kotagal, V. & Perlmutter, J.S. (2005) [18F]FDOPA PET and clinical features in parkinsonism due to manganism. *Mov Disord* Vol.20, No.4, (April 2005), pp. 492–496, ISSN 0885-3185

Ravina, B., Eidelberg, D., Ahlskog, J.E., Albin, R.L., Brooks, D.J., Carbon, M., Dhawan, V., Feigin, A., Fahn, S., Guttman, M., Gwinn-Hardy, K., McFarland, H., Innis, R., Katz, R.G., Kieburtz, K., Kish, S.J., Lange, N., Langston, J.W., Marek, K., Morin, L., Moy, C., Murphy, D., Oertel, W.H., Oliver, G, Palesch, Y., Powers, W., Seibyl, J., Sethi, K.D., Shults, C.W., Sheehy, P., Stoessl, A.J. & Holloway, R. (2005) The role of radiotracer imaging in Parkinson's disease. *Neurology* Vol.64, No.2, (January 2005), pp. 208–215, ISSN 0028-3878

Rosen, Y, & Lenkinski, R.E. (2007) Recent advances in magnetic resonance neurospectroscopy. *Neurotherapeutics* Vol.4, No.3, (July 2007), pp. 330–345, ISSN 1933-7213

Ross, A.J., Sachdev, P.S., Wen, W., Brodaty, H., Joscelyne, A. & Lorentz, L.M. (2006) Prediction of cognitive decline after stroke using proton magnetic resonance spectroscopy. *J Neurol Sci* Vol.251, No.1–2, (December 2006), pp. 62–69, ISSN 0022-510X

Sabatini, U., Boulanouar, K., Fabre, N., Martin, F., Carel, C., Colonnese, C., Bozzao, L., Berry, I., Montastruc, J.L., Chollet, F. & Rascol, O. (2000) Cortical motor reorganization in akinetic patients with Parkinson's disease: a functional MRI study. *Brain* Vol.123, No.2, (February 2000), pp. 394–403, ISSN 0006-8950

Seibyl, J.P., Marek, K.L., Quinlan, D., Sheff, K., Zoghbi, S., Zea-Ponce, Y., Baldwin, R.M., Fussell, B., Smith, E.O., Charney, D.S. & van Dyck, C. (1995) Decreased single-photon emission computed tomographic [123I]beta-CIT striatal uptake correlates with symptom severity in Parkinson's disease. *Ann Neurol* Vol.38, No.4, (October 1995), pp. 589–598, ISSN 0364-5134

Shinotoh, H., Snow, B.J., Hewitt, K.A., Pate, B.D., Doudet, D., Nugent, R., Perl, D.P., Olanow, W. & Calne, D.B. (1995) MRI and PET studies of manganese-intoxicated monkeys. *Neurology* Vol.45, No.6, (June 1995), pp. 1199–1204, ISSN 0028-3878

Shinotoh, H., Snow, B.J., Chu, N.S., Huang, C.C., Lu, C.S., Lee, C., Takahashi, H. & Calne, DB. (1997) Presynaptic and postsynaptic striatal dopaminergic function in patients with manganese intoxication: a position emission tomography study. *Neurology* Vol.48, No.4, (April 1997), pp. 1053–1056, ISSN 0028-3878

Spahr, L., Butterworth, R.F., Fontaine, S., Bui, L., Therrien, G., Milette, P.C., Lebrun, L.H., Zayed, J., Leblanc, A. & Pomier-Layrargues, G. (1996) Increased blood manganese in cirrhotic patients: relationship to pallidal magnetic resonance signal hyperintensity and neurological symptoms. *Hepatology* Vol.24, No.5, (November 1996), pp. 1116–1120, ISSN 0270-9139

Spahr, L., Vingerhoets, F., Lazeyras, F., Delavelle, J., DuPasquier, R., Giostra, E., Mentha, G., Terrier, F. & Hadengue, A. (2000) Magnetic resonance imaging and proton spectroscopic alterations correlate with parkinsonian signs in patients with cirrhosis. *Gastroenterology* Vol.119, No.3, (September 2000), pp. 774–781, ISSN 0016-5085

Strange, K., Emma, F., Paredes, A. & Morrison R. (1994) Osmoregulatory changes in myo-inositol content and Na+/myo-inositol cotransport in rat cortical astrocytes. *Glia* Vol.12, No.1, (September 1994), pp. 35–43, ISSN 0894-1491

Trope, I., Lopez-Villegas, D., Cecil, K.M. & Lenkinski, R.E. (2001) Exposure to lead appears to selectively alter metabolism of cortical gray matter. *Pediatrics* Vol.107, No.6, (June 2001), pp.1437–1442, ISSN 0031-4005

Vion-Dury, J., Meyerhoff, D.J., Cozzone, P.J. & Weiner MW. (1994) What might be the impact on neurology of the analysis of brain metabolism by in vivo magnetic resonance spectroscopy? *J Neurol* Vol.241, No.6, (May 1994), pp. 354–371, ISSN 0340-5354

Walker, R..C, Purnell, G.L., Jones-Jackson, L.B., Thomas, K.L., Brito, J.A. & Ferris EJ. (2004) Introduction to PET imaging with emphasis on biomedical research. *Neurotoxicology* Vol.25, No.4, (June 2004), pp. 533-542, ISSN 0161-813X

Weissenborn, K. & Kolbe, H. (1998) The basal ganglia and portal-systemic encephalopathy. *Metab Brain Dis* Vol.13, No.4, (December 1998), pp. 261–272, ISSN 0885-7490

Weisskopf, M.G. Magnetic resonance spectroscopy and environmental toxicant exposure. (2007) *Ann N Y Acad Sci* Vol.1097, (February 2007), pp. 179–182, ISSN 0077-8923

Weisskopf, M.G., Hu, H., Sparrow, D., Lenkinski, R.E. & Wright, R.O. (2007) Proton magnetic resonance spectroscopic evidence of glial effects of cumulative lead exposure in the adult human hippocampus. *Environ Health Perspect* Vol.115, No.4, (April 2007), pp. 519–523, ISSN 0091-6765

Wolters, E.C., Huang, C.C., Clark, C., Peppard, R.F., Okada, J., Chu, N.S., Adam, M.J., Ruth, T.J., Li, D. & Calne, D.B. (1989) Positron emission tomography in manganese intoxication. *Ann Neurol* Vol.26, No.5, (November 1989), pp. 647–651, ISSN 0364-5134

6

Extraction of Single-Trial Post-Movement MEG Beta Synchronization in Normal and Parkinson's Patient Using ICA-Based Spatiotemporal Approach

Po-Lei Lee[1,2,3], Yu-Te Wu[2] and Jen-Chuen Hsieh[2]
[1]Department of Electrical Engineering, National Central University,
[2]Institute of Brain Science, National Yang-Ming University,
[3]Center for Dynamical Biomarkers and Translational Medicine, National Central University,
Taiwan

1. Introduction

The human brain is a dynamic system that frequently changes functional mode (Lopes da Silva, 1991; Lopes da Silva, 1996). Spatiotemporal analysis of brain activities with regard to distinct spatial locations and frequency bands reveals task-specific brain activation which changes in a fraction of a second (Jensen & Vanni, 2002). At rest, Rolandic EEG and MEG rhythms are dominated by rhythmic activity around 10 (alpha band) and 20 (beta band) Hz. Electrocorticographic (Pfurtscheller et al., 1994) and neuromagnetic recordings have shown that the ~20-Hz rhythm mainly originates in the anterior bank of the central sulcus while the ~10-Hz rhythm is concentrated predominantly in the post-central cortex (Pfurtscheller & Lopes da Silva, 1999). These two frequency components appear to have different functional roles, with the ~20-Hz rhythm being more closely connected to movements and their termination and the ~10-Hz component behaving more like a classical "idling" rhythm (Salmelin et al., 1995). Voluntary movement is composed of three phases: planning, execution and recovery (Pfurtscheller et al., 1998a). It has been suggested that localized event-related alpha desynchronization (ERD) upon movement can be viewed as an EEG/MEG correlate of an activated cortical sensorimotor network, servicing planning and execution, while beta event-related synchronization (ERS) may reflect deactivation/inhibition during the recovery phase in the underlying cortical network (Pfurtscheller et al., 1996).

Movement-related ERD and ERS have been used as probes to study neurophysiology in normal brains and pathophysiology in the diseased (Tamas et al., 2003). It has been reported that the diagnostic features of patients with Parkinson's disease, in comparison with controls, are a slowing and suppression of the post-movement beta ERS independent of the amount of beta activity in the reference period (Pfurtscheller et al., 1998a). These findings imply that slowed and reduced recovery after the motor act impedes cortical preparation of the next movement (Pfurtscheller et al., 1996). Patients with Unverricht-Lundborg type myoclonic epilepsy demonstrate little rebound of beta activities contingent upon median nerve stimulation (Silen et al., 2000). The diminished beta ERS indicates that the myoclonic patients have sustained motor cortex reactivity which can be attributed to impaired cortical inhibition (Pfurtscheller & Lopes da Silva, 1999).

ERD and ERS activities are time-locked, but not phase-locked, to external stimuli or tasks (Andrew & Pfurtscheller, 1995; Kalcher & Pfurtscheller, 1995; Pfurtscheller & Lopes da Silva, 1999). Existing methods for extraction of ERD/ERS signals essentially measure power or amplitude changes of corresponding frequency bands as derived from the average of dozens or hundreds of trials. The band power method squares and averages filtered brain signals within a selected frequency band (Pfurtscheller & Aranibar, 1977), and an inter-trial variance method to remove the phase-locked portion in the band power method was reported by Klimesch et al. (1998). Likewise, autoregressive and spectral decomposition methods have been used to extract significant frequency components in rhythmic signals (Florian & Pfurtscheller, 1995). Salmelin's temporal-spectral evolution method rectifies and averages filtered MEG signals (Salmelin et al., 1995). To increase the temporal resolution of the ERD/ERS technique, Clochon et al. (1996) proposed an amplitude modulation (AM) method based on the Hilbert transform to detect the envelope of filtered signals by squaring and summing their real and imaginary parts. All these approaches presume stereotypical frequency and temporal characteristics across trials and require an average of many trials for the ERD/ERS using a preset frequency filter and time window to preprocess every trial. However, non-phase-locked rhythmic signals can vary from trial-to-trial contingent upon variations in a subject's performance and state, which may be linked to fluctuations in expectation, attention, arousal, and task strategy (Bastiaansen et al., 2001; Bastiaansen et al., 1999; Earle, 1988; Haig et al., 1995; Hoffman et al., 1991; Yabe et al., 1993). Since trial-to-trial variability in amplitude, latencies, or scalp distribution might carry important information on cognitive and physiological states (Jung et al., 2001), a method that permits the extraction and analysis of the oscillatory signal on a single-trial base is crucial for the study of subtle brain dynamics. Furthermore, such a method should require fewer trials for analysis and hence shorter experiment time, which is beneficial for patients with impairment of motor and/or cognitive performance (Muller-Gerking et al., 1999).

Single-trial multi-channel EEG analysis has been developed for time-locked, phase-locked, evoked brain activities (Jung et al., 2001; Tang et al., 2002). However, approaches to single-trial movement-related oscillatory changes are less explored. Independent component analysis (ICA), a data-driven method for multivariate data analysis, has been used to reveal temporally-independent neuronal activities of EEG measurements (Jung et al., 2001; Makeig et al, 1997; McKeown et al., 1998), MEG measurements (Wu et al., 2002; Wu et al., 2003; Tang et al., 2002), fMRI (Duann et al., 2002; McKeown et al., 1998) and recently perfusion MRI (Kao et al., 2003). The present study proposes a new approach using ICA and the Hilbert transformation for the single-trial detection of movement-related beta rhythmic activity during a self-paced right finger lifting task. This study focuses on beta activity and beta ERS, centered around 20 Hz, because it has been demonstrated that the movement-related short bursts of beta oscillation have higher task and movement specificity than alpha ERD (Pfurtscheller & Aranibar, 1979b; Pfurtscheller et al., 1996).

Since brain oscillation may be expressed alone in a specific frequency band independent of artifacts (Ermer et al., 2000; Lins et al., 1993a; Lins et al., 1993b; Mosher et al., 1992), ICA is applied to transform brain signals across all channels (in a single trial) into mutually independent components by means of an unmixing matrix in which each column represents a spatial map tailoring the weights of the corresponding temporal component at each MEG sensor. The spatial maps and temporal waveforms of decomposed independent components

Extraction of Single-Trial Post-Movement MEG Beta Synchronization in Normal and
Parkinson's Patient Using ICA-Based Spatiotemporal Approach

121

are categorized into task-related and task-unrelated groups respectively, based on temporal and spatial characteristics. This temporal template is the grand average of hundreds of vector-norm envelopes of the band-pass filtered, single-trial MEG measurements obtained from right index finger lifting. The spatial template can be derived from the spatial distribution at beta rebound activity either from the grand average of the generation group (for signal extraction) or from each individual (for verification). Correlations between the temporal template and component waveforms, as well as between the spatial template and spatial maps, are computed, and coupled component waveforms and spatial maps that conjointly survive with high correlation values are taken as task-related information and subjected to data reconstruction. In this way the phase and amplitude information of noise-free MEG beta activities can be preserved for profound studies of temporal and spectral variation across trials. Due to the high signal-to-noise ratio (SNR) in beta activities extracted through ICA, trial-specific reactive frequency ranges can be determined by means of the comparisons of two short time spectra between the reference and post-movement periods. Beta reactivity per single trial can be quantified using the amplitude modulation (AM) method (Clochon et al., 1996), and insignificant epochs can be determined using a nonparametric sign test (Brovelli et al., 2002). Source estimation and localization techniques can be successfully applied to single-trial epoch to estimate the source locations of beta modulation.

The current study presents: 1) a novel ICA-based spatiotemporal approach for single-trial analysis of event-related beta oscillatory modulations with a high extraction rate; 2) the prospect of trial-specific frequency bandpass filtering that takes into account subtle trial-by-trial brain dynamics; 3) the feasibility of using sophisticated source estimation/localization methods demanding high signal-to-noise ratio (SNR) on single trial data; and 4) a common template approach permitting an effective alternative in cases where lengthy procedures cannot be endured by participants or in clinical settings where patients have attention problems or are incapable of sustaining long experiments. The proposed ICA-based approach was applied to discover the mechanisms of beta ERS in one Parkinson's patient. It is helpful to investigate the reasoning of ERS vanishment due to suppression of post-movement beta rebound in each single-trial, rather than the cause of temporal jittering and/or loss of synchronization in Parkinson's disease.

2. Materials and methods

2.1 Subjects and task

The present study examined six healthy right-handed subjects (gender balanced), aged 24-30 years. Five of the healthy subjects were used in the model generation group, and MEG data from the last healthy subject were used for validation. Subjects performed self-paced lifting of the right index finger approximately once every 8 sec. Subjects were trained to perform the movement briskly for a duration of 200 to 300 ms, as monitored by surface electromyogram (EMG) on extensor digitorum communis, with a range of finger movement around 35~40°, while keeping their eyes open in order to suppress the occipital alpha rhythm. In addition, somatosensory evoked fields (SEFs) for right median nerve stimulation were measured to locate the primary sensorimotor area (SMI) in each subject as part of the procedure for the generation of a temporal template (see below). Informed written consent was obtained from all subjects. This study was approved by the Institutional Review Board of Taipei Veterans General Hospital. In addition, one 56-year-old patient with idiopathic Parkinson's disease in Hoehn and Yahr stage 1 was also recruited as a demonstration in this study.

2.2 Data recording

Cortical magnetic signals were recorded with a 306-channel (102 sensor unit) whole-head neuromagnetometer (band-pass, 0.05-250 Hz; digitized at 1kHz; Vectorview; Neuromag Ltd., Helsinki, Finland) with subjects in sitting position. Each sensor unit was composed of a pair of planar gradiometers and a magnetometer. The magnetometer measured magnetic flux (B_z), normal to the sensor unit, while the gradiometers measured two tangential derivatives of B_z ($\partial B_z / \partial x$ and $\partial B_z / \partial y$, mutually orthogonal). Only magnetic signals measured by the gradiometers were used in this study. Bipolar horizontal and vertical electro-oculograms (EOG) were recorded using electrodes placed below and above the left eye and at the bilateral outer canthi to monitor eye movement and blinks. The exact position of the head with respect to the sensor array was determined by measuring magnetic signals from four head position indicator (HPI) coils placed on the scalp. Coil positions were identified with a three-dimensional digitizer with respect to three predetermined landmarks (naison and bilateral preauricular points) on the scalp, and this data used to superimpose MEG source signals on individual MRI images obtained with a 3.0 T Bruker MedSpec S300 system (Bruker, Kalsrube, Germany). The anatomical image was acquired using a high-resolution T1-weighted, 3D gradient-echo pulse sequence (MDEFT: Modified Driven Equilibrium Fourier Transform; TR/TE/TI= 88.1ms/4.12ms/650ms, 128*128*128 matrix, FOV=250mm).

Empty room measurements were recorded for 3 minutes. Approximately 100 EOG-free trials of right index finger lifting were acquired and analyzed off-line. Since the focus was on beta-activities, the signals were further band-pass-filtered between 6-50 Hz (zero-phase, tenth-order, IIR Butterworth filter) to remove dc drifts and 60 Hz noise. The initial finger movement (movement onset; zero time) was registered with an optical switch (Taniguchi et al., 2000). Electromyographic (EMG) activity from the extensor digitorum communis (digitized at 1 KHz) was continuously recorded to monitor performance (see above). Each epoch comprised data points from –4s to 3s relative to the movement onset (Salmelin et al., 1995; Salmelin and Hari, 1994a) and epochs were subjected to further single-trial ICA analysis.

For SEF measurement, the right median nerve was electrically stimulated every 2 sec with constant current pulses (0.3 msec in duration) exceeding the motor threshold. Approximately 100 EOG-free trials were acquired and digitized at 1 kHz for off-line analysis.

2.3 Data analysis
2.3.1 Independent Component Analysis of the single-trial MEG epoch

We take the advantages of sensitivity and localizing power of superficial sources by planar gradiometers (Rosell et al., 2001; Kajola et al., 1991). Each single-trial MEG epoch contains m channels (m = 204, 102 pairs of gradiometers) and n time points (usually m < n). The paired gradiometer signals ($\partial B_z / \partial x$ and $\partial B_z / \partial y$) are arranged into two $\frac{m}{2} \times n$ sub-matrices $\mathbf{B_1}$ and $\mathbf{B_2}$ and concatenated into an $m \times n$ matrix $\mathbf{B}$. The ith rows ($i \le 102$) of $\mathbf{B_1}$ and $\mathbf{B_2}$ contain the measured gradiometer signals from the ith sensor location, and the jth column in $\mathbf{B}$ contains the measured data at the jth time point across all gradiometer channels.

Extraction of Single-Trial Post-Movement MEG Beta Synchronization in Normal and
Parkinson's Patient Using ICA-Based Spatiotemporal Approach

123

Mathematically, we can consider each row of **B** as samples generated from one random variable b_i, i = 1, 2, ..., m. In other words, matrix **B** is a realization of a random vector $b = [b_1 \ b_2 \ \cdots b_m]^T$.

The ICA techniques (Jung et al., 2001; Hyvarinen et al., 2001) seek to find a $p \times m$ ($p \leq m$) matrix, **W**, which converts the random vector b into another vector variable, s, consisting of p mutually independent random variables, thus:

$$
\underset{p \times 1}{\mathbf{S}} = \begin{bmatrix} s_1 \\ s_2 \\ . \\ . \\ . \\ s_p \end{bmatrix} = \underset{p \times m}{\mathbf{W}} \ \underset{m \times 1}{b} \tag{1}
$$

The mutual independence of s_i, for i = 1,..., p, implies that if $P(s_i)$ represents the probability distribution of the ith component, the joint probability distribution for all components can be factorized as:

$$
P(s_1, s_2, ..., s_p) = P(s_1)P(s_2)...P(s_p) \tag{2}
$$

The ICA techniques use this assumption of mutual independence to find the un-mixing matrix **W**.

All calculations in the present study were carried out using the FastICA algorithm which features high speed calculation (cubic convergence) and does not require selection of step size parameters or learning rate, unlike the gradient-based algorithm (Hyvarinen et al., 1997, 2001). The FastICA technique first removes means of row vectors in the **B** sample matrix such that each random variable bi has a zero mean, and then employs a whitening process using principal component analysis. After whitening, the covariance matrix of the whitened data becomes an identity matrix, and only the first p ($p \leq m$) most significant principal components are preserved in the FastICA calculation.

The next step is to look for a matrix that transforms the whitened data into a set of components as mutually independent as possible. Mutual information, as a measure of the independence of random variables, is used as the criterion for finding such a transformation. Mutual information can be expressed in terms of negentropy, an important measure of non-Gaussianity (Hyvarinen et al., 1997, 2001). Therefore, the problem of finding the independent components (s) and the transform matrix (**W**) can be translated into a search for linear combinations of the whitened data that maximize the negentropy of the distributions of s_i, for i = 1,..., p.

After applying FastICA to the pre-processed single-trial MEG epochs, matrix **B** can be factored into a (mixing) matrix **U** and an (independent source) matrix **S** as follows:

$$B_{mxn} = \begin{bmatrix} B_1 \\ B_2 \end{bmatrix} = U_{mxp}S_{pxn}$$

$$= \begin{bmatrix} \begin{bmatrix} u_{1,1} & \cdots & u_{1,p} \\ \vdots & & \vdots \\ u_{\frac{m}{2},1} & \cdots & u_{\frac{m}{2},p} \end{bmatrix} \\ \begin{bmatrix} u_{\frac{m}{2}+1,1} & \cdots & u_{\frac{m}{2}+1,p} \\ \vdots & & \vdots \\ u_{m,1} & \cdots & u_{m,p} \end{bmatrix} \end{bmatrix}_{mxp} \begin{bmatrix} \overrightarrow{s_1} \\ \overrightarrow{s_2} \\ \vdots \\ \overrightarrow{s_p} \end{bmatrix}_{pxn} \tag{3}$$

in which each row $\overrightarrow{s_i}$ of matrix $S \in \Re^{p \times n}$ represents samples of an independent component (IC) s_i, for $i = 1,..., p$ and $U \in \Re^{m \times p}$ is the pseudo-inverse of matrix $\mathbf{W}$ whose column vectors represent the weight distribution values of the corresponding ICs in S across all MEG gradiometer channels. In fact, matrix $\mathbf{U}$ is the "mixing matrix" that combines the p ICs to reconstruct signal $\mathbf{B}$. These temporal ICs can be categorized into task-related ICs and task-unrelated ICs. Since the elicited brain activities or artifacts can be distributed over multiple ICs, no one-to-one correspondence between IC and source information is projected (Makeig et al., 1997). To facilitate the selection of task-related ICs, a temporal and spatial template pair was constructed prior to selection (see below). Spatial map $\bar{x}_j$ of the jth IC was defined as the topographic display of all vector norms for weights of 102 gradiometer pairs in the jth column vector of U,

$$\bar{x}_j = \left[\sqrt{u_{1,j}^2 + u_{(\frac{m}{2}+1),j}^2} \quad \sqrt{u_{2,j}^2 + u_{(\frac{m}{2}+2),j}^2} \quad \cdots \quad \sqrt{u_{\frac{m}{2},j}^2 + u_{m,j}^2} \right]^T \tag{4}$$

in which $u_{i,j}$ is the entry in the ith row and jth column of $\mathbf{U}$ in Eq. (3). The spatial map is intended for component selection (see below).

2.3.2 Creation of a temporal template (VAMW$_{template}$) using amplitude modulation (envelope) of the MEG data

The recorded MEG signals at each gradiometer are filtered in the task-specific frequency band (Pfurtscheller & Lopes da Silva, 1999) and rectified by computing the AM waveform (envelope) using the amplitude modulation (AM) method (Clochon et al., 1996) as follows:

$$m(t) = \sqrt{M_{BP}(t)^2 + H(M_{BP}(t))^2} \tag{5}$$

in which $M_{BP}(t)$ is the band-passed MEG signal and $H(M_{BP}(t))$ is its Hilbert transform. The task-specific frequency band is determined by the contrast between two 1-s amplitude spectra calculated over about one hundred event-related EEG trials (Pfurtscheller and Lopes da Silva, 1999). One (serving as rest reference) is computed over the duration from 4s to 3s

Extraction of Single-Trial Post-Movement MEG Beta Synchronization in Normal and
Parkinson's Patient Using ICA-Based Spatiotemporal Approach

125

preceding the onset of movement, and the other (serving as reactive target) from 0.8s to 1.8s after the onset of movement (see Fig. 1a, b). All beta-frequency components with significant modulation in terms of post-movement amplitude increase (above 95% confidence level, i.e. Z>3.09, P<0.01) in the differential amplitude spectrum (see Fig. 1c) are taken as the task-specific frequency band for subsequent processing (Pfurtscheller G. and Berghold A., 1989).

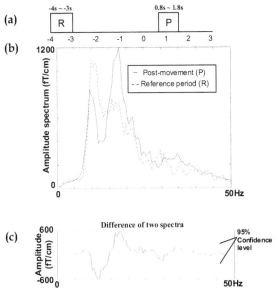

Fig. 1. Determination of task-specific frequency band using two 1-s amplitude spectra. (a) "R" represents the reference period from -4s to -3s preceding onset of movement and "P" represents the post-movement duration from 0.8s to 1.8s after onset of movement. (b) Two spectra computed over the reference (R) and post-movement periods (P), respectively. (c) The task-specific frequency band for beta-band VAMW is defined as the one where the difference between two spectra exceeds the 95% confidence level.

The vector norm of AM waveforms (VAMW) at each sensor site is computed using the square root of the AM waveforms of each gradiometer pair, i.e., $V(i,t)=\sqrt{m_x(i,t)^2+m_y(i,t)^2}$, in which $V(i,t)$ is the VAMW at the ith sensor location, and $m_x(i,t)$ and $m_y(i,t)$ are the AM waveforms in $\frac{\partial B_z}{\partial x}$ and $\frac{\partial B_z}{\partial y}$ directions of the ith sensor location. Event-related beta modulation is then computed as the difference in amplitude between the maximum amplitude of VAMW for each sensor site in the post-movement (0.8s to 1.8s) interval and mean activity between -2.5s and -2s (see Fig. 2a) (Leocani et al., 1997). Beta rebound (BR) is defined as the maximum amplitude of the computed event-related beta modulation from the subset of nine sensor sites in the vicinity of SMI (identified by SEF). The VAMWs of the BR calculation were averaged across the subjects (500 trials, 100 trials for each subject, 5 subjects pooled) to create the common temporal template, designated VAMW$_{template}$ (Fig. 2a).

2.3.3 Creation of a spatial template using topographical distribution of event-related beta modulation values

Individual spatial templates were first generated from the topographical distributions of event-related beta modulation values (see above). The five templates from the model generation group were then averaged to generate a common spatial template. In order to optimize conditions for spatial averaging, subjects' heads were carefully positioned before actual measurements to keep head positioning and orientation as similar as possible. Distances between head centers of the five subjects and the reference point (the origin of the MEG sensor array) in the horizontal plane were less than 4mm, and angles between the vertical axis of the helmet and that of the head (the normal vector of the plane constituted by the three landmark points, i.e., nasion, and both pre-auricular points) remained within $5.5°$ (maximum deviation $1.5°$) between subjects.

Only the left half of the spatial map (unshaded in Fig. 2b) was used as the spatial template because this study focused on beta event-related activities in the hemisphere contralateral to the side of finger lifting; however, the other half can be generated analogously to extract activities in the ipsilateral hemisphere. Correlations among individual spatial templates ranged from 0.92 to 0.68. Respective correlations between the common spatial template and the individual spatial templates were 0.973, 0.811, 0.881, 0.904, and 0.915. These high correlation values support the use of the spatial template in component selection for each individual's magnetic signals.

2.3.4 Selection of pertinent independent components for the reconstruction of reactive beta activities

A spatial map (Eq. (4)) and corresponding VAMWs of each IC were generated for the selection of task-related ICs. Since the original signals may be decomposed into multiple ICs, the spectrum of each IC may vary from the one in the original signal due to the decomposition process. When settings for band-pass filtering for VAMW computation cannot be optimally determined using two-spectrum comparison for the generation of a $VAMW_{template}$ (Pfurtscheller & Lopes da Silva, 1999), three standard beta bands, 12-16, 16-20 and 20-24 Hz (Pfurtscheller G., 1981), enclosing the event-related beta activities in motor task, were used to band-pass filter (zero-phase, tenth-order, IIR Butterworth filter) for each single-trial IC such that the three frequency-laden resultant $VAMW_{IC}$s (the VAMWs band-pass filtered in three frequency bands of each IC) retained all task-related information. These $VAMW_{IC}$s were subsequently used in the selection of task-related ICs, which must fulfill the following dual criteria: 1) at least one of three corresponding $VAMW_{IC}$s has a correlation with the $VAMW_{template}$ higher than 95% (Z>1.63, P<0.05) among $VAMW_{IC}$s of all the ICs for that single epoch, and 2) correlation between the spatial map and spatial template is above 95% (Z>1.63, P<0.05) for the spatial maps of all ICs. Data processed via 3-standard band filtering are not used in subsequent data reconstruction, but rather are used in conjunction with the dual-criteria only in the procedure "selecting" the pertinent ICs. Unselected columns, i.e., task-unrelated components, of mixing matrix $\mathbf{U}$ (Eq. (3)) are zeroed to produce a matrix $\hat{\mathbf{U}}$ such that task-related rhythmic signals are reconstructed by multiplying $\hat{\mathbf{U}}$ and $\mathbf{S}$ (Fig. 3). The reconstructed data in each trial are then filtered within a trial-specific frequency band to extract reactive beta activities.

Extraction of Single-Trial Post-Movement MEG Beta Synchronization in Normal and
Parkinson's Patient Using ICA-Based Spatiotemporal Approach

127

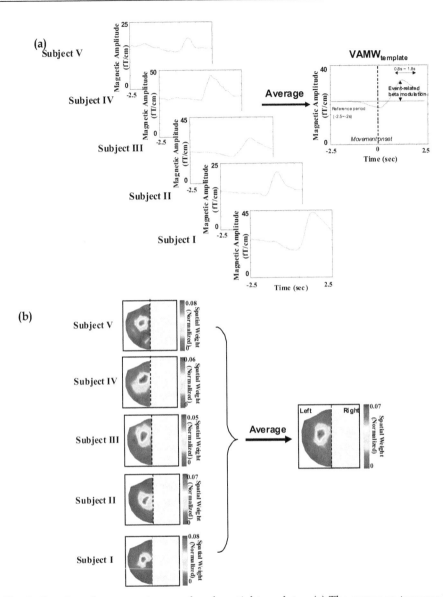

Fig. 2. Creation of common temporal and spatial templates. (a) The common temporal
template, VAMW$_{template}$, is created by averaging VAMWs (500 trials, 100 trials for each
subject, 5 subjects pooled). Event-related beta modulation is defined as the amplitude
difference between the mean amplitude of baseline activity (-2.5 to -2 s) and maximum
amplitude in the post-movement interval (0.8 to 1.8 s). (b) The common spatial template is
the average of the topographical distributions of event-related beta modulations of five
subjects from model generation group. Only the half the spatial map (unshaded)
contralateral to the side of finger lifting is used as the spatial template.

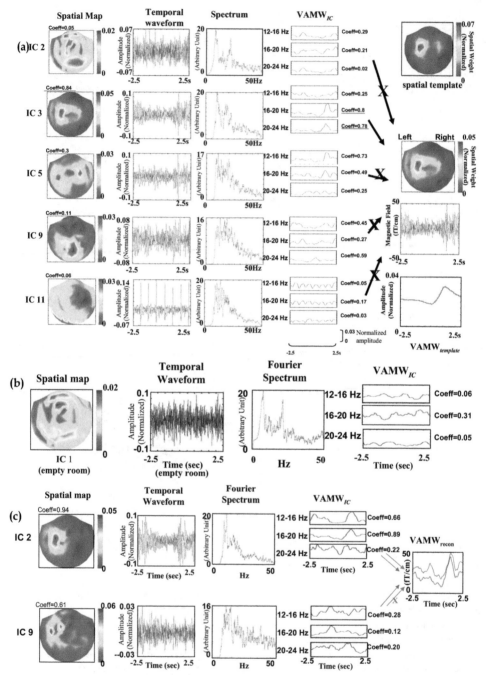

Fig. 3. Examples of IC-selection and signal reconstruction procedure. (a) Spatial maps, IC waveforms, Fourier spectra of IC waveforms and VAMW$_{ICs}$ of five ICs obtained from one

Extraction of Single-Trial Post-Movement MEG Beta Synchronization in Normal and
Parkinson's Patient Using ICA-Based Spatiotemporal Approach

129

single epoch by ICA. Only ICs fulfilling the dual criteria are selected for signal reconstruction. For example, IC 3 meets the dual criteria (underscored in red): i) correlation value between spatial map and spatial template is 0.84 (rank= 97%, Z= 1.89, P=0.03); ii) correlation value between 16-20Hz $VAMW_{IC}$ and 20-24 Hz $VAMW_{IC}$ with $VAMW_{template}$ is 0.8 (rank= 99%, Z=3.08, P=0.01) and 0.78 (rank= 97.8%, Z= 2.85, P=0.022), respectively. (b) Noise identification and removal. The deselected IC 2 in Fig. 2a may emanate from background noise since it resembles the IC 1 extracted from empty room measurement. (c) The impact of including task-unrelated IC into signal reconstruction. This figure illustrates (a different trial from Fig. 3a) that inclusion of task-unrelated IC (IC 9) with a high spatial correlation (correlation value=0.61, rank= 95.2%, Z=1.67, P=0.048) but poor temporal correlation (correlation value=0.28, rank=13%, Z=0.34, P=0.87) causes deterioration in the beta BR from 28.9 fT/cm (arrows and trace in red; IC9 eliminated from reconstruction) to 18.6 fT/cm (arrows and trace in blue; IC9 included for reconstruction).

2.3.5 Detection of task-laden trial-specific frequency band and extraction of reactive beta activities

The trial-specific frequency band detected in each trial is used to confine the reconstructed data within the most reactive beta band for further BR computation and source estimation. This frequency band is defined by the reactive beta band of the sensor site showing highest event-related beta modulation value (see creation of temporal template) over the nine SMI vicinal sensor sites (identified by SEF) and is identified using the aforementioned two-spectrum procedure which has been suggested as the best approach for the determination of reactive frequencies (Pfurtscheller & Lopes da Silva, 1999). Following data filtering with a trial-specific frequency band (zero-phase, tenth-order, IIR Butterworth filter), reactive beta activities in each single epoch can be extracted. The extracted reactive beta activities are then subjected to source estimation and beta rebound (BR) computations.

2.3.6 Calculation of $VAMW_{recon}$ of reactive beta activities and single-trial epoch selection using a nonparametric sign test

Movement-related beta rebound (BR) can be quantified from single-epoch reactive beta activities and $VAMW_{recon}$ (VAMW of reconstructed data) for reactive beta activity at each sensor site computed. The $VAMW_{recon}$ of highest event-related beta modulation (see creation of temporal template) among the nine sensor sites vicinal to SMI is designated as $VAMW_{recon\_max}$ and is used in turn for single-trial epoch selection and BR computation, as the sensor site expressing $VAMW_{recon\_max}$ did not change throughout the experiment in our observations. A deterministic procedure, modified from Brovelli's et al. (2002) approach, is used to select the significant trial. A nonparametric sign test is applied to the $VAMW_{recon\_max}$ designated for BR calculation in each single trial by computing the Z-score at each time point as $Z(t) = (N^+(t) - \frac{1}{2}N) / (\frac{1}{2}\sqrt{N})$, in which $N^+(t)$ denotes the number of trials whose magnitudes are larger than the median value of their baseline activities at time point t, and N the total number of trials. Time points with Z values greater than 3.09 (P<0.01) are defined as the time interval-of-interest (IOI). After the determination of IOI for each subject, another sign test is then applied to find epochs showing significant increases in amplitude (Z>1.63, P<0.05) using $Z_{IOI}(i) = (N_{IOI}^+(i) - \frac{1}{2}N_{IOI}) / (\frac{1}{2}\sqrt{N_{IOI}})$, in which $Z_{IOI}(i)$ is the Z value of the

i^{th} trial, $N_{IOI}^{+}(i)$ is the number of data points in post-movement IOI with values larger than the median of baseline activities of the ith trial, and N_{IOI} is the total number of time points in post-movement *IOI* (Brovelli et al., 2002). An example of single-trial epoch selection is given in Fig. 4 (Subject I). The first trial in Fig. 4 with a Z_{IOI} score equal to -4.53 is marked as an insignificant epoch and eliminated from further analysis.

2.3.7 Source estimation of the reactive beta activities

Source estimation of the MEG reactive beta activities was done using equivalent current dipole (ECD) analysis and minimum current estimation (MCE, Uutela et al., 1999; toolbox provided by Neuromag Ltd, Helsinki, Finland). A single dipole model was applied to explain the field every 1ms, and only dipoles showing goodness-of-fit (Jensen and Vanni, 2002) values higher than 80% were used for data explanation. In MCE, the lattice constant of the triangular grid was 10mm and locations closer than 30mm to the center of the conductor were excluded from current estimates. Both analyses used a realistic head model for each subject. Template generation and single-trial data processing procedure are schematized in Figs. 5a and 5b respectively. Epochs achieving significance in the increase of beta activities were chosen for subsequent BR calculation and dipole/source analysis.

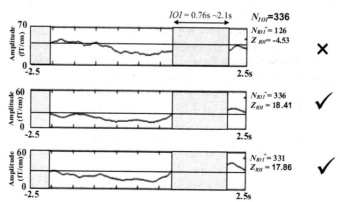

Fig. 4. Example of single-trial epoch selection based on a nonparametric sign test. Single-trial VAMW$_{recon\_max}$s of reconstructed data are examined through a nonparametric sign test. $Z_{IOI}(i)$ is the Z value of the ith trial, $N_{IOI}^{+}(i)$ is the number of data points in post-movement *IOI* with values larger than the median of baseline activities of the ith trial, and N_{IOI} is the total number of time points in post-movement *IOI*. Only epochs showing significant increase of beta activities are chosen for further analysis. The first trial with a Z_{IOI} score equal to -4.53 is marked as an insignificant epoch and eliminated from further analysis.

2.3.8 Validation of coupled common spatial and temporal templates for single-trial analysis

Since there are inevitably differences in head size and variations in head positions inside the MEG scanner among subjects, BR amplitude differences were compared using both individual spatial templates and the common spatial template. The use of a pair of common

Extraction of Single-Trial Post-Movement MEG Beta Synchronization in Normal and
Parkinson's Patient Using ICA-Based Spatiotemporal Approach

131

spatial and temporal templates for the extraction of individuals' neuromagnetic single-trial signals was further validated on one additional subject.

3. Results

Based on the known spatial location and temporal expression in terms of spatial and temporal templates, reactive beta activities were successfully extracted. Figure 3a shows that IC 3 meets the dual criteria: i) the correlation values between spatial map and spatial template is 0.84 (rank= 97%, Z= 1.89, P=0.03); ii) correlation values of 16-20Hz $VAMW_{IC}$ and 20-24 Hz $VAMW_{IC}$ vs. $VAMW_{template}$ are 0.8 (rank= 99%, Z=3.08, P=0.01) and 0.78 (rank= 97.8%, Z= 2.85, P=0.022), respectively. Fig. 3a illustrates that noise could also be identified and removed. IC2 in Fig. 3a correlates highly (=0.88) in spatial distribution with the IC1 extracted from empty room measurements (Fig. 3b), and is therefore rejected.

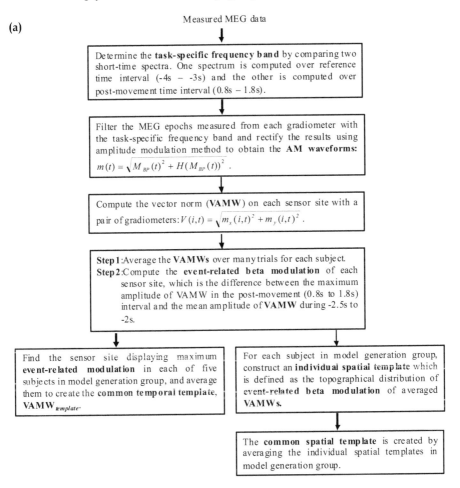

Fig. 5a. Flow chart for creation of common spatial and temporal templates.

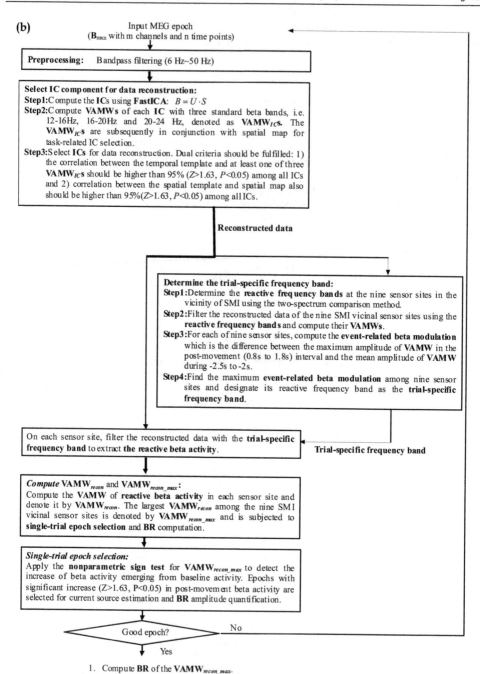

Fig. 5b. Flow chart for ICA-based single-trial analysis method.

Figure 6a depicts the single-trial VAMW$_{recon}$s of subject I filtered within the trial-specific frequency band (Fig. 6b). The conventional AM method on the average of 100 epochs reveals a bilateral post-movement rebound pattern with contralateral (left hemisphere) dominance, whereas the current ICA-based single-trial analysis (one hemisphere template) yields only activation (one trial) in the left hemisphere (Fig. 6a and 6c).

Epoch acceptance rates were 84% (65/78), 89% (83/91), 71% (60/85), 73% (68/93), and 87% (76/87), respectively for the model generation group and 81% (71/88) for the validation subject; the average for all six was 80.8%. The IOIs of significance were 0.76s - 2.1s, 0.66s - 1.5s, 0.8s - 1.75s, 0.46s - 1.49s, and 0.71s – 1.28s for the five subjects in the model generation group, and 0.88s – 1.67s for the validation subject. Averaged magnitude of BR was calculated from the reconstructed data on trials that survived the epoch-selection procedure.

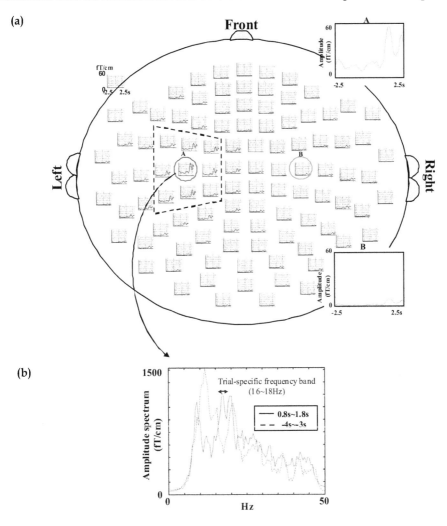

(c)

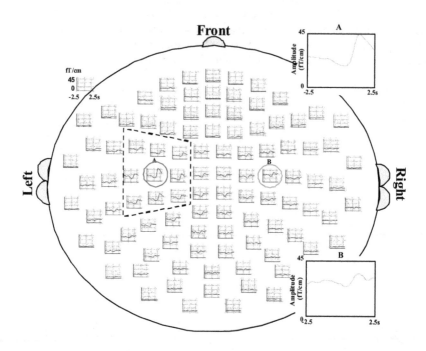

Fig. 6. Sensor-array display of VAMW$_{recon}$s and VAMWs. (a) One example of ICA single-trial VAMW$_{recon}$ of all sensor sites in subject I. The single-trial result shows only left sensorimotor area dominance of event-related activities, as the present study focuses on the area contralateral to movement side and only the left spatial template is used. The dashed trapezoid marks the nine SMI vicinal sensor sites and the VAMW$_{recon\_max}$ is marked with the red circle. (b) Trial-specific frequency band used for VAMW$_{recon}$s calculation in Fig. 6a. (c) VAMWs obtained from the conventional averaging method over 100 trials in subject I. This figure shows a bilateral beta rebound pattern with contralateral (left hemisphere) dominance.

The BR amplitudes computed from individual spatial templates were 20.9±7.1 (mean±sd), 18.1±10.3, 16.2±6.2, 23.2±10.89, and 6.2±2.7 for the first 5 subjects, respectively, and 27.6±11.1 fT/cm for the 6th subject (Table 1). Using the common spatial template, BR amplitudes were 21.1±7.97, 19.02±9.7, 15.5±5.3, 19.75±8.75, 5.91±3.2, and 27.1±10.2 fT/cm, respectively (Table 1). There was no significant difference between the results obtained with two approaches (p=0.88; unpaired two-tailed t test). BR amplitudes obtained with the conventional method of averaging on 100 trials were 18.2, 7.254, 12.92, 16.4, 2.9, and 23.12 fT/cm, respectively. Means for single-trial ICA-derived BRs, using either individual or common spatial templates, were significantly higher than those obtained using the conventional method of averaging (p<0.005; Matched-pair Wilcoxon test; Table 1). The comparisons of BR amplitude and task-specific frequency band between ICA-based single-trial and conventional methods are given in Table 1.

Extraction of Single-Trial Post-Movement MEG Beta Synchronization in Normal and
Parkinson's Patient Using ICA-Based Spatiotemporal Approach

135

The ICA-based single-trial approach shows remarkable latency jittering and inter-trial variability throughout the whole measurement process. Both factors can result in attenuation and smearing of averaged movement-related MEG responses. Figure 7a shows the raster plot of sixty-five normalized single-trial VAMW$_{recon\_max}$s which survived the

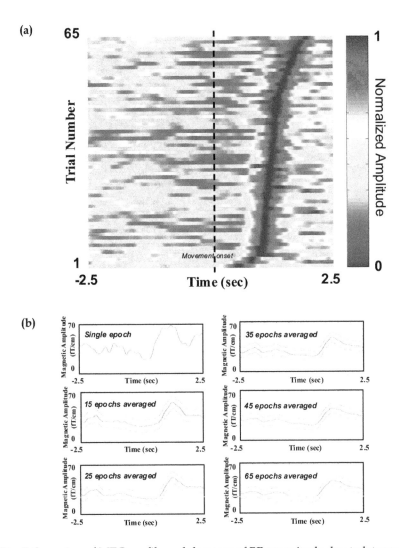

Fig. 7. Smearing of MEG profile and decrease of BR magnitude due to latency jittering. (a) Raster plot of normalized VAMW$_{recon\_max}$s as sorted by the latency measured between the time of peak beta rebound and the movement onset. Black dashed line indicates movement onset time. (b) Latency jittering resulting in a smearing of the MEG profile and a decrease of BR magnitude when more VAMW$_{recon\_max}$s are averaged, as is common in the conventional averaging method.

selection procedure for subject I, sorted by $VAMW_{recon\_max}$ peak latency as indexed to movement onset. The mean latency of peak beta rebound for the 65 trials was 1.41±0.43 s (mean±sd). With more epochs (random selection) averaged as with the conventional method of averaging, the averaged BR was attenuated (25.3, 24.6, 22.3, 21.5, 20.3 and 21.1 fT/cm for 1, 15, 25, 35, 45 and 65 trials averaged, respectively; values taken from the averaged $VAMW_{recon\_max}$s using common spatial template) and the time-activity plots smeared (Fig. 7b).

	ICA based single-trial method				Conventional AM method	
	BR amplitude (fT/cm)		Trial-specific frequency band (Hz)		BR amplitude	Task-specific
Subject index	Individual spatial template	Common spatial template	Individual spatial template	Common spatial template	(fT/cm)	frequency band (Hz)
I	20.9±7.1	21.1±7.97	16.67±2.77 ~ 21.22±2.44	15.57±3.21~ 22.17±3.3	18.2	15~21
II	18.1±10.3	19.02±9.7	18.04±2.62 ~ 22.18±3.12	17.92±2.3~ 21.9±2.72	7.25	17~20
III	16.2±6.2	15.5±5.3	16.2±1.89 ~ 20.49±2.3	16.8±23~ 20.91±2.22	12.92	15~19
IV	23.2±10.89	19.75±8.75	16.1±2.37 ~ 20.7±3.08	15.5±33~ 19.2±2.77	16.4	14~17
V	6.2±2.7	5.91±3.2	17.31±3.23 ~ 20.77±3.67	16.8±3.1~ 21.2±2.9	2.9	17~20
VI (validation)	27.6±11.1	27.1±10.2	16.32±2.83 ~ 19.94±2.68	16.81±2.72~ 20.14±3.1	23.12	16~20

Table 1. The comparison of BR amplitude and specific frequency bands for ICA-based single-trial and conventional methods.

Source estimation using ECD and MCE both showed a cluster of current sources centered (mean coordinates) in the anterior bank of the central sulcus (see Fig. 8e and 8f) on data points around the rebound peak of extracted reactive beta activities (see Fig. 8d, time interval between 1202ms – 1302ms of one single epoch of subject I). The ECD-located dipoles oscillate and span a sector. Furthermore, the center of MCE-estimated current sources (yellow dots) lies less than 2mm from the center of ECD-estimated dipoles (red dots) (see Fig. 8f). These results cross-verify the validity of the ICA-based single-trial method.

Figure 10 depicts the time-frequency plot of a normal subject and a Parkinson's disease patient at an MEG channel in the vicinity of left sensorimotor area. Clear suppression of post-movement ERS (red circle) and an attenuated ERD (yellow circle) are observed in the Parkinson's disease patient. The VAMWs was significantly larger both in alpha band and beta band in the normal subject than in the Parkinson's patient. These imply the slowed and reduced recovery after motor act may impede cortical preparation of the next movement.

Extraction of Single-Trial Post-Movement MEG Beta Synchronization in Normal and
Parkinson's Patient Using ICA-Based Spatiotemporal Approach

137

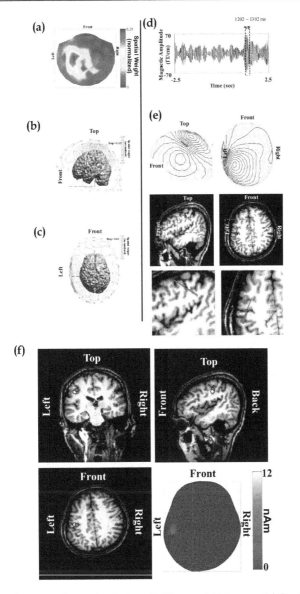

Fig. 8. Overlay of extracted reactive beta activities on MR image. (a) Spatial map

reconstructed using $\vec{x}_{recon} = \sum_{j=1}^{k} \vec{x}_j$ (see Method Section). (b) and (c): Different views of

superposition of the isocontour spatial map on the segmented MRI brain. (d) Representative
trace of reconstructed reactive beta activities in the vicinity of SMI. (e) Upper panels are
isocontour maps of reconstructed neuromagnetic signals at 1202 ms post movement. Lower
panels show that all dipoles (from 1202 to 1302 ms after movement onset as box-framed in

(d)) are located in the primary motor area and oscillate accordingly. (f) The center of the MCE-estimated current sources (yellow dot) overlays the source location determined using the equivalent current dipole method (ECD) (red dot). Upper-left panel: coronal view. Upper-right panel: sagittal view. Lower-left panel: axial view. Lower-right panel: distribution of MCE estimated current sources.

Examining the single-trial variability using the proposed ICA-based method (Fig. 11), subtle dynamics of the beta rhythmic activities can be further studied. Figure 11 shows the ongoing trial-by-trial variabilities in amplitudes and latencies over 60 ICA de-noised post-movement ERS trials. With the utilization of ICA-based single-trial analysis, it is possible to investigate the reasoning of ERS vanishment is due to suppression of post-movement beta rebound in each single-trial, rather than the cause of temporal jittering and/or loss of synchronization. Even though the patient could perform lifting behavior well, his neuron activities show distinct sensorimotor patterns from normal subject, regardless of movement performance.

4. Discussion

The movement-related oscillatory modulations (ERD/ERS of alpha, beta and gamma) have been reported to be spatially extended (Babiloni et al., 1999; Crone et al., 1998a; Crone et al., 1998b; Leocani et al., 1997; Neuper and Pfurtscheller, 2001; Salmelin and Hari, 1994a; Taniguchi et al., 2000; van Burik et al., 1998). Source localizations using conventional filtering have also been reported to disperse among several regions (Salmelin & Hari, 1994a). However, our results strongly indicate that proper treatment when trial-by-trial dynamics can be accounted for yields clustered localizations congruent to neuroanatomical representations.

The present ICA-based spatiotemporal approach for single-trial analysis study is dedicated to the extraction of neuromagnetic measurements of event-related beta oscillatory activities. One distinct feature of the current ICA-based method as compared with other single-trial approaches (Guger et al., 2000; Ioannides et al., 1993; Jung et al., 2001) is the simultaneous use of a spatial template and a temporal template for component selection. The spatial template provides a priori spatial information for brain signals, while the temporal template contains temporal characteristics of event-related responses. Using the paired criteria for component selection, identification specificity of task-related components for signal reconstruction is significantly improved. As shown in Fig. 3c, the inclusion of IC 9 with high spatial correlation (correlation value=0.61, rank= 95.2%, Z=1.67, P=0.048) but devoid of temporal congruence (correlation value =0.28, rank=13%, Z=0.34, P=0.87) causes beta BR to deteriorate from 28.9 fT/cm (red curve) to 18.6 fT/cm (blue curve). The ICA-preprocessed dataset yields cleaner field maps (Fig. 9a), which result in circumscribed localizations (Figs. 9b-9c and 9e-9f., Salmelin and Hari, 1994a).

Significantly, the current method also makes possible the analysis of the reactive frequency band for every single trial once task-related rhythmic activities are extracted. The conventional method discounts this subtle but potentially important information. Notwithstanding, the idea of using a fixed window for signal filtering is neurophysiologically not optimal. We emphasize the precise identification of reactive trial-specific frequencies for BR calculation, since task-related frequency modulation might exist in one or multiple bands (Pfurtscheller & Lopes da Silva, 1999). The three-standard frequency band procedure is used for generation of $VAMW_{ICS}$ to recover all possible task-related information and is followed by a two short-time spectra

Extraction of Single-Trial Post-Movement MEG Beta Synchronization in Normal and
Parkinson's Patient Using ICA-Based Spatiotemporal Approach

139

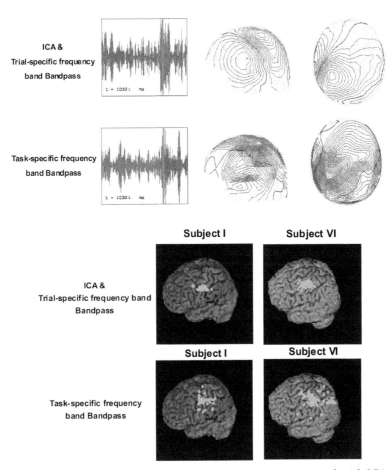

Fig. 9. Comparisons of magnetic fields and source locations preprocessed with ICA-bandpass trial specific (upper panel) and task-specific bandpass filtering (lower panel). (a) Neuromagnetic field maps. Data preprocessed with ICA-trial specific bandpass filter (15.57±3.21~22.17±3.3 Hz) gives a much less noisy neuromagnetic field pattern than that processed with the task-specific bandpass filtering method (15~21 Hz) (Pfurtscheller et al. 1999). Black vertical lines in the tracings of the left column denote time points of the corresponding field maps in the right column. (b) Source localizations by ECD model. Only dipoles in post-movement IOI (interval-of-interest) with goodness-of-fit higher than 80% are accepted. The one with highest goodness-of-fit value out of each trial is rendered onto the subjects' 3D MRI surfaces. The estimated source positions preprocessed by ICA-bandpass filtering (upper panel) are (x, y, z)= (-45±4.45, -3.9±6.33, 80.7±3.63mm; goodness-of-fit= 97.5±3.7%) in subject I (65 trials) and (x, y, z)=(-35.3±3.5, 5.7±6.02, 88.7±5.61mm; goodness-of-fit= 96.9±3.7%) in subject VI (71 trials), whereas task specific bandpass filtering (lower panel) yields (x, y, z)=(-46.3±11.6, -9.99±10.3, 84.51±6.7; goodness-of-fit=89.7±3.4%) in subject I (65 trials) and (x, y, z)=(-31.8±8.13, 0.5±14.01, 87.9±12.54mm; goodness-of-fit=87.2±4.5%) in subject VI (71 trials), respectively. The ICA-trial specific bandpass procedure yields better

results in terms of much focused source locations and higher goodness-of-fit. x, y, and z denote the dipole location in the head coordinate system as anchored by the HPI (head position indicator) coils. The x-axis passes through the preauricular points, pointing to the right; the positive y-axis traverses the nasion and is normal to the x-axis; the positive z-axis points upward and normal to the xy-plane.

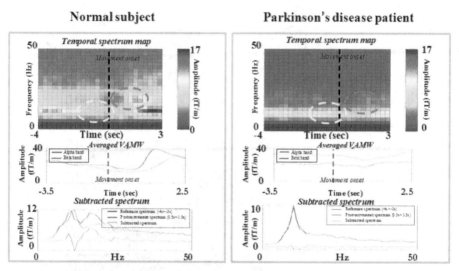

Fig. 10. The comparion of neural activity via time-frequency, VAMW and spectrum analysis obtained from one normal subject and a parkinson's disease patient. The ensemble averaging results reflect the ERD attenuation (yellow circle) and the ERS disappearance (red circle) in the pakinson's patient.

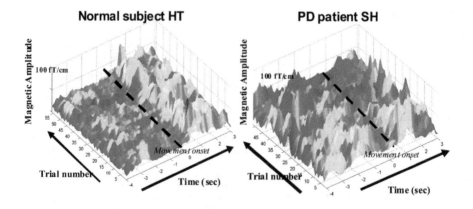

Fig. 11. Trial-by-trial comparison of VAMWs could be performed via the proposed ICA-based approach between the normal subject and the Parkinson's disease patient.

Extraction of Single-Trial Post-Movement MEG Beta Synchronization in Normal and
Parkinson's Patient Using ICA-Based Spatiotemporal Approach

141

comparison procedure (Pfurtscheller & Lopes da Silva, 1999) for the identification of the optimal reactive trial-specific frequency band in the reconstructed epochs. The present approach not only extracts the specific reactive frequencies but also retains phase information on a trial-by-trial basis. The trial-specific frequency band of post-movement beta modulation anchors mainly (~85% of all trials) in the lower beta band (16Hz~20Hz) and less frequently (~15%) in the higher beta band (20~24Hz). Great variation of BR values is also seen, as reflected in large SD (Table 1). The revealed trial-by-trial dynamics provide a possibility for future profound study of subtle brain dynamics.

It is noteworthy that not all the data reconstructed from the selected ICs survives the statistical threshold. We have carefully monitored online and thoroughly checked offline the EMG measurements in terms of EMG onset (p=0.61, unpaired two-tailed t- test), termination (p=0.53, unpaired two-tailed t-test) and the EMG duration (p=0.573, unpaired two-tailed t-test) during finger lifting between significant and insignificant trials as indexed to the movement registration by the optic pad (Abbink et al., 1998). The data indicate an absence of prominent behavioral difference commensurate to the differential neuromagnetic responses. Some epochs with a fluctuating baseline, e.g., non-task-related spontaneous bursts of beta oscillatory activities, may manifest high baseline activity, which in turn results in a decrease in BR readout leading to exclusion after statistical manipulation (Fig 4). It has been suggested that baseline spontaneous activities may carry important information relevant to attention level, wakefulness, task difficulty, etc. (Buser & Rougeul-Buser, 1999; Sterman, 1999). The jittering of the neuromagnetic beta ERS is likewise interesting and may be also physiological. A zero-phase Butterworth filter was used to bandpass filter the raw data. The symmetric property of the zero-phase filter means that processed signals have precisely zero phase distortion and therefore no time shift of peak beta rebound was introduced. Hence, fluctuations of significance level and the jittering of central processing despite similar behavioral performance may be ascribed to the subject's variant cognitive states or the degree of training (Buser & Rougeul-Buser, 1999; Sterman, 1999; Flotzinger et al., 1992; Wolpaw et al., 1994; Bastiaansen et al., 2001; Bastiaansen et al., 1999; Earle, 1988; Haig et al., 1995; Hoffman et al., 1991; Yabe et al., 1993). The exploration of underlying mechanisms mandates more meticulous designs in the future. Using the conventional method of averaging, certain diseases, such as Parkinson's and Unverricht-Lundborg myoclonic epilepsy, have been observed to show either attenuated, prolonged or abolished ERS responses (Silen et al., 2000; Tamas et al., 2003). Such cases can be further examined using the current ICA-based single-trial method for the time course and trial-by-trial dynamics to disclose hitherto unexplored mechanisms underlying these phenomena.

A concern with any data driven method is that prominent artifacts or noise can be intermingled with task-specific information (Ermer et al., 2000; Lins et al., 1993a; Lins et al., 1993b). However, previous ICA reports (Makeig et al., 2002; Mckeown & Radtke, 2001) indicate that brain rhythmic signals generated from different sources usually have their own oscillatory frequencies with distinct phases and are located in specific brain regions with patterns that are distinct from artifacts or noise (see also Fig. 3). This endorses the feasibility of using ICA to separate targeted rhythmic signals from irrelevant ones. The high epoch-acceptance rate (~80%) can be attributed to an improved SNR as compared to other studies on single-trial approaches to sensorimotor oscillatory activities (Brovelli et al., 2002; Wolpaw and McFarland, 1994). For instance, the spatial map of IC2 in Fig. 2a correlates highly (0.88) with the spatial map of IC1 from empty room measurement as shown in Fig. 3b; this suggests that the neuromagnetic signal IC2, deselected for subsequent processing, can be accounted for by background noise in the shielding room. IC11 in Fig. 3a has a stationary cycle around 1.2 Hz, and its spatial map has higher weights at the outer rim of the MEG sensor array, which suggests a plausible connection with cardiac cycles. It was also observed (Fig. 3) that rhythmic activities in left and right SMIs as well as the occipital areas could be extracted into separate ICs that can be reminiscent of various mechanisms and time courses of different brain oscillatory activities (Pfurtscheller & Lopes da Silva, 1999; Pfurtscheller et al., 1997; Pfurtscheller et al., 1998b; Stancak and Pfurtscheller, 1996a; Stancak & Pfurtscheller, 1996b; Andrew & Pfurtscheller, 1999).

Since most task irrelevant signals, e.g., internal and external noises, can be removed by proper de-selection of ICs, it is possible to reconstitute the representative spatial map of all

contributing ICs using $\bar{x}_{recon} = \sum_{j=1}^{k} \bar{x}_j$, in which $\bar{x}_{recon}$ is the reconstructed spatial map, k is the

number of selected ICs and $\bar{x}_i$ is the spatial map of the ith selected IC in Fig. (4) (Fig. 8a).

This spatial map of reconstructed signals, which is a topographical distribution of weighting factors on the sensor array, can be overlaid with the segmented MRI brain (Fig. 8b & 8c; ASA program, ANT Software, Dutch). The highest weight is shown to project over the SMI area, which demonstrates that the high SNR of the ICA-extracted rhythmic activities of each trial has made possible the use on single-trial data of source estimation methods that require high SNR on input data for processing, e.g., the equivalent current dipole technique (ECD), minimum current estimation (MCE), and minimum norm estimation (MNE) (Delorme et al., 2001; Delorme et al., 2002; Jung et al., 2001; Makeig et al., 1997; Mckeown et al., 2001). Conventionally, these estimation methods exploit averaged data out of a large amount of trials.

Another reason why the intricate phase-unlocked signal can be preserved is the fact that no averaging procedure is needed; such a procedure would otherwise inherently distort the embedded information. Accordingly, as shown in Fig. 8d, source modeling with a moving dipole on a msec by msec basis on the reconstructed oscillatory beta signals during the rebound period (Brovelli et al., 2002) of a single-trial epoch results in a focused clustering of dipole foci at the pre-central area, i.e., the primary motor cortex (Fig. 8e). Figure 8 shows the result of MCE modeling (Uutela et al, 1999), where the center of MCE-estimated current sources (yellow dot) is very close (< 2mm distance) to the dipole location as estimated using the ECD approach (red dot).

It can be argued that one can first localize the generator area and then build a spatial filter for extracting single-trial data so that the subsequent analysis can be conducted on the source level instead of the sensor level. One premise and justification of using a source-area-generated spatial filter is that the source area can be precisely localized for the generation of a spatial filter (Tesche et al., 1995). The very first step is to filter the signals to obtain a presupposed reactive frequency band. However, using conventional simple filtering techniques, ambient noise with ~20Hz components cannot be optimally removed, and this will cause localization uncertainty for the probed sources (Fig 9). However, ICA pre-processing decomposes the compound neuromagnetic signals into various independent task-related and task-unrelated/noise components so that ~20Hz activities not related to the a priori spatiotemporal profile will not confound the selected ones. Furthermore, our ICA-based method differs from other spatial filtering techniques, e.g., signal space projection (SSP) which is a fixed spatial filter for signal extraction (Tesche et al., 1995). The ICA-based method blindly decomposes the MEG epochs (B) into a spatially distributed map (U) multiplied by temporal signals (S), i.e. $B=U \cdot S$, on the basis of independency among sources (Vigario & Oja, 2000), whereas SSP mandates a pre-defined spatial filter (U_{-sf}) for recovering signals (S), i.e. $S=U_{-sf}^+ \cdot B$, where + denotes pseudo inverse, based on orthogonal projection. When ambient noise and the spatial filter are not mutually orthogonal, the SSP has difficulty in resolving the two. Subsequent application of ICA following SSP does not ensure finer signal extraction or further noise removal since the data recovered from SSP are already linear mixtures of components out of a pre-defined spatial filter, which is a constraint drag on the optimal performance of ICA designed for blind decomposition.

Left and right sensorimotor rhythms can be decomposed into two distinct ICs (IC3 and IC5 in Fig. 3), implying possible independent modulatory mechanisms between the two hemispheres. This view is corroborated by an event-related coherence study (Andrew and Pfurtscheller, 1999) that reports a lack of interhemispheric coherence in human post-movement beta activities. Movement-related beta oscillatory activities of the right hemisphere can be extracted in the same way using spatial and temporal templates for right sensorimotor rhythm. The source locations for extracted right hemispheric beta activities were mainly in the right premotor area (data not shown), which agrees with previous studies (Brovelli et al., 2002; Ilmoniemi, R. J., 1991). Event-related beta activities in SMA and posterior parietal cortical areas (Brovelli et al., 2002; Joliot et al., 1999) are not observed in our data, possibly due to the fact that the contributing sources here are radial in orientation and thus could not be optimally detected by MEG (Salmelin and Hari, 1994b).

The agreement between the values of BR amplitude obtained with the common spatial/temporal templates and the individually generated ones (Table 1) promises a flexibility in both experimental design and analytical strategy. The proposed ICA-based spatiotemporal approach for single trial analysis can also be applied on fewer trials (Fig 7b), which is a great advantage over conventional methods. Given meticulous head positioning (see above the Method Section), common spatial and temporal templates can be used to extract pertinent movement-related neuromagnetic signals from subjects, which may shorten the overall time needed to run an experiment. We have no preference for the use of a grand averaged template over individual ones. On the contrary, the use of an individual template is suggested for any profound individual–based ERD/ERS study. However, the feasibility of using a grand averaged template provides an effective alternative in cases where lengthy procedures cannot be endured by the participants. This is particularly true for clinical settings where patients have attention problems or are incapable of sustaining long experiments so that individual templates cannot be optimally obtained. Nevertheless, caution should be exercised when applying the current ICA-based single-trial method for clinical studies. For patients whose heads cannot be properly positioned in the center of the MEG helmet, the use of a common spatial template may fail, making a customized individual spatial template mandatory for IC selection. For patients whose motor performance deviates significantly from normal, e.g., victims of motor stroke or severe movement disorders, the use of the common temporal template might not be justified since the time courses of event-related brain activities may be significantly altered due to primary deficit or secondary plasticity. Accordingly, in such situations, an individual spatial template can be applied without a temporal template as an aid to component selection. Our future investigations will combine the current dual-template approach with a source estimation method so that a spatial filter of better precision and higher dimensions can be designed, which will make possible sophisticated analysis on the source level instead of the sensor level, eliminating the positioning problem.

Degeneration of the dopaminergic neurons in substania nigra pars compacta (SNc) in Parkinson's patients result in abnormal projection in thalamo-cortical pathway which causes an abnormal projection from thalamus to supplementary motor area (SMA). Pfurtscheller et al. (1998) also have demonstrated that Parkinson's patients have delayed ERD and abolished post-movement ERS and speculated there is dysfunction in subcortico-cortical connections in Parkinson's patients. In this study, we analyzed post-movement ERS in one Parkinson's patient. The present ICA-based approach may be helpful for disclosing the mechanism of movement-related brain rhythms which could be used as a clinical index for diagnosing Parkinson's patients.

5. Conclusions

The present novel ICA-based spatiotemporal approach for single trial analysis features a paired-template matching for stringent component selection. The spatial template provides a priori spatial information for targeted brain signals while the temporal template contains temporal characteristics of event-related responses. The method promises not only a high extraction rate of post-movement beta synchronization but also better localization of the corresponding sources. Various source modeling methods commanding high SNR can now be applied to single trial data as extracted using the ICA-spatiotemporal procedure. Our method takes into account subtle trial-by-trial dynamics. The reconstructed MEG brain signals per trial unravel the temporal information and inter-trial variations of reactive oscillatory activities, which in turn may shed light on the subtle dynamics of brain processing. The embodied common template approach permits an effective alternative in cases where lengthy procedures cannot be endured by the participants or in clinical settings where patients have attention problems or are incapable of sustaining long experiments.

6. Acknowledgment

This study was funded by the National Central University, Center for Dynamical Biomarkers and Translational Medicine (99-2911-1-008-100), National Science Council (99-2628- E-008-003, 99-2628- E-008-012, 100-2628-E-008-013, 100-2628-E-008-001, 100-2613-E-008-006-D), and Veterans General Hospital University System of Taiwan Joint Research Program (VGHUST96-P4-15, VGHUST97-P3-11, VGHUST98-98- P3-09).

7. References

Andrew, C. & Pfurtscheller G. (1995). Event-related coherence during finger movement: a pilot study, *Biomedizinische Technik*, Vol. 40, pp. 326-332.

Andrew, C. & Pfurtscheller, G. (1999). Lack of bilateral coherence of post-movement central beta oscillations in the human electroencephalography, *Neuroscience letters*, Vol. 273, pp. 82-89.

Bastiaansen, M. C. M.; Bocker, K. B. E.; Cluitmans, P. J. M. & Brunia, C. H. M. (1999). Event-related desynchronization related to the anticipation of a stimulus providing knowledge of results, *Clinical Neurophysiology*, Vol. 110, pp. 250-260.

Bastiaansen, M. C. M.; Bocker, K. B. E. & Brunia, C. H. M. (2001). Event-related
    desynchronization during anticipatory attention for an upcoming stimulus: a
    comparative EEG/MEG study, *Clinical Neurophysiology*, Vol. 112, pp. 393-403.
Brovelli, A.; Battaglini, P. P.; Naranjo, J. R. & Budai, R. (2002). Medium-range oscillatory
    network and the 20-Hz sensorimotor induced potential, *Neuroimage*, Vol. 16, pp.
    130-141.
Buser, P. & Rougeul-Buser A. (1999). EEG synchronization in cat, monkey and human
    during attentive states: a brief survey, In: *Event-related desynchronization. Handbook of
    electroencephalography and clinical neurophysiology*, G. Pfurtscheller & F. H. Lopes da
    Silva, 13-32, Elsevier, Amsterdam.
Clochon, P.; Fontbonne, J. M. & Etevenon, P. (1996). A new method for quantifying EEG
    event-related   desynchronization: amplitude   envelope   analysis,
    Electroencephalography and Clinical Neurophysiology, Vol. 98, pp. 126-129.
Delorme, A.; Makeig, S.; Fabre-Thorpe, M. & Sejnowske, T. 2001. From single-trial EEG to
    Brain Area dynamics, *Neurocomputing*, Vol. 44, pp. 1057-1064.
Delorme, A. & Makeig, S. (2003). EEG changes accompanying learned regulation of 12-Hz
    EEG activity, *IEEE transactions on rehabilitation engineering*, Vol. 11, pp. 133-137.
Earle, J. B. (1988). Task difficulty and EEG alpha asymmetry: an amplitude and frequency
    analysis, *Neuropsychobiology*, Vol. 20, pp. 95-112.
Ermer, J. J.; Mosher, J. C.; Huang, M. & Leahy, R. M. (2000). Paired MEG data set source
    localization using recursively applied and projected (RAP) MUSIC, *IEEE
    Transactions on Biomedical Engineering*, Vol. 47, pp. 1248-1260.
Florian, G. & Pfurtscheller, G. (1995). Dynamic spectral analysis of event-related EEG data,
    Electroencephalography and Clinical Neurophysiology, Vol. 95, pp. 393-396.
Flotzinger, D.; Kalcher, J. & Pfurtscheller, G. (1992). EEG classification by learning vector
    quantization, *Biomedizinische Technik*, Vol. 37, pp. 303-309.
Guger, C.; Ramoser, H. & Pfurtscheller, G. (2000). Real-time EEG analysis with subject-
    specific spatial patterns for a brain-computer interface (BCI). *IEEE Transactions on
    Rehabilitation Engineering*, Vol. 8, pp. 447-456.
Haig, A. R.; Gordon, E.; Rogers, G., & Anderson, J. (1995). Classification of single-trial ERP
    sub-types: application of globally optimal vector quantization using simulated
    annealing, *Electroencephalography and Clinical Neurophysiology*, Vol. 94, pp. 288-297.
Hoffman, R. E.; Buchsbaum, M. S.; Escobar, M. D.; Makuch, R. W.; Nuechterlein, K. H. &
    Guich, S. M. (1991). EEG coherence of prefrontal areas in normal and schizophrenic
    males during perceptual activation, *Journal of Neuropsychiatry and Clinical
    Neurosciences*, Vol. 3, pp. 169-175.
Hyvarinen, A.; Karhunen, J. & Oja, E. (2001). *Independent component analysis*. John Wiley and
    Sons, New York.
Hyvarinen, A & Oja, E. (1997). A fast fixed-point algorithm for independent component
    analysis, *Neural Computation*, Vol. 9, pp. 1483-1492.
Ilmoniemi, R. J. (1991). Estimates of neuronal current distributions, *Acta Otolaryngol*, Vol.
    49(Suppl.), pp. 80–87.
Ioannides, A. A.; Singh, K. D.; Hasson, R.; Baumann, S. B.; Rogers, R. L.; Guinto, F. C. &
    Papanicolaou, A. C. (1993). Comparison of current dipole and magnetic field
    tomography analyses of the cortical response to auditory stimuli, *Brain Topography*,
    Vol. 6, pp. 27-34.

Jensen, O. & Vanni, S. (2002). A new method to identify multiple sources of oscillatory activity from magnetoencephalographic data, *Neuroimage*, Vol. 15, pp. 568-574.

Joliot, M.; Papathanassiou, D.; Mellet, E.; Quinton, O.; Mazoyer, N.; Courtheoux, P. & Mazoyer, B. (1999). FMRI and PET of self-paced finger movement: comparison of intersubject stereotaxic averaged data, *Neuroimage*, Vol. 10, pp. 430-447.

Jung, T. P.; Makeig, S.; Westerfield, M.; Townsend, J.; Courchesne,E. & Sejnowski, J. T. (2001). Analysis and Visualization of Single-Trial Event-Related Potentials, *Human Brain Mapping*, Vol. 14, pp. 166-185.

Kajola, M.; Ahonen, A.; Hamalainen, M. S.; Knuutila, J.; Lounasmaa, O. V.; Simola, J. & Vilkman, V. (1991). Development of multichannel neuromagnetic instrumentation in Finland, *Clinical Physics & Physiological Measurement*, Vol. 12, pp. 39-44.

Kao, Y. H.; Guo, W. Y.; Wu, Y. T.; Liu, K. C.; Chai, W. Y.; Lin,C. Y.; Hwang, Y. H.; Liou, A. J. K.; Cheng, H. C.; Yeh, T. C.; Hsieh, J. C. & Teng, M. M. H. (2003). Hemodynamic segmentation of MR brain perfusion images using independent component, thresholding and Bayesian estimation, *Magnetic Resonance in Medicine*, Vol. 49, pp. 885-894.

Kalcher, J. & Pfurtscheller, G. (1995). Discrimination between phase-locked and non-phase-locked event-related EEG activity, *Electroencephalography and Clinical Neurophysiology*, Vol. 94, pp. 381-384.

Klimesch, W.; Russegger, H.; Doppelmayr, M. & Pachinger, T. (1998). A method for the calculation of induced band power: implications for the significance of brain oscillation, *Electroencephalography and Clinical Neurophysiology*, Vol. 108, pp. 123-130.

Leocani, L.; Manganotti, C. T.; Zhuang, P. & Hallett, M. (1997). Event-related coherence and event-related desynchronization/synchronization in the 10 Hz and 20 Hz EEG during self-paced movements, *Electroencephalography and clinical neurophysiology*, Vol. 103, pp. 199-206.

Lins, O. G.; Picton, T. W.; Berg, P. & Scherg, M. (1993a). Ocular artifacts in EEG and event-reated potentials. I. Scalp topography, *Brain Topography*, Vol. 6, pp. 51-63.

Lins, O. G.; Picton, T. W.; Berg,P. & Scherg, M. (1993b). Ocular artifacts in recording EEGs and event-related potentials. II. Source dipoles and source components, *Brain Topography*, Vol. 6, pp. 65-78.

Lopes da Silva, F. H. (1991). Neural mechanisms underlying brain waves: from neural membranes to networks, *Electroencephalography and Clinical Neurophysiology*, Vol. 79, pp. 81-93.

Lopes da Silva, F. H. (1996). The generation of electric and magnetic signals of the brain by local networks, *Comprehensive human physiology*, Vol. 1, pp. 509-531.

Makeig, S.; Jung, T. P.; Bell, A. J.; Ghahremani, D. & Sejnowski, T. (1997). Blind separation of auditory event-related brain responses into independent components, *Proceedings of the National Academy of Sciences of the United States of America*, Vol. 94, pp. 10979-10984.

McKeown, M. J.; Makeig, S.; Brown. G. G.; Jung. T. P.; Kindermann. S. S.; Bell. A. J & Sejnowski, T. J. (1998). Analysis of fMRI data by blind separation into independent spatial components, *Human Brain Mapping*, Vol. 6, pp. 160-188.

Mckeown, M. & Radtke, R. (2001). Phasic and tonic coupling between EEG and EMG demonstrated with independent component analysis, *Journal of clinical neurophysiology*, Vol. 18, pp. 45-57.

Mosher, J. C.; Lewis, P. S. & Leahy, R. M. (1992). Multiple dipole modeling and localization from spatio-temporal MEG data, *IEEE Transactions on Biomedical Engineering*, Vol. 39, pp. 541-557.

Muller-Gerking, J.; Pfurtscheller, G. & Flyvbjerg, H. (1999). Designing optimal spatial filters for single-trial EEG classification in a movement task, *Clinical Neurophysiology*, Vol. 110, pp. 787-798.

Pfurtscheller, G. & Aranibar A. 1(977). Event-related cortical desynchronization detected by power measurements of scalp EEG, *Electroencephalography and Clinical Neurophysiology*, Vol. 42, pp. 817-826.

Pfurtscheller, G. & Aranibar A. (1979a). Evaluation of event-related desynchronization (ERD) preceding and following voluntary self-paced movement, *Electroencephalography and Clinical Neurophysiology*, Vol. 46, pp. 138-146.

Pfurtscheller, G. & Aranibar A. (1979b). Evaluation of event-related desynchronization (ERD) preceding and following voluntary self-paced movements, *Electroencephalography and Clinical Neurophysiology*, Vol. 46, pp. 138-146.

Pfurtscheller, G. (1981). Central beta rhythm during sensorimotor activities in man, *Electroencephalography and Clinical Neurophysiology*, Vol. 51, pp. 253-264.

Pfurtscheller, G. & Berghold, A. (1989). Patterns of cortical activation during planning of voluntary movement, *Electroencephalography and Clinical Neurophysiology*, Vol. 72, pp. 250-258.

Pfurtscheller, G.; Pregenzer M. & Neuper C. (1994). Visualization of sensorimotor areas involved in preparation for hand movement based on classification of alpha and central beta rhythms in single EEG trials in man, *Neuroscience Letters*, Vol. 181, pp. 43-46.

Pfurtscheller, G.; Stancak A., Jr. & Neuper C. (1996). Post-movement beta synchronization: a correlate of an idling motor area?, *Electroencephalography and Clinical Neurophysiology*, Vol. 98, pp. 281-293.

Pfurtscheller, G.; Neuper C.; Flotzinger D. & Pregenzer M. (1997). EEG-based discrimination between imagination of right and left hand movement, *Electroencephalography and Clinical Neurophysiology*, Vol. 103, pp. 642-651.

Pfurtscheller, G.; Pichler-Zalaudek K.; Ortmayr B.; Diez J. & Reisecker F. (1998a). Postmovement beta synchronization in patients with Parkinson's disease, *Journal of Clinical Neurophysiology*, Vol. 15, pp. 243-250.

Pfurtscheller, G.; Zalaudek K. & Neuper C. (1998b). Event-related beta synchronization after wrist, finger and thumb movement, *Electroencephalography and Clinical Neurophysiology*, Vol. 109, pp. 154-160.

Pfurtscheller, G. & Lopes da Silva F. H. (1999). Event-related EEG/MEG synchronization and desynchronization: basic principles, *Clinical Neurophysiology*, Vol. 110, pp. 1842-1857.

Rosell, J.; Casanas, R. & Scharfetter H. (2001). Sensitivity maps and system requirements for magnetic induction tomography using a plannar gradiometer, *Physiological Measurement*, Vol. 22, pp. 121-130.

Salmelin, R. & Hari, R. (1994a). Characterization of spontaneous MEG rhythms in healthy adults, *Electroencephalography and Clinical Neurophysiology*, Vol. 91, pp. 237-248.

Salmelin, R. & Hari, R. (1994b). Spatiotemporal characteristics of sensorimotor neuromagnetic rhythms related to thumb movement, *Neuroscience*, Vol. 60, pp. 537-550.

Salmelin, R.; Hamalainen, M.; Kajola, M. & Hari, R. (1995). Functional segregation of movement-related rhythmic activity in the human brain, *Neuroimage*, Vol. 2, pp. 237-243.

Silen T.; Forss, N.; Jensen, O. & Hari, R. (2000). Abnormal Reactivity of the ~20-Hz Motor Cortex Rhythm in Unverricht Lundborg Type Progressive Myoclonus Epilepsy, *Neuroimage*, Vol. 12, pp. 707-712.

Stancak, A. Jr. & Pfurtscheller G. (1996a). The effects of handedness and type of movement on the contralateral preponderance of mu-rhythm desynchronization, *Electroencephalography and Clinical Neurophysiology*, Vol. 99, pp. 174-182.

Stancak, A. Jr. & Pfurtscheller G. (1996b). Mu-rhythm changes in brisk and slow self-paced finger movements, *Neuroreport*, Vol. 7, pp. 1161-1164.

Sterman, M. B. (1999). Event-related EEG response correlates of task difficulty, sleep deprivation and sensory distraction, In: *Event-related desynchronization. Handbook of electroencephalography and clinical neurophysiology*. G. Pfurtscheller & F. H. Lopes da Silva, 233-242, Elsevier, Amsterdam.

Tamas, G.; Szirmai, I.; Palvolgyi, L.; Takats, A. & Kamondi, A. (2003). Impairment of post-movement beta synchronization in parkinson's disease is related to laterality of tremor, *Clinical Neurophysiology*, Vol. 114, pp. 614-623.

Tang, A. C.; Pearlmutter, B. A.; Malaszenko, N. A. & Phung, D. B. (2002). Independent components of magnetoencephalography: single-trial response onset times, *Neuroimage*, Vol. 17, pp. 1773-1789.

Taniguchi, M.; Kato, A.; Fujita, N.; Hirata, M.; Tanaka, H.; Kihara, T.; Ninomiya, H.; Hirabuki, N.; Nakamura, H.; Robinson, S. E.; Cheyne, D. & Yoshimine, T. (2000). Movement-related desynchronization of the cerebral cortex studied with spatially filtered magnetoencephalograpy, *Neuroimage*, Vol. 12, pp. 298-306.

Tesche, C. D.; Unsitalo M. A.; Ilmoniemi R. J.; Huotilainen M.; Kajola M. & Salonen O. (1995). Signal-space projections of MEG data characterize both distributed and well-localized neuroal sources, Electroencephalography and Clinical Neurophysiology, Vol. 95, pp. 189-200.

Uutela, K.; Hamalainen, M. & Somersalo, E. (1999). Visualization of magnetoencephalography data using minimum current estimates, *Neuroimage*, Vol. 10, pp. 173-180.

Wolpaw, J. R. & McFarland, D. J. (1994). Multichannel EEG-based brain-computer communication, *Electroencephalography and clinical Neurophysiology*, Vol. 90, pp. 444-449.

Wu, Y. T.; Lee, P. L.; Chen, L. F.; Yeh, T. C. & Hsieh, J. C. (2002). Single-trial quantification of imagery beta-band Mu rhythm in finger lifting task using independent component analysis (ICA). *Proceeding of BioMag 13th international conference on biomagnetism*, pp. 1045-1047.

Wu, Y. T.; Lee, P. L.; Chen, L. F.; Yeh, T. C. & Hsieh, J. C. (2003). Quantification of movement-related modulation on beta activity of single-trial magnetoencephalography measuring using independent component analysis (ICA). *Proceeding of the 1st international IEEE EMBS conference on neural engineering*, pp. 396-398.

Yabe, H.; Satio, F. & Fukushima, Y. (1993). Median method for detecting endogenous event-related brain potentials, *Electroencephalography and clinical Neurophysiology*, Vol. 87, pp. 403-407.

7

Minor and Trace Elements in Cerebrospinal Fluid of Parkinson's Patients – Suggestions After a Critical Review of the Analytical Data

Margherita Speziali[1] and Michela Di Casa[2]
[1]CNR-IENI (Institute for Energetics and Interphases),
Department of Pavia, University of Pavia, Pavia,
[2] Department of Chemistry, University of Pavia, Pavia,
Italy

1. Introduction

Patients suffering from neurodegenerative diseases are known to present, in comparison to controls, variations on the contents of minor and trace elements in body tissues and fluids. For individuals affected by Parkinson's disease (PD), some findings, regarding brain and serum, are cited hereafter. BRAIN. Various brain areas were characterized for trace element levels and some alterations were observed in patients. Higher concentrations of aluminum were determined by Yasui et al. (1992) in different sites; increased levels of copper were detected by Riederer et al. (1989) in raphe plus reticular formation, whereas diminished amounts were found in substantia nigra by Rajput et al. (1985) and Dexter et al. (1989). Dexter et al. (1991) and Griffits et al. (1999) observed an iron enrichment in substantia nigra; regarding to zinc, Dexter et al. (1989) found more elevated amounts in a few areas, while Riederer et al. (1989) noticed lower contents in raphe formation. Variations of aluminum, copper, iron and zinc levels in definite brain sites of PD patients were reviewed by Speziali & Orvini (2003). SERUM. For PD patients, trace element changes were observed also in serum. Several studies were carried out at the Italian Istituto Superiore di Sanità (ISS) by Bocca et al. (2004, 2006), Forte et al. (2004, 2005), Alimonti et al. (2007a). A decreasing trend for aluminum was observed by Bocca et al. (2004) and Forte et al. (2004), as well as by Hedge et al. (2004) and Pande et al. (2005). Copper resulted elevated in these last two works and in a paper by Mindadse & Tschikowani (1967); in other investigations, by Bocca et al. (2006), Forte et al. (2004) and Tan et al. (2007), copper resulted diminished. Hedge et al. (2004), Pande et al. (2005), Forte et al. (2005), Alimonti et al. (2007a) detected lower iron concentrations, whereas Tan et al. (2007) reported a higher amount. In the case of zinc, a slight increase was noticed by Tan et al. (2007), whereas Hedge et al. (2004), Pande et al. (2005), Forte et al. (2005), Alimonti et al. (2007a) observed a significant decrease. A lower mercury content was found by Gellein et al. (2008).

From this survey, it emerges that disagreeing findings for the same element are quite frequent. In the case of brain, we can suppose that the discrepancies among the various trials are related to the different areas examined. The less expected controversial findings for serum stimulated us to examine the up to date knowledge about the CSF of PD subjects. We have already published a short review on this topic (Speziali & Di Casa, 2009). In this

Chapter we present in a series of tables, for the first time, all the original values retrieved, along with several parameters that can influence the results. Here we discuss more extensively the role of all the factors affecting the results, which are the parameters reported in the tables along with the criteria for the enrollment of subjects, the analytical procedures and the statistical tests used. Finally, we propose with wider completeness several suggestions useful for possible future studies.

C = Controls	Et-AAS = Electrothermal Atomic
PD = Parkinson's disease patients	Absorption Spectrometry
PD (On) = PD with positive response to the therapy	ICP-AES = Inductively Coupled Plasma - Atomic Emission Spectometry
PD (On/Off) = PD without positive response to the therapy	DCP-AES = Direct Current Plasma -AES
PDCN = PD cognitively normal patients	SF-ICP-MS = Sector Field – Inductively Coupled Plasma – Mass
PDD = PD demented patients	Spectrometry
SD = Standard Deviation	S = significant or highly significant
M = male	difference
F = female	NS = non-significant difference

Table 1. Captions for the tables

2. Aim

We performed an investigation on the minor and trace element amounts, available in the literature, regarding the CSF of PD patients and paired controls. Our purpose was to obtain a comprehensive picture of the element concentrations and to verify possible imbalances in the CSF of the diseased individuals.

3. Data presentation

We considered only studies where: a) both patients and controls were examined in the same investigation; b) the concentration values determined were reported as numbers; c) statistical tests were employed to verify the significance of potential changes of element amounts in the CSF of patients. The scientific publications were retrieved through the data bank Medline along with the Personal Alert Service of Thomson Reuters, Philadelphia, PA. From the bibliographies of the recruited papers further references were derived. The concentration data we recruited in the literature were published from 1987 to 2008. Values of Al, Ba, Be, Bi, Ca, Cd, Co, Cr, Cu, Fe, Hg, Li, Mg, Mn, Mo, Ni, Pb, Sb, Se, Si, Sn, Sr, Tl, V, W, Zn and Zr were found. In Tab. 1 we set out the captions useful for all our tables. In Tab. 2 - 11 we report the mean concentration values, along with the standard deviations; we also show several parameters affecting the results: number, gender and age of the subjects enrolled, analytical technique employed, significance of possible differences between concentration values for patients and controls. The simultaneous availability of all these factors allows scientists to evaluate immediately the reliability of each trial findings. From the tables, indications can be also deducted on the possibility (or not) to compare directly the results of different trials; increasing or decreasing element trends in patients are evident right away. Finally, in Tab. 12 we sum up some indications recorded in other publications of interest.

Minor and Trace Elements in Cerebrospinal Fluid of Parkinson's Patients – Suggestions After
a Critical Review of the Analytical Data

151

Ele-ment	Subjects	Mean	SD	N. of subjects (Gender)	Age, y	Technique	Signif-icance	References
Ca	C	24.696	1.997	13 (6 M + 7 F)	63.8 ± 13.7	ICP-AES	NS	Forte et al., 2004
	PD	27.911	4.964	26 (24 M + 2 F)	64.9 ± 10.8			
	C	26.956 {median: 25.579}	5.515	20 (17 M + 3 F)	66.2 ± 14.7	ICP-AES	NS	Alimonti et al., 2007b
	PD	27.312 {median: 27.301}	3.385	42 (36 M + 6 F)	64.5 ± 10.7			
Mg	C	21.229	3.160	13 (6 M + 7 F)	63.8 ± 13.7	ICP-AES	NS	Forte et al., 2004
	PD	20.913	2.024	26 (24 M + 2 F)	64.9 ± 10.8			
	C	21.868 {median: 22.665}	3.509	20 (17 M + 3 F)	66.2 ± 14.7	ICP-AES	NS	Alimonti et al., 2007b
	PD	23.693 {median: 22.365}	4.263	42 (36 M + 6 F)	64.5 ± 10.7			

Table 2. Calcium and magnesium in Controls and Patients (mg/L)

Subjects	Mean	SD	N. of subjects (Gender)	Age, y (Range)	Technique	Signif-icance	References
C	75.9	153.6	22 (20 M + 2 F)	age-matched	Et-AAS		Gazzaniga et al., 1992
PD tot	181	75.1	11 (10 M + 1 F)	64.9 (49-78)		NS	
PD untreated	28.3 *	141.5*	6	63.1 (49-78)		NS	
PD treated	266.4	183.6	5	67 (59-77)		NS	
C	210	150	37 (16 M + 21 F)	62.4 ± 17.8	Et-AAS		Jiménez-Jiménez et al., 1998
PD	170	170	37 (14 M + 23 F)	65.7 ± 8.8		NS	
C	73.3	72.7	13 (6 M + 7 F)	63.8 ± 13.7	ICP-AES		Forte et al., 2004
PD	33.0	29.4	26 (24 M + 2 F)	64.9 ± 10.8		NS	
C	237	37	21 (13 M + 8 F)	62 ± 11	Et-AAS		Qureshi et al., 2005 and 2006
PD (On)	345	47	17 (10 M + 7 F)	70 ± 15		S >	
PD (On/Off)	397	50	19 (13 M + 6 F)	72 ± 17		S >	
C	45.0	30.2	18 (10 M + 8 F)	63.8 ± 13.8	ICP-AES		Bocca et al., 2006
PD	28.2	14.6	91 (64 M + 27 F)	65.5 ± 9.7		S <	
C	35.5 {median: 36.8}	5.03	20 (17 M + 3 F)	66.2 ± 14.7	ICP-AES		Alimonti et al., 2007b
PD	28.2 {median: 24.4}	14.6	42 (36 M + 6 F)	64.5 ± 10.7		S <	

* these two values are incoherent

Table 3. Iron in Controls and Patients (μg/L)

4. Considerations on factors influencing the results

As already pointed out in the **Introduction,** many factors affect the results, conditioning then the comparability among the findings of the various studies. We describe now in details the influence of each factor as it emerged in the examined publications.

4.1 Criteria for subject enrollment
4.1.1 Health conditions

In the subject enrollment, the criteria for inclusion/exclusion are fundamental and should absolutely include health conditions along with age and gender. Ideally, exposures due to environmental pollution or occupational activities and diet should also be considered.

In the reviewed papers, only a few teams give full details of the selection criteria used. The researchers of the Italian Istituto Superiore di Sanità (ISS), Bocca, Forte, Alimonti and coworkers, along with the Spanish scientists (Jiménez-Jiménez et al. 1998 and Aguilar et al. 1998) are among the few authors who describe extensively the criteria employed. The diseases affecting the individuals recruited as patients or controls are often not precisely described, mainly in the less recent works. In some publications, incongruities appear within the text or among the text and the data presented in the tables. It is not always clear whether the patients were affected by comorbidities. Due to the fact that severe illnesses of heart, liver, kidney and also tumors are known to affect the levels of trace elements in human fluids and tissues, an exhaustive health report is also necessary in the case of controls. For these subjects, very heterogeneous situations have been observed. In Bourrier-Guerin et al. (1985) - see Tab. 12 - controls were not enrolled at all. Mindadse & Tschikowani (1967) - see Tab. 12 - employed blood donors. In Qureshi et al. (2005, 2006) control individuals, simply defined "healthy", were affected by tension headache, ischemic cerebrovascular disease or polyneuropathy. The Spanish group selected "healthy" subjects with suspected subarachnoid hemorrhage or pseudotumor cerebri, oculomotor palsies, etc. The scientists of the ISS enrolled individuals not suffering from any central neurological disease. Kjellin (1967a and 1967b - see Tab. 12) assumed psychoneurotic outpatients as representative of the "normal" condition. It is evident that, in the diverse investigations, were enrolled as controls subjects in really different health conditions. It is worth considering that, differently from blood, the samples of CSF are not easily available; therefore, the control specimens are mostly withdrawn from subjects undergoing lumbar puncture for clinical analyses. In the case of patients, the differences among the groups enrolled in the diverse studies are amplified by some clinical variables, as duration and severity of the disease along with medical treatments and possible comorbidities. Regarding duration and severity of the disease, in the trial by Aguilar et al. (1998) Se and Cr levels showed no correlation with age at onset and duration of the illness. On the other hand, Alimonti et al. (2007b) detected in patients a negative association of Cr amount and severity and duration of the illness; in the same study, Pb appeared to be negatively related to the severity of the disorder, while Sn resulted to be negatively associated with the duration of the disease. The authors also found that age at onset did not affect the concentration of Fe and of the other elements that resulted significantly different between controls and patients (Co, Cr, Pb, Si, Sn). Bocca et al. (2006) observed that duration and severity of the disease appeared not to be correlated with Al, Ca, Cu, Fe, Mn, Si and Zn amounts; on the other hand, Mg level decreased with the duration and severity of the illness. Concerning medical treatments, the therapies followed by patients are described by

Minor and Trace Elements in Cerebrospinal Fluid of Parkinson's Patients – Suggestions After
a Critical Review of the Analytical Data

153

Subjects	Mean	SD	N. of subjects (Gender)	Age, y (Range)	Technique	Signif- icance	References
C	19.2 (range: 10 – 33)	5.8	21		DCP-AES	NS	Belliveau et al., 1990
PD	18.7 (range: 7 – 30)	6.3	16				
C	64.9	14.4	22 (20 M + 2 F)	age-matched	Et-AAS	NS	Gazzaniga et al., 1992
PD tot	67.7	19.9	11 (10 M + 1 F)	64.9 (49 – 78)		NS	
PD untreated	63.2	11.5	6	63.1 (49 – 78)		NS	
PD treated	67.0	18.5	5	67 (59 – 77)			
C	109.1	88.2	37 (16 M + 21 F)	62.4 ± 17.8	Et-AAS	NS	Jiménez-Jiménez et al., 1998
PD	104.9	86.3	37 (14 M + 23 F)	65.7 ± 8.8			
C	22.5	4.76	13 (6 M + 7 F)	63.8 ± 13.7	ICP-AES	NS	Forte et al., 2004
PD	23.7	10.5	26 (24 M + 2 F)	64.9 ± 10.8			
C	132	17	21 (13 M + 8 F)	62 ± 11	Et-AAS	NS	Qureshi et al., 2005 and 2006
PD (On)	119	18	17 (10 M + 7 F)	70 ± 15		NS	
PD (On/Off)	109	19	19 (13 M + 6 F)	72 ± 17			
C	21.9 {median: 2.2}	4.77	20 (17 M + 3 F)	66.2 ± 14.7	ICP-AES	NS	Alimonti et al., 2007b
PD	19.4 {median: 17.0}	7.97	42 (36 M + 6 F)	64.5 ± 10.7			
C	19.6	1.3	32	85.2 ± 1.0		NS	Sparks et al., 2008
PDCN	17.4	4.3	12	85.3 ± 1.4		NS	
PDD	10.0	1.1	5	78.6 ± 2.2			

Table 4. Copper in Controls and Patients ($\mu g/L$)

many authors, as Gazzaniga et al. (1992), Qureshi et al. (2005, 2006), Aguilar et al. (1998), Jimenez-Jimenez et al. (1998), Bocca et al. (2004, 2006), Forte et al. (2004), Alimonti et al. (2007b) along with Campanella et al. (1973) and Takahashi et al. (1994). Aguilar et al. (1998) carried out studies about the influence of antiparkinsonian treatment with various drugs on Se and Cr levels; in the entire group of PD patients, Se showed a non significant increase compared to controls, but the elevation attained the significance when only patients not treated with levodopa were considered. This interesting observation is just recorded in the article text. Jimenez-Jimenez et al. (1998) studied the effects of the same drugs on the concentrations of Fe, Cu, Zn and Mn; they did not observe any significant influence. Gazzaniga et al. (1992), confronting long-term levodopa treated and untreated patients, did not find any significant differences in the amounts of Cu, Fe and Mn. Qureshi et al. (2005, 2006) determined the amounts of Cu, Fe, Se and Zn in patients treated with levodopa, who were divided into two groups (PD On and PD On/Off), depending on the positive or negative response to the therapy. Fe and Se were found to be markedly higher than in controls in both kinds of patients; Zn resulted instead significantly reduced in both groups. Bocca et al. (2006) evaluated that the type of therapy did not influence the concentrations of all the elements studied (Al, Ca, Cu, Fe, Mg, Mn, Si, Zn). Alimonti et al. (2007b) observed that diverse drugs did not affect the concentration of Fe; on the contrary, they influenced the amounts of the elements which resulted significantly different between controls and patients (Co, Cr, Pb, Si, Sn). Takahashi et al. (1994 - see Tab. 12) found that the Mg concentration in both untreated and treated (with levodopa) patients was lower than in controls.

4.1.2 Age

The subject age is known to influence the amounts of some elements in tissues and fluids. In serum, it has been documented for Cu by Ghayour-Mobarhan et al. (2005) and Kouremenou-Dona et al. (2006); for Se by Lopes et al. (2004). In brain, Markesbery et al. (1984), Ongkana et al. (2010) and Tohno et al. (2010) found age-related changes for several

Subjects	Mean	SD	N. of subjects (Gender)	Age, y	Technique	Signif- icance	References
C	170	140	37 (16 M + 21 F)	62.4 ± 17.8	Et-AAS	S <	Jiménez-Jiménez
PD	100	60	37 (14 M + 23 F)	65.7 ± 8.8			et al., 1998
C	32.9	8.85	13 (6 M + 7 F)	63.8 ± 13.7	ICP-AES	NS	Forte et al., 2004
PD	27.3	10.5	26 (24 M + 2 F)	64.9 ± 10.8			
C	161	31	21 (13 M + 8 F)	62 ± 11	Et-AAS	S <	Qureshi et al.,
PD (On)	117	19	17 (10 M + 7 F)	70 ± 15		S <	2005 and 2006
PD (On/Off)	96	11	19 (13 M + 6 F)	72 ± 17			
C	32.3 {median: 33.5}	11.4	20 (17 M + 3 F)	66.2 ± 14.7	ICP-AES	NS	Alimonti et al.,
PD	27.7 {median: 27.8}	9.01	42 (36 M + 6 F)	64.5 ± 10.7			2007b

Table 5. Zinc in Controls and Patients (µg/L)

Subjects	Mean	SD	N. of subjects (Gender)	Age, y (Range)	Technique	Signif- icance	References
C	0.97 ♥	0.34 ♥	29		Et-AAS	NS	Pall et al., 1987
PD	0.96 ♥	0.36 ♥	9				
C	5.7	1.8	22 (20 M + 2 F)	age-matched	Et-AAS	NS	Gazzaniga et al.,
PD tot	5.4	3.9	11 (10 M + 1 F)	64.9 (49 - 78)		NS	1992
PD untreated	6.0	1.3	6	63.1 (49 - 78)		NS	
PD treated	5.4	2.4	5	67 (59 - 77)			
C	0.88	0.76	37 (16 M + 21 F)	62.4 ± 17.8	Et-AAS	NS	Jiménez-Jiménez
PD	1.20	0.98	37 (14 M + 23 F)	65.7 ± 8.8			et al., 1998
C	0.85 {median: 0.91}	0.36	13 (6 M + 7 F)	63.8 ± 13.7	SF-ICP-MS		Bocca et al., 2004
PD	0.63 {median: 0.54}	0.43	26 (24 M + 2 F)	64.9 ± 10.8		NS	and Forte et al., 2004
C	0.95	0.39	18 (10 M + 8 F)	63.8 ± 13.8	SF-ICP-MS	NS	Bocca et al., 2006
PD	0.69	0.42	91 (64 M + 27 F)	65.5 ± 9.7			
C	0.95 {median: 1.02}	0.39	20 (17 M + 3 F)	66.2 ± 14.7	SF-ICP-MS	NS	Alimonti et al.,
PD	0.69 {median: 0.58}	0.42	42 (36 M + 6 F)	64.5 ± 10.7			2007b

♥ data converted from nmol/L

Table 6. Manganese in Controls and Patients (µg/L)

elements. All authors who studied CSF and published element concentration values also for patients reported the mean age of each subject group; Gazzaniga et al. (1992) specified also the age range. Regarding element changes with age, Aguilar et al. (1998) found that Se and Cr levels were not correlated with the age of PD patients. Bocca et al. (2006) found no Zn changes in patients (no data given); in controls, they observed a significant Zn increment in subjects elder than 70 years in comparison with younger individuals, but these differences disappeared in patients.

4.1.3 Gender

This parameter also influences trace element levels. For changes of Se, Cu and Zn in serum, see Lopes et al. (2004) and Ghayour-Mobarhan et al. (2005). For Zn variations in brain, see Ongkana et al. (2010). Regarding CSF, Bocca et al. (2006) noticed lesser Fe amounts in PD males than in females, whereas the opposite was found in controls. They also report that Si concentration resulted significantly lower in patients than in controls and that in PD females it was two-times lower than in males. This remarkable observation could come out because the authors calculated distinct values, not published, for the two genders.

Minor and Trace Elements in Cerebrospinal Fluid of Parkinson's Patients – Suggestions After
a Critical Review of the Analytical Data

155

Ele-ment	Subjects	Mean	SD	N. of subjects (Gender)	Age, y	Technique	Signif-icance	References
Cr	C	14.6	6.3	43 (19 M + 24 F)	65.2 ± 13.0	Et-AAS	NS	Aguilar et al., 1998
	PD	14.5	7.4	28 (11 M + 17 F)	65.5 ± 9.1			
	C	1.39 {median: 1.47}	0.64	13 (6 M + 7 F)	63.8 ± 13.7	SF-ICP-MS	S <	Bocca et al., 2004
	PD	0.60 {median: 0.54}	0.47	26 (24 M + 2 F)	64.9 ± 10.8			
	C	1.28 {median: 1.39}	0.59	20 (17 M + 3 F)	66.2 ± 14.7	SF-ICP-MS	S <	Alimonti et al., 2007b
	PD	0.65 {median: 0.55}	0.46	42 (36 M + 6 F)	64.5 ± 10.7			
Se	C	13.5	8.2	43 (19 M + 24 F)	65.2 ± 13.0	Et-AAS	NS	Aguilar et al., 1998
	PD	17.9	12.3	28 (11 M + 17 F)	65.5 ± 9.1			
	C	14.2	1.8	21 (13 M + 8 F)	62 ± 11	Et-AAS	S >	Qureshi et al., 2006
	PD (On)	19.7	1.9	17 (10 M + 7 F)	70 ± 15		S >	
	PD (On/Off)	22.7	2.1	19 (13 M + 6 F)	72 ± 17			

Table 7. Chromium and selenium in Controls and Patients ($\mu g/L$)

Ele-ment	Subjects	Mean	SD	N. of subjects (Gender)	Age, y	Technique	Signif-icance	References
Pb	C	1.06 {median: 1.0}	0.34	13 (6 M + 7 F)	63.8 ± 13.7	SF-ICP-MS	S <	Bocca et al., 2004
	PD	0.42 {median: 0.30}	0.38	26 (24 M + 2 F)	64.9 ± 10.8			
	C	0.91 {median: 0.84}	0.36	20 (17 M + 3 F)	66.2 ± 14.7	SF-ICP-MS	S <	Alimonti et al., 2007b
	PD	0.46 {median: 0.43}	0.24	42 (36 M + 6 F)	64.5 ± 10.7			
Si	C	105	39.3	13 (6 M + 7 F)	63.8 ± 13.7	ICP-AES	S <	Forte et al., 2004
	PD	66.9	49.7	26 (24 M + 2 F)	64.9 ± 10.8			
	C	95.0	38.0	18 (10 M + 8 F)	63.8 ± 13.8	ICP-AES		Bocca et al., 2006
	"	92.5	44.3	1 F				
	PD	58.4 •	44.8	91 (64 M + 27 F)	65.5 ± 9.7		S <	
	"	63.9	46.5	1 M			S <	
	"	28.9	13.7	1 F			S <	
	C	95.0 {median: 96.3}	38.3	20 (17 M + 3 F)	66.2 ± 14.7	ICP-AES	S <	Alimonti et al., 2007b
	PD	58.4 {median: 52.3}	44.8	42 (36 M + 6 F)	64.5 ± 10.7			

• For gender difference, see text (section 4.1.3 Gender)

Table 8. Lead and silicon in Controls and Patients ($\mu g/L$)

4.1.4 Number of subjects examined

In the reviewed papers, the authors usually publish the total number of controls and patients, and even the numbers of males and females; however, they frequently do not report the information actually needed, that is the number of individuals really tested for each element. In our review, we observed that Be, Cd, Hg, and V were determined in two investigations by the team of ISS (Bocca et al. 2004 and Alimonti et al. 2007b). In the previous one, where a lower number of individuals was considered, the element decrements in patients were evaluated as significant; in the second trial, where more subjects were enrolled, the variations came out to be not significant. Fe resulted decreased in patients at the limits of significance (p = 0.052) in a trial carried out by Forte et al. (2004); in two successive investigations by the same team (Bocca et al. 2006 and Alimonti et al. 2007b), with a higher number of individuals, Fe was found to be significantly reduced. The control and patient groups of successive trials by the same authors probably included the corresponding groups already examined in the previous ones; the disagreeing findings could be due to the

Element	Subjects	Mean	SD	N. of subjects (Gender)	Age, y	Technique	Significance	References
Co	C	0.15 {median: 0.16}	0.04	13 (6 M + 7 F)	63.8 ± 13.7	SF-ICP-MS	S <	Bocca et al., 2004
	PD	0.04 {median: 0.03}	0.04	26 (24 M + 2 F)	64.9 ± 10.8			
	C	0.13 {median: 0.13}	0.05	20 (17 M + 3 F)	66.2 ± 14.7	SF-ICP-MS	S <	Alimonti et al., 2007b
	PD	0.09 {median: 0.06}	0.09	42 (36 M + 6 F)	64.5 ± 10.7			
Ni	C	8.01 {median: 7.54}	1.39	13 (6 M + 7 F)	63.8 ± 13.7	SF-ICP-MS	NS	Bocca et al., 2004
	PD	4.37 {median: 1.07}	5.61	26 (24 M + 2 F)	64.9 ± 10.8			
	C	5.40 {median: 6.44}	3.33	20 (17 M + 3 F)	66.2 ± 14.7	SF-ICP-MS	NS	Alimonti et al., 2007b
	PD	3.34 {median: 1.53}	3.61	42 (36 M + 6 F)	64.5 ± 10.7			

Table 9. Cobalt and nickel in Controls and Patients (μg/L)

Element	Subjects	Mean	SD	N. of subjects (Gender)	Age, y	Technique	Significance	References
Be	C	0.87 {median: 0.85}	0.33	13 (6 M + 7 F)	63.8 ± 13.7	SF-ICP-MS	S <	Bocca et al., 2004
	PD	0.44 {median: 0.44}	0.13	26 (24 M + 2 F)	64.9 ± 10.8			
	C	0.70 {median: 0.55}	0.37	20 (17 M + 3 F)	66.2 ± 14.7	SF-ICP-MS	NS	Alimonti et al., 2007b
	PD	0.56 {median: 0.54}	0.21	42 (36 M + 6 F)	64.5 ± 10.7			
Cd	C	0.06 {median: 0.06}	0.02	13 (6 M + 7 F)	63.8 ± 13.7	SF-ICP-MS	S <	Bocca et al., 2004
	PD	0.03 {median: 0.03}	0.01	26 (24 M + 2 F)	64.9 ± 10.8			
	C	0.05 {median: 0.05}	0.03	20 (17 M + 3 F)	66.2 ± 14.7	SF-ICP-MS	NS	Alimonti et al., 2007b
	PD	0.04 {median: 0.4}	0.02	42 (36 M + 6 F)	64.5 ± 10.7			
Hg	C	1.20 {median: 1.19}	0.50	13 (6 M + 7 F)	63.8 ± 13.7	SF-ICP-MS	S <	Bocca et al., 2004
	PD	0.67 {median: 0.74}	0.32	26 (24 M + 2 F)	64.9 ± 10.8			
	C	1.05 {median: 0.85}	0.46	20 (17 M + 3 F)	66.2 ± 14.7	SF-ICP-MS	NS	Alimonti et al., 2007b
	PD	0.73 {median: 0.81}	0.32	42 (36 M + 6 F)	64.5 ± 10.7			
V	C	0.12 {median: 0.11}	0.06	13 (6 M + 7 F)	63.8 ± 13.7	SF-ICP-MS	S <	Bocca et al., 2004
	PD	0.07 {median: 0.08}	0.03	26 (24 M + 2 F)	64.9 ± 10.8			
	C	0.09 {median: 0.10}	0.03	20 (17 M + 3 F)	66.2 ± 14.7	SF-ICP-MS	NS	Alimonti et al., 2007b
	PD	0.07 {median: 0.07}	0.03	42 (36 M + 6 F)	64.5 ± 10.7			

Table 10. Berillium, cadmium, mercury and vanadium in Controls and Patients (μg/L)

different number of the considered subjects. In the case of Co, Cr, Pb and Si, the outcomes for significance are always the same when the number of subjects, in both control and patient groups, is either lower or higher. We wonder whether the changes in patients of these elements are so marked that result noticeable in every case. As a general consideration, it is obvious that the higher is the number of the subjects examined, the higher is the representativeness of the results obtained.

4.2 Analytical procedures

When determining elements at trace levels, the entire analytical process is critical. Sampling and storage should be carried out in an appropriate way to minimize contamination and losses, following the recognized requirements in the field. The chemical treatments needed by each method should be as standardized as possible. The analytical technique employed must assure high sensitivity and good reproducibility.

In the reviewed studies, the preanalytical steps were described with more or less details; the techniques employed were cited by all authors, except Sparks et al. (2008). A careful description of the method is generally available in the most recent papers, that sometimes refer to previous publications. The techniques used for the most studied elements were principally electrothermal   atomic absorption spectrometry (Et-AAS) and inductively coupled plasma atomic emission spectrometry (ICP-AES). For some elements, sector field inductively coupled plasma mass spectrometry (SF-ICP-MS) was also employed by the team of ISS. All these analytical techniques are widely used for trace element determination in human samples.

Element	Subjects	Mean	SD	Median	Significance
Al	C	2.64	0.51	2.72	NS
	PD	2.15	1.03	2.05	
Ba	C	0.35	0.15	0.31	NS
	PD	0.26	0.13	0.24	
Bi	C	0.10	0.07	0.09	NS
	PD	0.08	0.05	0.06	
Li	C	0.52	0.13	0.52	NS
	PD	0.82	0.53	0.65	
Mo	C	0.45	0.27	0.43	NS
	PD	0.33	0.17	0.27	
Sb	C	0.08	0.02	0.09	NS
	PD	0.06	0.04	0.07	
Sn	C	0.32	0.07	0.31	S <
	PD	0.26	0.11	0.24	
Sr	C	30.0	8.69	27.7	NS
	PD	24.6	8.66	22.6	
Tl	C	0.01	0.01	0.01	NS
	PD	0.01	0.007	0.01	
W	C	0.04	0.02	0.04	NS
	PD	0.03	0.02	0.03	
Zr	C	0.06	0.05	0.06	NS
	PD	0.04	0.03	0.04	
N. of subjects (Gender)			Age, y		
C 20 (17 M + 3 F)			66.2 $\pm$ 14.7		
PD 42 (36 M + 6 F)			64.5 $\pm$ 10.7		
Technique: SF-ICP-MS					

Table 11. Other trace elements in Controls and Patients ($\mu g/L$); (modified from Alimonti et al., 2007b)

4.3 Statistical tests
In this kind of studies, statistical tests of various types are required for diverse appraisals. Within each study and for each element considered, tests are applied at first to evaluate whether the concentrations found for controls and patients are significantly different or not. In the same trial, other tests can reveal non negligible dissimilarities among the control and patient groups, regarding one or more factors affecting the results. When a significant

discrepancy is disclosed, the comparison between the mean concentration values   for controls and those for patients results rather inappropriate.

A crucial point, worth of a close investigation by the scientists of the field, is to assess at what extent the outcomes for significance of the various tests applied are the same. When comparing the results of different investigations, the diversity of the statistical tests applied in each one causes an amplification of the general inhomogeneity.

In the reviewed papers, the statistical tests used to verify the difference between the results for controls and patients are generally indicated. Some authors checked also possible differences, for one or more variability factors, among the various subject groups; their information is therefore more accurate.

5. Summary of the retrieved data

The retrieved data are non numerous, being the withdrawal of the fluid unpleasant; the control samples are taken from individuals undergoing lumbar puncture for neurological exams. Some values have been found for Cu, Fe, Mn and Zn, whereas only few results have been retrieved for Cr and Si. As far as other elements are concerned, the data are absolutely scarce or determined only once, mainly by the scientists of ISS.

Examining the collected values, regarding **copper** - see Tab. 4 - no significant variations for patients as compared to controls were found in trials performed by diverse teams; nevertheless, in other papers (not showing analytical data for Cu), Pall et al. (1987) and Pan et al. (1997) - see Tab. 12 - assess to have observed a remarkable elevation. In the case of **manganese** too – see Tab. 6 - no changes were observed in the different investigations; of note, the levels determined by Gazzaniga et al. (1992) are higher than those found by the other author groups. Concerning **calcium** and **magnesium** - see Tab. 2 - no significant alterations are reported; however, Takahashi et al. (1994) - see Tab. 12 - assess to have found a lesser Mg level in patients. As for **zinc** - see Tab. 5 - Forte et al. (2004) and Alimonti et al. (2007b) observed in PD a slight diminution, which in the trials by Jiménez- Jiménez et al. (1998) and Qureshi et al. (2005 and 2006) attained the significance. Aguilar et al (1998) found for PD subjects a non significant **selenium** increment - see Tab. 7; a significant elevation resulted instead in all the patients, with both positive and negative response to the therapy, enrolled by Qureshi et al. (2006). **Lead** - see Tab. 8 - was found to be significantly reduced in patients by the team of ISS (Bocca et al. 2004 and Alimonti et al. 2007b), that obtained the same finding also for **silicon** (Forte et al. 2004, Bocca et al. 2006, Alimonti et al. 2007b) - see Table 8. In the case of **iron** - see Tab. 3 - the most interesting element for PD, discordant results were unfortunately recruited. A significant depletion was found by Bocca et al. 2006 and Alimonti et al. 2007b; for a detailed description, see the paragraph 4.1.4. An elevation, also significant, was seen by Qureshi et al. (2005 and 2006); other scientists as Gazzaniga et al. (1992) and Jiménez- Jiménez et al. (1998) did not observe noticeable variations. The values determined by the ISS team appear to be remarkably lower than those published by the other groups. Dealing with **chromium** - see Tab. 7 - Aguilar et al. (1998) found similar amounts in the CSF of patients and controls; differently, Bocca et al. (2004) and Alimonti et al. (2007b) obtained much lower values and noticed a significant decrement in patients. **Al, Ba, Be, Bi, Co, Li, Mo, Ni, Sb, Sn, Sr, Tl, V, W** and **Zr** were determined only by the scientists of ISS - see Tab. 9, 10, 11. No variations were observed, except significant decreases of Co and Sn. Regarding the results for Be and V, see the paragraph 4.1.4, where are described also the findings for **Cd** and **Hg**; the values for these last four elements are shown in Tab. 10.

Minor and Trace Elements in Cerebrospinal Fluid of Parkinson's Patients – Suggestions After
a Critical Review of the Analytical Data
159

Bourrier-Guerin et al. 1985 report values for 13 elements in 70 patients (34 M and 36 F) affected by different neurodegenerative diseases; patients were grouped all together. Si and Zn resulted to be significantly higher in men than in women.

Campanella et al. 1973 enrolled 18 individuals (5 controls; 7 untreated patients; 6 patients treated with dopaminergic drugs), age > 39 y, no gender given. They published the Cu mean amount found for each subject. For both patients groups, the range of the mean values was wider than for controls.

Kjellin 1967a and 1967b reported Cu and Fe amounts in the CSF of a female patient (69 y) suffering from parkinsonism.
Cu and Fe resulted respectively higher and lesser in comparison to a unique control, who was probably in both cases a male of 65 y.

Mindadse & Tschikowani 1967 found that Au amount in PD patients was 66 µg/g, about the double than in controls. The Au concentration in controls (blood donors) is however not reported.

Pall et al. 1987 found in patients (24) with untreated, idiopathic PD, a higher Cu concentration than in controls (34) with various other neurological diseases. For Fe, they did not observe a difference between patients (26) and controls (33).

Pan et al. 1997 observed that Cu increased significantly in PD patients; on the other hand, the amounts of Cd, Fe, Mn and Zn did not change.

Takahashi et al. 1994 evaluated Br, Cu, Fe, Se, Zn and Mg levels in 25 controls and 20 PD patients (13 untreated and 7 treated with L-dopa). The mean Mg concentration in both treated and untreated parkinsonians was found to be lower than in controls.

Woodbury et al. 1968 determined in one PD patient a Mg amount overlapping the mean value found for controls (11). Always in one patient, these authors determined a higher zinc concentration than in controls (2).

Table 12. Additional information

6. Conclusion

Regarding the matrix CSF, the first remark we make is that the element concentration values available in the literature are non numerous, probably due to the rareness of the samples. Among the recruited papers, the range of values was recorded only in that by Belliveau et al. (1990). Knowing the ranges for controls and patients would allow to establish a range of normalcy for each element and, as a consequence, to individuate in patients a possible shift towards elevation or diminution. Examining the retrieved data, it is evident that for some elements the results obtained by the various research groups are of different levels. For Cu, the values published by the different teams vary from less than two decades to more than a hundred of µg/L. For Fe and Zn, the scientists of ISS determined concentrations much lesser than the other teams. For Cr, Aguilar et al. (1998) found values an order of magnitude higher than those reported by the team of ISS. The discrepancies regarding the element levels are difficult to explain. The mean values retrieved have often very large standard deviations. In the case of Be, Cd, Cr Hg, Se, Si, V, the SDs are sometimes as high as the half of the mean. A similar situation resulted for Mn and Cu in the study by Jiménez-Jiménez et al. (1998). Dealing with Fe, Jiménez-Jiménez et al. (1998) and Forte et al. (2004) detected SD values very close to the mean. SDs close to the mean were also found for Co and Pb by the researchers of ISS; they report, for Ni, SDs even higher. The large SDs can be due to the individual variability and/or to the low number of the subjects enrolled; they are not surprising also when the element concentration level is very low (a few µg/L or less). In the case of Cr and Se, and mostly in that of Fe and Si, high SDs are less expected. Obviously, they make it really difficult to evaluate the significance of the difference among the results.

In this review, we have verified the influence, on the results, of number, age, gender of the subjects enrolled; health conditions (with regard also to clinical variables as duration and severity of the disease and pharmacological therapies) were demonstrated to be other influencing factors. The importance of adequate analytical procedures and statistical tests has been previously described (see the respective paragraphs).

At this point, we can suggest that, in a trial, attention should be paid to match, as far as possible, age and health conditions of the subjects belonging to the same group; this is more difficult to obtain in the case of patients. Concerning gender, separate male and female groups could reveal possible unexpected information. A similar number of individuals in the various groups should be enrolled; anyway, we are aware that, in the clinical practice, the scarceness of the CSF control samples and the prevalent number of male PD patients (Alimonti et al. 2007b) make these requirements not always achievable. In addition, all the previously mentioned factors should be not too different when confronting the results of the various studies, to allow a proper comparison. It is evident that this is a truly unattainable task.

In our opinion, a real upgrading in this field could actually be achieved if many specific indications were recorded in the single studies. Regarding every subject enrolled, information as age, gender, health condition, lifestyle and environmental exposure should be clearly reported; for each individual, also the results obtained for every element should be published. A detailed description of the various steps of sampling and analytical procedures should also be given; the single steps should be performed according to the indications most recently standardized.

Following all these suggestions, a database useful for diverse kind of investigations would be obtained; retrospective studies as meta-analyses, based on single factors affecting the results, could be derived; even findings not detectable at the moment could arise.

Minor and Trace Elements in Cerebrospinal Fluid of Parkinson's Patients – Suggestions After
a Critical Review of the Analytical Data
161

7. References

Aguilar, M.V.; Jimenez-Jimenez, F.J.; Molina, J.A.; Meseguer, I.; Mateos-Vega, C.J.;
Gonzalez-Munoz, M.J.; de Bustos, F.; Gomez-Escalonilla, C.; Ortí-Pareja, M.;
Zurdo, M. & Martinez-Para, M.C. (1998). Cerebrospinal fluid selenium and
chromium levels in patients with Parkinson's disease. *J. Neural Transm.*, Vol.105,
pp. 1245-1251

Alimonti, A.; Ristori, G.; Giubilei F.; Stazi, M.A.; Pino, A.; Visconti, A.; Brescianini, S.; Sepe
Monti, M.; Forte, G.; Stanzione, P.; Bocca, B.; Bomboi, G.; D'Ippolito, C.; Annibali,
V.; Salvetti, M. & Sancesario, G. (2007a). Serum chemical elements and oxidative
status in Alzheimer's disease, Parkinson disease and multiple sclerosis.
Neurotoxicol., Vol.28, pp. 450-456

Alimonti, A.; Bocca, B.; Pino, A.; Ruggieri, F.; Forte, G. & Sancesario, G. (2007b). Elemental
profile of cerebrospinal fluid in patients with Parkinson's disease. *J. Trace Elem.
Med. Biol.*, Vol.21, pp. 234-241

Belliveau, J.F.; Friedman, J.H.; O'Leary, G.P. Jr. & Guarrera, D. (1990). Evaluation of
increased copper levels in the cerebrospinal-fluid of Parkinson's patients, In: *Metal
Ions in Biology and Medicine,* P. Collery, L.A. Poirier, M. Manfait & J.C. Etienne,
(Eds.) 89-91, John Libbey Eurotext, London-Paris

Bocca, B.; Alimonti, A.; Petrucci, F.; Violante, N.; Sancesario, G.; Forte, G. & Senofonte, O.
(2004). Quantification of trace elements by sector field inductively coupled plasma
mass spectrometry in urine, serum, blood and cerebrospinal fluid of patients with
Parkinson's disease. *Spectrochim. Acta Part B*, Vol.59, pp. 559-566

Bocca, B.; Alimonti, A.; Senofonte, O.; Pino, A.; Violante, N.; Petrucci, F.; Sancesario, G. &
Forte, G. (2006). Metal changes in CSF and peripheral compartments of PD patients.
J. Neurol. Sci., Vol.248, pp. 23-30

Bourrier-Guerin, L.; Mauras, Y.; Truelle, J.L. & Allain, P. (1985). CSF and plasma
concentrations of 13 elements in various neurological disorders. *Trace Elem. Med.*,
Vol.2, pp. 88-91

Campanella, G.; Carrieri, P.; Romito, D. & Pasqual-Marsettin, E. (1973). Ferro, transferrina,
rame e ceruloplasmina del siero e del liquor nelle malattie extrapiramidali e nelle
miopatie primitive. [Iron, transferrin, copper and ceruloplasmin of the serum and
cerebrospinal fluid in extrapyramidal diseases and primary myopathies]. *Acta
Neurol.* (Napoli), Vol.28, pp. 1-34

Dexter, D.T.; Wells, F.R.; Lees, A.J.; Agid, F.; Agid, Y.; Jenner, P. & Marsde, C.D. (1989).
Increased nigral iron content and alterations in other metal ions occurring in brain
in Parkinson's disease. *J. Neurochem.*, Vol.52, pp. 1830-1836

Dexter, D.T.; Carayon, A.; Javoy-Agid, F.; Agid, Y.; Wells, F.R.; Daniel, S.E.; Lees, A.J.;
Jenner, P. & Marsden, C.D. (1991). Alterations in the levels of iron, ferritin and
other trace metals in Parkinson's disease and other neurodegenerative diseases
affecting the basal ganglia. *Brain,* Vol.114, pp. 1953-1975

Forte, G.; Bocca, B.; Senofonte, O.; Petrucci, F.; Brusa, L.; Stanzione, P.; Zannino, S.;
Violante, N.; Alimonti, A. & Sancesario, G. (2004). Trace and major elements in
whole blood, serum, CSF and urine of patients with PD. *J. Neural Trans.*, Vol.111,
pp. 1031-1040

Forte, G.; Alimonti, A.; Pino, A.; Stanzione, P.; Brescianini, S.; Brusa, L.; Sancesario, G.; Violante, N. & Bocca, B. (2005). Metals and oxidative stress in patients with Parkinson's disease. *Ann. Ist. Super. Sanità*, Vol.41, pp. 189-195

Gazzaniga, G.C.; Ferraro, B.; Camerlingo, M.; Casto, L.; Viscardi, M. & Mamoli, A. (1992). A case control study of CSF copper, iron and manganese in Parkinson disease. *Ital. J. Neurol. Sci.*, Vol.13, pp. 239-243

Gellein, K.; Syversen, T.; Steinnes, E.; Nilsen, T.I.; Dahl, O.P.; Mitrovic, S.; Duraj, D. & Flaten, T.P. (2008). Trace elements in serum from patients with Parkinson's disease - A prospective case-control study - The Nord-Trøndelag Health Study (HUNT). *Brain Res.*, Vol.1219, pp. 111-115

Ghayour-Mobarhan, M.; Taylor, A.; New, S.A.; Lamb, D.J. & Ferns, G.A. (2005). Determinants of serum copper, zinc and selenium in healthy subjects. *Ann. Clin. Biochem.*, Vol.42, pp. 364-375

Griffiths, P.D.; Dobson, B.R.; Jones, G.R. & Clarke, D.T. (1999). Iron in the basal ganglia in Parkinson's disease. An in vitro study using extended X-ray absorption fine structure and cryo-electron microscopy. *Brain*, Vol.122, pp. 667-673

Hegde, M.L.; Shanmugavelu, P.; Vengamma, B.; Rao, T.S.; Menon, R.B.; Rao, R.V. & Rao, K.S. (2004). Serum trace element levels and the complexity of inter-element relations in patients with Parkinson's disease. *J. Trace Elem. Med. Biol.*, Vol.18, pp. 163-171

Jimenez-Jimenez, F.J.; Molina, J.A.; Aguilar, M.V.; Meseguer, I.; Mateos-Vega, C.J.; Gonzalez-Munoz, M.J.; de Bustos, F.; Martínez-Salio, A.; Ortí-Pareja, M.; Zurdo, M. & Martinez-Para, M.C. (1998). Cerebrospinal fluid levels of transition metals in patients with Parkinson's disease. *J. Neural Transm.*, Vol.105, pp. 497-505

Kjellin, K.G. (1967). Trace elements in the cerebrospinal fluid, In: *Nuclear Activation Techniques in The Life Sciences*, A. Ericson, (Ed.), 517-532, IAEA Proc. Series SM-91/3

Kjellin, K.G. (1967). The CSF iron in patients with neurological diseases. *Acta Neurol. Scand.*, Vol.43, pp. 299-313

Kouremenou-Dona, E.; Dona, A.; Papoutsis, J. & Spiliopoulou, C. (2006). Copper and zinc concentrations in serum of healthy Greek adults. *Sci. Total Environ.*, Vol.359, pp. 76-81

Lopes, P.A.; Santos, M.C.; Vicente, L.; Rodrigues, M.O.; Pavão, M.L.; Nève, J. & Viegas-Crespo, A.M. (2004). Trace element status (Se, Cu, Zn) in healthy Portuguese subjects of Lisbon population: a reference study. *Biol. Trace Elem. Res.*, Vol.101, pp. 1-17

Markesbery, W.R.; Ehmann, W.D.; Alauddin, M. & Hossain, T.I. (1984). Brain trace element concentrations in aging. *Neurobiol. Aging*, Vol.5, pp. 19-28

Mindadse, A.A. & Tschikowani, T.I. (1967). Über die Verteilung von Spurenelementen (Mangan, Kupfer, Zink und Gold) im Serum und Liquor bei Epilepsie und Parkinsonsyndrom [On the distribution of trace elements (manganese, copper, zinc, and gold) in serum and cerebro-spinal fluid in epilepsy and parkinsonism]. *Dtsch Gesundheitsw.*, Vol.22, pp. 1746-1748

Ongkana, N.; Tohno, S.; Tohno, Y.; Suwannahoy, P.; Mahakkanukrauh, P.; Azuma, C. & Minami, T.(2010). Age-related changes of elements in the anterior commissures and the relationships among their elements. *Biol. Trace Elem. Res.*, Vol.135, pp.86-97

Pall, H.S.; Williams, A.; Blake, D.R.; Lunec, J.; Gutteridge, J.M.; Hall, M. & Taylor, A. (1987). Raised cerebrospinal-fluid copper concentration in Parkinson's disease. *Lancet*, Vol.2, pp. 238-241

Pan, B.Y.; Cheng, Q.L.; He, Z.X. & Su, C.C. (1997). Transition metals in serum and CSF of patients with Parkinson's disease. *Mov. Disord.*, Vol.12 (Suppl.), p. 33

Pande, M.B.; Nagabhushan, P.; Hegde, M.L.; Rao, T.S. & Rao, K.S. (2005). An algorithmic approach to understand trace elemental homeostasis in serum samples of Parkinson disease. *Comput. Biol. Med.*, Vol.35, pp. 475-493

Qureshi, G.A.; Qureshi, A.A.; Memon, S.A.; Sarwar, M. & Parvez, S.H. (2005). The role of iron, copper and zinc and their effects in on/off Parkinson's patients on L-dopa therapy. *Biogenic Amines*, Vol.19, pp. 257-267

Qureshi, G.A.; Qureshi, A.A.; Memon, S.A. & Parvez, S.H. (2006). Impact of selenium, iron, copper and zinc in on/off Parkinson's patients on L-dopa therapy. *J. Neural Transm.*, Vol.71, (Suppl.), pp. 229-236

Rajput, A.H.; Uitti, R.J.; Rozdilsky, B. & Yuen, W.K. (1985). Distribution of metals in Parkinson's disease and control brains. *Neurol.*, Volo.35 (Suppl. 1), p. 224.

Riederer, P.; Sofic, E.; Rausch, W.D.; Schmidt, B.; Reynolds, G.P.; Jellinger, K. & Youdim, M.B. (1989). Transition metals, ferritin, glutathione and ascorbic acid in parkinsonian brains. *J. Neurochem.*, Vol.52, pp. 515-520

Sparks, D.L.; Ziolkowski, C.; Connor, D.; Beach, T.; Adler, C. & Sabbagh, M. (2008). Copper and cognition in Alzheimer's disease and Parkinson's disease. *Cell Biol. Toxicol.*, Vol.24, pp. 426-430

Speziali, M. & Orvini, E. (2003). Metals distribution and regionalization in the brain, In: *Metal Ions and Neurodegenerative Disorders*, P. Zatta (Ed.) 15-65,World Scientific Publishing Co., Singapore-New Jersey

Speziali, M. & Di Casa, M. (2009) Copper, iron, zinc and other element concentrations in cerebrospinal fluid of Parkinson's disease patients – considerations on literature data. *Trace Elem. Electrol.*, Vol.26, pp. 171-176

Takahashi, S.; Takahashi, J.; Osawa, N.; Abe, T.; Yonezawa, H.; Sera, K. & Tohgi, H. (1994). Trace elements analysis of serum and cerebrospinal fluid with PIXE - Effect of age and changes in parkinsonian patients. *Nippon Ronen Igakkai Zasshi*, Vol.31, pp. 865-871

Tan, X.; Luo, Y.; Pan, J.; Huang, B. & Wang P.Q. (2007). Serum Cu, Fe, Mn, and Zn levels and Parkinson's disease. *Parkinsonism Rel. Dis.* Vol.13 (Suppl.), p. S134

Tohno, Y.; Tohno, S.; Ongkana, N.; Suwannahoy, P.; Azuma, C.; Minami, T. & Mahakkanukrauh, P. (2010). Age-related changes of elements and relationships among elements in human hippocampus, dentate gyrus, and fornix. *Biol. Trace Elem. Res.* ,Vol.138, pp. 42-52.

Woodbury, J.; Lyons, K.; Carretta, R.; Hahn, A. & Sullivan, J.F. (1968). Cerebrospinal fluid and serum levels of magnesium, zinc, and calcium in man. *Neurol.*, Vol.18, pp. 700-705

Yasui, M.; Kihira, T. & Ota, K. (1992). Calcium, magnesium and aluminum concentrations in Parkinson's disease. *Neurotoxicol.*, Vol.13, pp. 593-600.

8

Language Processing in Parkinson's Disease Patients Without Dementia

Katrien Colman and Roelien Bastiaanse
University of Groningen
The Netherlands

1. Introduction

One of the major pathophysiological features in Parkinson's disease, from now on referred to as PD, is the loss of dopaminergic neurons in the substantia nigra, which in turn results in dysfunction of the cortico-striato-cortical circuits (Bartels & Leenders, 2009). In PD the components of the cortico-striato-cortical circuits are not in an optimal interaction, leading to insufficient engagement of for example the frontal and prefrontal lobes. Motor symptoms of tremor, bradykinesia, and rigidity are the clinical hallmark of PD (Wolters & Bosboom, 2007), however, non-motor symptoms are often present (Dubois & Pillon, 1995, 1997). In particular cognitive impairments in the domain of executive functioning have frequently been observed, both in late and also in very early stages of PD (Muslimovic et al., 2005). The term 'executive functioning' is used as a blanket term referring to a set of abilities that allow individuals to achieve goal-oriented behavior. These aspects of behavior can be regarded as top-down processes, in contrast to bottom-up processes that only represent stimulus-driven processing. Strauss et al. (2006) defined executive functioning as a collection of processes that are responsible for guiding, directing, and managing cognitive, emotional and behavioral functions, particularly during active, novel problem solving. As PD progresses, more severe cognitive impairments or dementia can occur (Aarsland et al., 2003). The dementia in PD exhibits normal or only slightly decreased performance in gnosis and praxis functions, and is typically characterized by a progressive dysexecutive syndrome with disturbed memory functions and attention (Dubois & Pillon, 1997).

In addition, it has repeatedly been shown that language functions in PD patients with dementia are affected. Demented PD patients show reduced verbal fluency, poor confrontation naming abilities, decreased word list generation, and difficulties in word-finding (Dubois & Pillon, 1997; Pahwa et al., 1998). However, prior to dementia, PD patients also evidence subtle language impairments. The question whether the language system itself is impaired, as for example in aphasia, or whether language performance is disrupted because of non-linguistic executive function disorders in PD is still unanswered. We assume that, intact executive functioning is a prerequisite for normal language functioning. Therefore, language processing deficits in PD will always be associated with executive function deficits. Under this view, the language faculty is not considered to be totally modular in nature, but thought to depend on other cognitive functions, since, for example, comprehending a sentence demands that a listener flexibly guides his/her attention to relevant linguistic information, maintains information in working memory during the incremental development of the sentence interpretation and inhibits prepotent or incorrect parsing. This raises the question which aspect(s) of executive functioning are most important for language comprehension.

The studies described in this review reported on PD patients' production and comprehension in several languages (English, French, German, Greek and Dutch). From the literature it is clear that PD disrupts the processes involved in both language production and language comprehension.

In the present chapter, we will use Levelt's framework for sentence processing (1983, 1989) to clarify production and comprehension of spoken language. This includes implementation of the distinction between controlled and automatic cognitive processing. Figure 1 depicts Levelt's "Blueprint for the speaker" and shows the complex architecture of the various processes involved in speech production and comprehension.

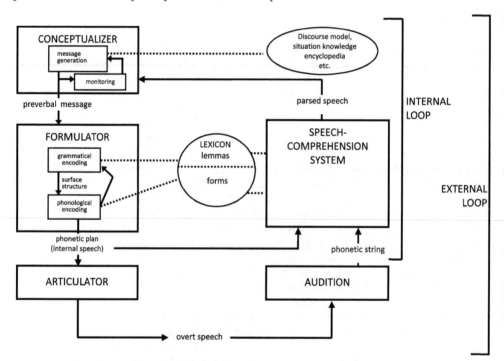

Fig. 1. Blueprint for the speaker (Adapted from Levelt, 1989)

In this figure, the boxes represent processing components and the circle as well as the ellipse represent knowledge stores. The framework consists of two subsystems, one for production and one for comprehension. The Production System is further divided into a Conceptualizer, a Formulator and an Articulator. When a speaker produces speech, he starts with an idea that he intends to communicate in the Conceptualizer. Conceptualizing demands working memory (Levelt, 1989), since during this stage an intention needs to be conceived and relevant information needs to be retrieved from long-term memory and ordered while keeping track of the discourse. In short, the Conceptualizer provides an interface between thought and language and produces a pre-verbal message. Then, using two steps, the Formulator translates this pre-verbal message into a linguistic structure. In a first step, the Grammatical Encoder must access lemma information[1] from the mental lexicon (i.e., declarative knowledge) and activate syntactic building procedures stored in the Grammatical Encoder (i.e., procedural knowledge). Based on the properties of the message, the Grammatical Encoder will assign grammatical functions to the words and build a phrasal representation (e.g., verb phrases or noun phrases), specifying the hierarchical relation between syntactic constituents and their linear order. In a second step, the Phonological Encoder fills in the word forms in the structure that was generated by the Grammatical Encoder. It then constructs a phonetic plan, which is transformed into a spoken utterance by the Articulator. Formulation is "a largely automatic process" (Levelt, 1989, p. 21), implying that lexical retrieval and syntactic planning during production do not rely much on executive functions. However, declarative and procedural memory are both not disconnected from executive functions. For example, during the course of syntactic structure building the selected lemmas from declarative memory need to be maintained and updated by executive functions until the process is terminated.

On the right-hand side in Fig. 1, the Speech Comprehension System is depicted. During comprehension, a spoken utterance is mapped to a phonetic string by the Audition component, from which the Speech Comprehension System computes parsed speech, a representation of the input in terms of phonological, morphological, syntactic, and semantic composition. This representation is further processed by the Conceptualizer. Sentence parsing during comprehension is constrained by working memory capacity (Caplan & Waters, 1999; Just & Carpenter, 1992; Just et al., 1996; Waters & Caplan, 1996).

Speakers inspect their overt and covert speech for errors, thereby allowing themselves to inhibit and repair erroneous utterances. As Levelt (1989, p. 13) says, "a speaker is his own listener". Levelt localizes the central Monitor in the Conceptualizer (see Fig. 1). Very much simplified, Levelt's framework proposes that during language production the speaker monitors production through the Comprehension module. This proposal is known as the 'perceptual loop theory of speech monitoring', and claims that a speaker's phonetic plan is processed by the Speech Comprehension System during speech production, which allows the speaker to compare the comprehension of what he is about to say ('the internal loop') to what he originally intended to express. Speakers are also hypothesized to listen to their own overt speech, giving them another chance to detect errors ('the external loop'). In that case, they use the Audition component to analyze their own speech. Both feedback loops will reach the Monitor located in the Conceptualizer, which checks whether the parsed speech matches the intended speech. Upon error detection, the Monitor signals the speech production system to interrupt speech and to plan a repair process. The Monitor in Levelt's framework has been described as being a central, conscious process that oversees end products of speech production (Postma, 2000). Analogously to the monitoring system in speech production, Van Herten (2006), Van Herten et al. (2006), Vissers (2008), and Van de Meerendonk et al. (2009) proposed a monitoring process during comprehension inspired by the conflict monitoring theory of Botvinick et al. (2001). In the same line, Kuperberg (2007) suggested a monitoring process embedded in her non-syntactocentric, dynamic model of language processing.

---

[1] The lemma of a word contains the semantic and syntactic information, necessary for the construction of the syntactic structure of the sentence. A lemma is still very abstract and distinct from the word forms, that are stored at a different level in the Lexicon

This chapter presents an overview of the extensive and still growing literature examining the underlying mechanisms of the subtle language impairments in non-demented PD patients. The connectivity of the basal ganglia with especially the frontal cortical regions explains why language processing is a vulnerable cognitive function in the course of PD. We start with reviewing what is known about language production deficits in non-demented patients with PD, followed by a summary of the receptive language deficits in PD. This review will not be limited to deficits at the sentence level, but will also consider deficits at the word and discourse level. Over the years, a variety of methodologies have been used, and recently functional imaging in PD patients has begun to add information to the neural instantiation of the patients' language impairments. Studying language processing in PD allows researchers to analyze the effects of poorly functioning, yet still engaged cortico-striato-cortical circuitry during language performance. Some of the studies reviewed in this chapter aimed at examining language processing in PD, to ultimately define the role of the basal ganglia in language processing (e.g., Ullman et al., 1997; Friederici et al., 2003; Grossman et al., 2003; Kotz et al., 2003). In the final section of this chapter, advice for communication guidelines that would guarantee a better quality of life for patients suffering from PD is given. The chapter will be concluded with suggestions for future research on language processing in PD.

2. Language production in PD

2.1 Spontaneous speech

Spontaneous speech in PD patients is often characterized by hypokinetic dysarthria and hypophonia, joined in the term 'dysarthrophonia' (Ackermann & Ziegler, 1989). Some PD patients in the advanced disease stage produce repetitions of speech, which are also labeled as stuttering, speech iterations, or palilalia (Benke et al., 2000). The major complaints reported by PD patients are not as much related to the acoustic, perceptual and physiological changes to their speech, but are related to the effect of these changes on communication overall, their view of themselves and the detrimental effects of the effort required to overcome physical and mental limitations (Miller et al., 2006). Also, PD patients' prosody, facial expression and gestures are abnormal, probably because these are influenced by the cardinal motor impairment.

One of the focuses of this review on language processing is grammatical effects in the spontaneous speech of PD patients, which were first reported by Illes et al. (1988). The sentences produced by the moderately impaired PD patients were syntactically simple. The pattern may reflect an adaptive, compensatory mechanism to reduce speech-motor difficulty, or may actually be evidence of a language impairment intrinsic to the disease process. Illes and colleagues (Illes, 1989; Illes et al., 1988) favored the adaptation hypothesis, stating that as the severity of the disease and, hence, the dysarthria increases, PD patients adapt to or compensate for their motor speech difficulties. Using a verbal picture description task, Murray (2000) observed compromised grammar and informativeness of spoken language in PD patients. Furthermore, a relationship between syntactic changes in production and concomitant cognitive changes was found. While analyzing conversational speech, Murray and Lenz (2001) found that patients with greater cognitive deficits and dysarthria performed more poorly on syntactic measures than patients with either more intact cognitive abilities or more intelligible speech. They suggested that PD patients show syntax limitations in production, but only under certain task requirements or related to other cognitive deficits. This conversational speech analysis showed that changes in language production in PD reflect concomitant cognitive and motor speech impairments, rather than being a pure language deficit. Ellis et al. (2006, see also Ellis, 2006 and Ellis & Rosenbek, 2007) analyzed narrative discourse in individuals with PD and in healthy control speakers. According to Ellis et al. (2006) the analysis of narrative discourse is as a method to differentially characterize expressive language form versus use[2]. They concluded that patients with mild to moderate PD demonstrate deficits in language use while maintaining spared language form.

Earlier, McNamara et al. (1992) suggested that mildly to moderately impaired PD patients have a reduced capacity to simultaneously speak and monitor one's own speech resulting in self-monitoring impairments during narrative discourse. To test overt speech monitoring in narrative discourse of patients with PD, they used the procedures of the Cookie Theft picture description task of the Boston Diagnostic Aphasia Examination (BDAE, Goodglass & Kaplan, 1972). The number and the distribution of uncorrected errors and two repair types were tallied. The results showed that PD patients made three times more errors than the age-matched control speakers and used both repair strategies, but relatively less often than the control speakers. According to the authors, this significant unawareness of speech errors is related to attentional dysfunctioning in PD. They furthermore suggested that PD patients display reduced sensitivity to context, which may complicate their language comprehension. In order to explicitly evaluate PD patients' pragmatic skills[3], McNamara and Durso (2003) used a formal pragmatic communication skills protocol (Prutting & Kirchner, 1987). The pragmatic communication skills were also rated on the basis of the assessment of (self-)awareness of the problem by individual PD patients and their spouses. It was concluded that PD patients were significantly impaired on measures of pragmatic communication abilities and were less aware of their communication problems. In line with Levelt's framework (1989, see Fig. 1) it is concluded that PD patients have a problem in their monitoring system and, thus, are not aware of their errors or, in other words, do not detect the mismatch when comparing their intentions and the actual speech output.

2.2 Verb production in sentence context

In 1997, Ullman and colleagues obtained evidence for a role of the basal ganglia in morphosyntactic production. Ullman et al. (1997) reported the results of a sentence completion task, which required the participants to read aloud randomly ordered sentence pairs and to fill in a past tensed verb. The authors found a correlation between right-side hypokinesia and the impaired production of rule-generated (regular) past tense forms in PD. The authors concluded that PD leads to the suppression of both motor activity and grammatical rule application. In essence, Ullman et al. (1997) and Ullman (2001) proposed that the frontal basal ganglia system, which is damaged in PD, constitutes the procedural memory system that regulates grammar (Grammatical Encoder in Fig. 1) and that the

---

[2] In defining 'what is language', Bloom and Lahey (1978) divided language into three different, but overlapping aspects: content, form and use. In brief, language content includes factors such as semantics, including word knowledge and world knowledge, and vocabulary. Language form refers to the grammar of the language, while language use is akin to the area of pragmatics.

[3] Pragmatic skills involve the ability to use and interpret verbal and nonverbal language appropriately within the social context in which communication occurs, requiring a degree of inference and interpretation (Perkins, 2005).

mental lexicon depends on declarative memory (see Fig. 1), embedded in the temporal lobe, which is largely intact in PD. Set in Levelt's framework (Fig. 1), it is proposed that PD patients have a deficit in grammatical encoding. As a result, PD patients are not able to produce the past tense form of regular verbs.

In the following years, the vast majority of studies on verbal morphosyntactic production in PD focused on testing the Declarative-Procedural hypothesis of Ullman et al. (1997), but the PD data of the Ullman study could not be replicated (Almor et al., 2002; Longworth et al., 2003; Longworth et al., 2005; Penke et al., 2005; Terzi et al., 2005). Longworth et al. (2005) found a tendency in English-speaking PD patients (among other patients with striatal damage) to perseverate on the cue (i.e., verb stem) rather than to produce past tense verbs as requested. Longworth et al. (2005) argued against an isolated grammatical deficit in PD and suggested that the striatum plays a general (i.e., not specific to language), inhibitory role in the later, controlled stages of language comprehension and production. The deficits in PD may reflect impairment of inhibition of competing alternatives during the later controlled processes involved in both comprehension and production (Longworth et al., 2005). Related is our evidence for executive dysfunctions being correlated to deficits in verb production in sentence context (Colman et al., 2009). Contrary to the findings of Ullman et al. (1997), but consistent with the findings of Longworth et al. (2005), no influence of regularity on verb production in sentence context was detected in the Dutch-speaking PD patients. In a study on verb production in sentence context, we showed that a deficit with regular inflection is not a characteristic for Dutch-speaking PD patients (Colman et al., 2009). We furthermore suggested that because of failing automaticity, PD patients relied more on the cortically represented executive functions. Unfortunately, due to the disturbed intimate relation between the basal ganglia and the frontal cortex, these executive functions are also dysfunctional. We manipulated the grammatical features of the test sentences, in order to simultaneously test verb retrieval and sentence integration processes in a group of PD patients compared to a control group consisting of age and education matched healthy participants. All subjects were assessed on both verb production in sentence context as well as on cognitive functions relevant for sentence processing. The verb production performances of the PD patients were correlated to their scores on executive function tasks. Analyses of PD patients' performance revealed that they have set-switching deficits and decreased sustained visual attention. The performance on verb production of PD patients was associated with the set-switching deficits, suggesting that PD patients who show poor set-switching have more difficulties with verb production. Many verb tense errors were made in sentences targeting the present tense. In our verb production task participants were instructed to inflect the verb in the past tense only in the presence of a temporal adverb referring to the past (e.g., 'yesterday') and in the present tense if the adverbial time phrase was absent. It is therefore suggested that the test materials and associated instructions provoked the tense errors. Due to the absence of a temporal adverb, PD patients were unable to switch to the present tense and showed 'stuck-in-set perseverations' which were evoked by the previous sentences. Evidence for self-monitoring deficits has earlier been reported by McNamara et al. (1992). While monitoring their performance, PD patients seemed to forget the instruction, especially in the longer subordinate sentences where working memory was challenged more than in the short main clauses. Hence, in Colman et al. (2009) set-switching impairments played a major role in performing the task assessing verb production in sentence context. These set-switching impairments reduce PD patients' performance seriously. Although the PD patients in our study did not show a decreased working memory capacity compared to healthy speakers, verb production was associated with working memory in PD patients. In healthy speakers, the production of verbs is a rather automatic language processing task, which is confirmed by the fact that no association was found between verb production and working memory in healthy controls. Automatic behavior is thought to be mediated by the basal ganglia (Saling & Phillips, 2007). Since PD is characterized by a dopaminergic dysfunction of the basal ganglia, we assume that PD patients cannot produce verbs in a rather automatic way as well as healthy speakers and, therefore, they need to rely more on their working memory, which we consider to be a compensatory mechanism.

2.3 Single word production tasks
The tests of word fluency that were employed in the studies that will be discussed in the next paragraphs all test, apart from semantic memory, aspects of executive functioning. In a standard word fluency task the subjects are asked to name as many words as possible within a given semantic category (known as semantic or category fluency) or starting with a certain letter (known as phonemic or letter fluency) during a restricted time period. During an alternating fluency task, subjects have to generate words alternately using two fluency probes, which could either be from the same domain (i.e., letter-letter or category-category) or from different domains (i.e., category-letter). In a standard fluency task, planning abilities are evaluated, while in an alternative fluency task, set shifting abilities are evaluated.

Impairments in non-demented PD patients have been reported in both semantic and phonemic fluency, but the most consistent finding is impaired performance in semantic fluency (e.g., Flowers et al., 1995; Grossman, Carvell et al., 1992, Grossman et al., 1993; Gurd & Ward, 1989; Van Spaendonck et al., 1996).

Henry and Crawford (2004) did a meta-analysis of 68 studies published between 1983 and 2002 which included more than 4600 PD participants. One of the aims was to find out if the word fluency deficit associated with PD predominantly reflects executive dysfunction, or problems with semantic memory, which is related to declarative memory. The outcome of the analysis was that, although PD was associated with deficits upon tests of phonemic and semantic fluency for studies that assessed both measures, the semantic fluency deficit was significantly larger than the phonemic fluency deficit. Moreover, since the confrontation naming deficit for the Boston Naming Test (BNT; Kaplan et al., 1983), a measure that imposes only minimal demands upon cognitive speed and effortful retrieval, was equivalent in magnitude to the deficits of these two types of fluency, Henry and Crawford concluded that PD is associated with a particular deficit in semantic memory. However, tests of alternating fluency were associated with slightly larger deficits than standard measures of fluency, which supports evidence for a specific deficit in cognitive set-shifting (Henry & Crawford, 2004). Some PD patients evidenced impairments in semantic knowledge, which correlate with their executive dysfunctions (Portin et al. 2000). The exact underlying nature of the semantic deficits has yet to be determined.

Interestingly, Auriacombe et al. (1993) examined the traditional semantic and phonemic fluency tasks, but also examined fluency performance in the non-verbal modality (i.e., design fluency and category drawing task). They found that PD patients' performance on the non-verbal fluency task was comparable to healthy speakers, and confirmed the discrepancy between relatively intact phonemic fluency and impaired semantic fluency. It is not necessary to retrieve a word form during category drawing, since knowledge of the concept underlying a target superordinate (i.e., vegetable) and the exemplars that contribute to a superordinate is sufficient. To check the hypothesis that PD patients are impaired in the retrieval of semantic information, Auriacombe et al. (1993) also administered a supraspan verbal learning task. A large proportion of the PD patients showed difficulties with free recall, but these patients were accurate at recognition, which is consistent with a retrieval deficit, and not an impairment of semantic memory itself. PD patients thus have difficulties retrieving the phonological form that is the label of an exemplar (Levelt et al., 1991).

In addition, in PD, action naming is often found to be more impaired than object naming (Bertella et al., 2002; Cotelli et al., 2007), a phenomenon also observed in agrammatic/Broca's aphasic patients. Related to this, Signorini and Volpato (2006) found that PD patients were impaired on an action fluency task but not on semantic and phonemic fluency tasks. However, analysis of spontaneous speech production of PD patients did not show the expected discrepancy between nouns and verbs, which supports the hypothesis that it is not the representation of verbs, but rather the utilization of the verb emerging under specific task demands that is troublesome (Pignatti et al., 2006). Moreover, verb fluency scores also discriminate between demented PD patients and non-demented PD patients and healthy elderly control participants, whereas tests of letter or category verbal fluency do not (Piatt et al., 1999a and 1999b). Piatt et al. (1999a, 1999b) concluded that verb fluency was particularly sensitive to the fronto-striatal pathophysiology of PD patients with dementia. According to these authors, verb fluency reflects the underlying integrity of frontal lobe circuitry, and problems on verbal fluency tasks could therefore indicate deficits in executive functioning.

Péran et al. (2003) developed a French word generation task that requires a semantic and grammar driven selection of single words over a limited time period. Compared to healthy control participants, non-demented PD patients made more grammatical errors in the noun-verb-generation task than in the verb-noun-generation task. Péran et al. (2003) suggested that this discrepancy was due to the combined effect of impaired set switching and a specific grammatical impairment in verb production. The authors assume that in the verb-noun task, the impact of impaired switching is compensated by the easier noun production, whereas in the noun-verb task both the switching and production of the verb were dysfunctional.

However, the argument that PD specifically affects verb processing was contradicted in a recent word generation study in PD conducted by Crescentini et al. (2008). Behavioral tasks already showed before that the Reaction Times (RTs) and accuracy of word generation both depend on the number of possible responses (response selection) and on the strength of association between cues and responses (associative strength) (Cheng & Martin, 2005; Martin & Cheng, 2006; Thompson-Schill & Botvinick, 2006). Based on these findings, Crescentini et al. (2008) controlled the response selection demands and association strength of the verb and the noun stimuli during a word generation task. The critical condition for PD patients was the one with a weak association between the stimulus and the response as opposed to the grammatical class. Crescentini et al. (2008) suggested that the verb generation problem in PD is caused by the fact that nouns are typically more associated with other nouns than with verbs in the semantic network. During the noun-verb condition, PD patients seem to have problems with both switching to task-relevant representations (i.e., verbs) and with inhibiting the task-irrelevant and more strongly activated options (i.e., nouns). Based on these findings, the authors proposed a non-language-specific involvement of the basal ganglia in the controlled rather than the routine semantic processes required during lexical retrieval.

One explanation for the discrepancy between verb and noun retrieval is that verb retrieval is more demanding than noun retrieval in terms of executive functioning (e.g., Péran et al., 2003; Piatt et al., 1999a and 1999b). The idea is that retrieving the name of an object elicits a more automatic lexical retrieval response than retrieval of the action name, which demands a more controlled retrieval. In other words, impaired action naming is seen as a result of executive function impairment. According to Levelt's framework (see Fig. 1), the lemmas contain information about word meaning, and word class. The lemmas of verbs additionally contain information on thematic roles, argument structure, and subcategorisation frame. Comparable to what was found for individuals with Broca's aphasia (Bastiaanse & Van Zonneveld, 2004), we suggest that for PD patients verbs are more difficult to produce than nouns, because verb lemmas contain simply more grammatical information than noun lemmas.

An alternative hypothesis for the discrepancy between verb and noun retrieval is that the link between representation of action words and representation of motor acts per se in the human motor and premotor cortex is damaged, leading to verb retrieval problems. The existence of a similar verb-naming deficit in other motor disorders, such as corticobasal degeneration (CBD) and progressive supranuclear palsy (PSP) (Cotelli et al., 2006), has provided a major argument for the idea that semantic mechanisms concerning the verb are grounded in the motor system of the brain. To test whether the motor system comes into play during the processing of verbs, Boulenger et al. (2008) compared lexical decision latencies for action verbs and concrete nouns of non-demented PD patients (off and on dopaminergic medication) using a masked priming paradigm. Priming effects for action verbs, but not for concrete nouns, were nearly absent in PD patients off treatment, confirming that processing lexico-semantic information of action words depends on the integrity of the motor system. As a follow up to their earlier French verb generation task, Péran et al. (2009) explored the relationship between the motor deficit in PD patients and brain activation in noun and verb generation tasks conducting a functional neuroimaging study. Although they did not find differences between the brain activity during the production of object-related action words and of object names, they did observe a clear relationship between brain activity and the severity of the motor deficit (as assessed by the Unified Parkinson's Disease Rating Scale (UPDRS), Fahn et al., 1987) in PD. This relation was particularly found during generation of action verbs in response to manipulable biological objects, in the pre- and post-central gyri bilaterally, left frontal operculum, left supplementary motor area and right superior temporal cortex. The impairment in the motor cortico-striato-cortical circuits in PD may result in the recruitment of a wider cortical network designed to alleviate the disturbed motor representations during the demanding generation of action verbs in response to manipulable objects.

3. Receptive language functions in PD

In the following section, receptive language functions in PD, with a particular focus on sentence comprehension of non-canonical sentences, will be discussed.

3.1 Comprehension of non-canonical sentences

From the early nineties of the last century, off-line tasks such as sentence-to-picture matching and grammaticality judgment have revealed that comprehension of complex syntactic structures (i.e., non-canonical structures such as passives) is vulnerable in individuals with PD (see Grossman, 1999 and Murray, 2008 for an extensive review). Sentences are defined as syntactically complex when the thematic roles are not in base (or canonical) word order and therefore require extra grammatical operations. The following examples are given of an active (a) and a passive (b) sentence in Dutch. Important to note is that base word order in Dutch is Subject-Object-Verb (SOV).

a. De kinderen plukken de appels
    'The children pick the apples'
b. De appels$_i$ worden door de kinderen t$_i$ geplukt
    'The apples are by the children picked'

In passive constructions, the *grammatical roles* are in base order. In sentence (b) the subject ('the apples') precedes the finite verb ('are') which precedes the prepositional phrase ('by the children'). However, the *thematic (semantic) roles* are not in their base position. The theme ('apples'), precedes the finite verb, whereas the agent ('children') follows the finite verb.

Lieberman et al. (1990) were among the first to find a comprehension deficit that could not be attributed to compensatory motor strategies, which had been claimed to be responsible for the sentence production deficits in PD till then (Illes et al., 1988; Illes, 1989). Lieberman et al. (1990) attributed the sentence comprehension errors in PD to "some deterioration of the patient's ability to make use of the syntactic 'rules' involved in English" (1990, p. 364). Similarly, researchers have attributed the sentence comprehension deficit to an impairment of some aspects of grammatical processing as such (Cohen et al., 1994; Natsopoulos et al., 1991, 1993). However, according to Lieberman et al. (1990), the cognitive impairments and syntactic comprehension deficits in PD have a common physiological basis; they are both caused by disruption of the cortico-striato-cortical circuits. Lieberman et al. (1990, 1992) do not regard grammatical processing and executive functions as separate mechanisms. They take the position that syntax comprehension is achieved by the operations of non-domain-specific executive functions over language-specific knowledge. Consistent with this view, some researchers claim that it is not syntax itself, but rather the interaction with executive dysfunction that might reflect the sentence comprehension deficits in PD (see for example Colman, 2011; Colman et al., 2006; Geyer & Grossman, 1994; Grossman, Carvell et al., 1992; Hochstadt et al., 2006, 2009; Kemmerer, 1999; Lieberman et al., 1990, 1992). In addition, some researchers reported deficits in lexical-semantic processing during sentence comprehension. For example, Angwin et al. (2005) reported a general semantic processing deficit, but also reported that PD patients with comprehension deficits for non-canonical sentences showed a delayed time course of semantic activation. This finding added evidence to the proposal that slowed information processing is one of the causes of the sentence processing deficits in patients with PD (Grossman, Zurif et al., 2002; Lee et al., 2003).

Grossman, Lee et al. (2002) administered both a traditional off-line sentence processing task and an on-line word detection task to the same PD patients. Subjects were instructed to press a button as soon as they heard the target word in an auditorily presented sentence. Half of the sentences contained a grammatical agreement violation (e.g., subject-verb agreement violation) prior to the target word. In healthy persons, responses to the target word were slowed down when they immediately followed a morphosyntactic error. The off-line measure of sentence comprehension required subjects to answer a simple question about a semantically unconstrained sentence. In addition to the language tasks, a battery of executive function tests was also run. Off-line, PD patients were significantly impaired on non-canonical sentences and their comprehension was correlated with the executive measures. However, PD patients and healthy control participants were equally sensitive to violations of grammatical agreements during on-line word detection. The comprehension impairment on the traditional measure in PD was argued to be related to impairments in inhibition and planning, emphasizing the important influence of task requirements on sentence comprehension in PD.

In the same year another study by Grossman and colleagues was published, using a different on-line methodology, that is, a list priming task (Grossman, Zurif et al., 2002). Those PD patients who had problems comprehending sentences with a non-canonical structure when measured off-line (e.g., "The boy that the girl chased was friendly") showed delayed lexical retrieval during the priming task. This was reported earlier for Broca's aphasic patients (Swinney et al., 1996; Zurif et al., 1993).

The Grossman group gained additional information on the connection between slowed lexical activation and sentence comprehension deficits in PD by applying the same word detection methodology as before, but by using a different violation type. Based on previous observation of PD patients' difficulty detecting phonetic errors in grammatical morphemes (Grossman, Carvell et al., 1992), the researchers tested phonetic errors in free grammatical morphemes and words as violation type (Lee et al., 2003). PD patients were insensitive to phonetic errors in free grammatical morphemes and showed a slowed sensitivity to words located in the non-canonical sentences. This delayed sensitivity was correlated with the measure of planning, which was seen as evidence for the fundamental contribution of executive functions to sentence comprehension. Lee et al. (2003) concluded that sentence comprehension impairments are due to limitations in specific executive resources such as attention to grammatical morphemes and delayed lexical retrieval of words, rather than being a pure linguistic deficit.

Hochstadt et al. (2006) conducted the first off-line study that also tested the inter-relationship between the distinct executive functions. The authors concluded that limits on sequencing and/or verbal working memory (i.e., executive component and articulatory rehearsal) are responsible for the sentence comprehension deficits in PD. Later, Hochstadt (2009) used eye-tracking to minimize the extraneous executive demands during off-line sentence-picture matching. Some of the PD patients in this study showed difficulties comprehending passive sentences and they looked toward a distractor picture before giving a response. One of the proposed explanations by Hochstadt (2009) for the errors in passive sentences is the exaggerated agent-first bias pointing to a reliance on heuristics to compensate for impaired syntax processing. However, this explanation did not hold for passives in general, since there was no evidence that the bias differed between patients with high and low error rates in final passive trials as compared to center passive trials.

To further explore the hypothesis that executive dysfunctions are involved in the comprehension deficits of passive sentences in PD (Lieberman et al., 1992), we recently tested Dutch-speaking PD patients on the comprehension of sentences that were varied for phrase structure complexity and sentence length (Colman, 2011) to see whether there was a relation between the processing of the sentences and relevant executive function deficits. In general, the PD patients showed slightly poorer sentence comprehension compared to healthy control participants. However, the difficulties encountered by PD patients were not limited to one specific grammatical aspect. Decreased set-switching, inhibition, and working memory abilities were all associated with comprehending non-canonical passive sentences, rather than one specific executive function being primarily associated with the comprehension difficulties. Deficits in sustained visual attention appear to underlie PD patients' overall comprehension performance, possibly due to the demands of the picture-sentence matching task. Generally, our study confirms that the language faculty is not independent from executive functioning.

Several studies using Positron Emission Tomography (PET) and functional Magnetic Resonance Imaging (fMRI) have investigated the pattern of brain activation during sentence processing in non-brain-damaged individuals. However, only a few imaging studies have investigated the underlying neural activity during sentence processing in PD patients. In an fMRI study, Grossman et al. (2003) found striatal activation in exclusively the brains of healthy senior volunteers for long sentences, relative to short sentences. Moreover, PD patients engaged significantly more brain regions associated with working memory than healthy participants to achieve the same level of comprehension accuracy as the control subjects. According to Grossman et al. (2003) the striatum contributes to cognitive resources such as working memory and information-processing speed. PD patients' sentence comprehension difficulties have been ascribed to their limited striatal recruitment, which causes an interruption of a large scale network important for cognitive resources that can interfere with sentence processing (Grossman et al., 2003).

Using Event Related Potential (ERP) studies, Friederici and colleagues have demonstrated that degeneration of the basal ganglia due to PD influences language-related ERP components dramatically and correlates with different aspects of language processing during comprehension (for an overview see Kutas & Van Petten, 1994; Osterhout & Holcomb, 1995) . In a study by Kotz et al. (2002) and by Friederici et al. (2003), the PD patients included showed an intact ELAN (reflecting highly automatic first-pass parsing processes), but a strongly reduced P600. The P600 is an ERP component that is controlled by attention and is explained as indicating secondary syntactic processes such as reanalysis and repair (Friederici & Mecklinger, 1996), or as reflecting syntactic integration processes in general (Kaan et al., 2000). According to Friederici et al. (2003), the alteration in the P600 reflected distortions of the late controlled syntactic integration processes in PD. This reduction in amplitude points to a failure in the activation of the generators of this ERP component in PD patients. The reduction in PD patients' P600 amplitude points to a lack of integrity of the cortico-striato-cortical circuits responsible for the P600 generation. The patient studies by Friederici and colleagues suggest that the frontal cortex and the basal ganglia are differently involved in sentence processing or are active during different stages of auditory sentence processing. The left frontal cortex and the left anterior temporal cortex both contribute to the early automatic processing underlying the (E)LAN, whereas the left basal ganglia contribute to the late controlled syntactic integration processes underlying the P600. The difficulties with syntactic integration processes as described by Friederici et al. suggest that the language system itself is disrupted in PD patients.

In a recent fMRI study, we evaluated the patterns of activation during the comprehension of sentences in which canonicity and grammaticality were manipulated in fifteen patients with PD compared to fifteen healthy older adults (Colman, 2011). Here we focus on the activation patterns related to the processing of the passives by the PD patients and healthy control participants. Our intergroup analysis contradicted the expectation of compensatory cortical activation (Grossman et al., 2003). However, PD patients showed significant increased activation for passive versus active sentences in the left medial/superior frontal gyrus compared to healthy control participants. Three possible explanations for the activation in this frontal area during the processing of passive sentences are suggested. PD patients may rely on working memory, lexical semantics or higher-level semantic processes involved in evaluation of plausibility to compensate for the lack of activation seen in the healthy control participants when dealing with non-canonical passive sentences. First, Carpenter et al. (1994) hypothesized that working memory load is directly related to sentence complexity. As mentioned before, higher sentence complexity is related to the non-canonical order of roles (such as in passives). All in all, non-canonical sentences impose a higher demand on working memory than canonical sentences (King & Just, 1991). The PD patients possibly relied more on their intact working memory allocated in the prefrontal cortex to compensate for their difficulties to process the non-canonical passive sentences (for a review see Wager & Smith, 2003). Secondly, examining ambiguity resolution, Stowe et al. (2004) reported a similar left medial prefrontal area as in our study, which they linked to supporting higher-level semantic processes involved in evaluation of plausibility. Finally, it is suggested that the exclusive activation of the prefrontal cortex in PD patients for passive sentences reflects a lexical-semantic strategy for dealing with word order information, which was probably not always a guarantee for successful comprehension.

3.2 Lexical and semantic processing

Semantic priming tasks are a straightforward measure for the evaluation of lexical and semantic processes in patients with PD. In healthy participants, RTs to the target word are faster if the prime and the target are semantically related (doctor-NURSE) as compared to when the prime and target are not related (doctor-FLOWER) (see Neely, 1991 for extensive review on priming tasks). Copland (2003) found that PD patients are unable to suppress the infrequent meaning of homophones (bank-RIVER) and proposes therefore that the selective attentional engagement of the semantic network is impaired. Thus, PD compromises the controlled aspects of semantic processing rather than the automatic processes. During sentence comprehension tasks, lexical-semantic processing has been found to be abnormal in PD patients as well (Angwin et al., 2005). Angwin et al. (2004, 2006) also found that semantic processing deficits in PD are related to striatal dopamine deficiency since automatic semantic activation was compromised in PD patients when off medication .

Spicer et al. (1994) were the first to evidence a unique increased semantic priming effect in PD patients as compared to the normal control subjects, which they called 'hyperpriming'. This hyperpriming was suggested to be caused by slowness in the unrelated prime-target conditions. Spicer et al. (1994) suggested two possible levels of the deficit, either the pre-lexical level or the post-lexical level. Somewhat later, the same research group (McDonald et al., 1996) revised their theory and concluded that PD patients show poor performance whenever the task requires switching between response sets or different semantic categories. However, rather than hyperpriming reflecting a switching problem between semantically unrelated words, Mari-Beffa et al. (2005) suggested that a lack of lexical-semantic inhibitory control in participants with PD is responsible for it. This idea was confirmed by Castner er al. (2007), who furthermore concluded that subthalamic nucleus stimulation restored these inhibitory processes. Consequently, it is concluded that the basal ganglia are involved in both the automatic and controlled aspects of semantic priming and thus support both the involved facilitation and inhibition processes.

3.3 Verb processing

Using receptive tasks, the existence of a specific verb processing deficit in PD was found. Grossman et al. (1994) reported impaired verb learning. They taught PD patients and healthy age-matched controls the grammatical and semantic information of a new verb ('to wamble'). The semantic and grammatical information of the new verb was probed by sentence judgment and picture classification. Significant impairment in recalling some aspects of the new verb was seen in 55% of the PD patients. These patients demonstrated a language-sensitive deficit in "appreciating grammatical information represented in the new verb" (Grossman et al., 1994, p. 413). However, a small number of PD patients responded randomly to probes of all information about the new verb, which suggests a memory impairment in these patients. More recently, Whiting et al. (2005) evaluated verb and context processing in PD by using a self-paced stop making sense task. The participants had to pace themselves through a sentence that was preceded by a context, which made the thematic role of the verb plausible or implausible. They found that PD patients were impaired in thematic role mapping, which was consistent with previous findings of Geyer and Grossman from 1994. Whiting et al. (2005) proposed that PD participants in their study processed sentences "on a more superficial level" than control subjects and concluded that the PD patients' performance was caused by both global discourse comprehension difficulties and impaired working memory.

3.4 Perceptive pragmatic language abilities
In daily life, healthy individuals interpret the intended meaning of language appropriate to the social context. Another line of research in receptive language functions has been focusing on the pragmatic language skills of PD patients. Pragmatic language use entails the ability to interpret nonliteral elements of language such as metaphors, proverbs, idioms, etc. Berg et al. (2003) conducted a survey of pragmatic language abilities and reported that PD patients exhibit impairments in making inferences,, comprehending metaphors and lexical ambiguities. The study by Whiting et al. (2005) showed that PD patients were less accurate than the control participants in using previously encountered discourse antecedents when deciding that a sentence stopped making sense. This is in line with the finding of Grossman, Crino et al. (1992) in which PD participants displayed an impaired ability to answer questions about previously encountered discourse elements compared to control participants. In addition, patients with PD have these problems also when resolving lexical ambiguities (Copland et al., 2001).
Monetta and Pell (2007) investigated how PD patients process metaphors using a timed property verification task (by Gernsbacher et al., 2001) compared to healthy control participants. The impact of PD on metaphor comprehension varied as a function of working memory ability, meaning that PD patients with a reduced working memory capacity were impaired in the comprehension of metaphors, whereas PD participants at a similar stage of disease but without working memory difficulties performed as good as the healthy control participants (Monetta & Pell, 2007). In a follow-up, similar resutls were found for inference generation (Monetta et al., 2008) and irony comprehension (Monetta et al., 2009). McKinlay et al. (2009) related pragmatic language skills to cognitive functions and suggested that processing speed was a stronger determiner of pragmatic language performance than working memory.
Research relating the pragmatic language problems of PD to their executive function deficits might be influenced by the research investigating morphosyntactic processes during sentence comprehension in PD patients.

4. Impact of language processing deficits on the daily life of PD patients

The subtle deficits in language comprehension and production in PD will lead to communication problems that may result in decreased socialization and participation in society. Miller et al. (2006) investigated the impact of particularly 'speech and voice' deficits on the life of the individual with PD and their family. To this purpose, a group of PD patients was interviewed to explore the onset of speech changes, their impact and patients' strategies to manage these changes. In general, the changes in PD patients' speech and voice had an effect on the overall communication, roles and relationships of those confronted with the disease. It was shown that alterations in speech do not need to be severe to have a significant impact. However, in addition to the speech and voice problems some of the interviewees reported difficulties with word retrieval, sentence formulation and comprehension. This suggests the necessity to refer all newly diagnosed PD patients to speech and language therapy. According to us, this preventive therapy will not only serve articulation and intelligibility abilities, but should also focus on the assessment and remediation of language problems. From our review it is clear that some PD patients suffer from unawareness of the extent of their communicative problems. During social conversations, deficit in the monitoring system influenced turn taking abilities and topic maintenance (McNamara et al., 2003). This unawareness or self-monitoring deficit can prevent the development of adaptive coping strategies, provokes feelings of frustration and might lead to complete withdrawal from communication. PD patients can profit from insights in their language disorders, for example it can help them to use effective compensation strategies or to simply inform the other speech partner of the impact of their disease on communication. From our clinical experience it is clear that patients and their caregivers are often surprised to hear that not only motor symptoms, but also language processing can be affected in the course of the disease. This review on language problems in PD may help in bringing the topic under the attention of those confronted with the disease, meaning that professionals need more up-to-date information. Up-to-date knowledge on the language problems on the part of the patients' environment will facilitate successful communication and, thus, support good family relations. Hence, including routine screening for cognitive decline and language problems early in the disease, in addition to supplying information on PD patients' language problems to caregivers and professionals could keep the PD patients from becoming socially isolated. Examples of communication advice for caregivers could be to simplify and avoid redundancy of information. Speech and language therapy must provide information in tune with the patient's individual limitations and whishes towards language and speech, which in turn can facilitate patients and their environment to implement coping strategies when communicative contexts are arising. In addition, we expect that intensive training of cognitive functions and strategies in PD patients will positively influence processing in the language domain. In the near future a therapy effectiveness study will be developed, which will remediate language problems in combination with executive function deficits in PD.

5. Suggestions for future research

Medication with levodopa is well known to improve the motor symptoms. However, the effects on cognitive functions are more complex: both positive as well as negative effects have been observed. According to Cools (2006), these contrasting effects of levodopa are due to the spatio-temporal progression of dopamine (DA) depletion in PD. PD starts in the dorsal striatum (tail of the Caudate nucleus) and progresses to the ventral striatum (head of the Caudate nucleus). Levodopa in early stages of the disease may improve cognitive functions of the dorsal striatum while simultaneously 'over-dosing' functions of the ventral striatum. This effect of over-dosing is related to the base level of DA in underlying cortico-striato-cortical circuitry and the task instructions. Therefore, in future research, to control for the influence of dopaminergic medication on cognitive processing, we suggest conducting experiments in the practically defined 'off state'. This is typically following an overnight fast from the patient's anti-Parkinson medications. More positive results are expected in this 'off state', but we also expect more influence of other factors such as frustrations with task performance and tremors and rigidity making testing in the MRI scanner impossible. Ultimately, conducting experiments in drug naïve 'de novo' patients is preferred, but clinically these patients are not always willing to participate in research. Apart from the important effects of medication on language processing, the variables of disease duration and age of onset of PD should be taken in consideration in future research.

Future studies on the influence of set-shifting and working memory on sentence processing in PD can benefit from the use of better-controlled and better-understood methods than the clinical accepted neuropsychological tests which were used in the studies reported above. For example, reading span tasks have been used as tests of working memory because they require active manipulation of information and concurrent item retention (Just & Carpenter, 1992). However, reading span tasks rely on many of the same processes as reading comprehension tasks (Engle et al., 1992), which makes it difficult to draw any strong conclusions in terms of the mediating value of working memory for exactly that language process.

In the near future, the nature of the connectivity between the inferior frontal gyrus and the basal ganglia can be further explored. A functional connectivity analysis can provide functional evidence for a basal ganglia-frontal cortical network during the comprehension of sentences in which the variables of canonicity and grammaticality are crossed. However, it is generally known that in fMRI, temporal resolution is inferior and that it cannot index neural activity that is specifically time-locked to the critical word itself. The temporal coarseness of the fMRI method probably blurred the linguistic processes. Simultaneous ERP/fMRI may allow improved localization of neural generators as well as enhanced temporal resolution of BOLD activation foci. Functional connectivity analysis can be used to examine the degree of collaboration between language-specific cortical areas and the basal ganglia, when processing violated compared to non-violated sentences. In on-line behavioral tasks, the impact of executive functions necessary for syntactic processes per se and the executive functions necessary for the task can potentially be disentangled. Therefore, a valuable technique for obtaining on-line data from sentence-picture matching is the eye-tracking method as suggested by Hochstadt (2009).

Finally, as evidenced by this review, there exists an extensive amount of literature on language processing in PD, but language processing in other motor syndromes has received little attention. The existence of a similar verb naming deficit in other movement disorders, such as CBD and PSP (Cotelli et al., 2006) has provided a major argument for the theory that semantic characteristics of the verb are grounded in the motor system of the brain. It will be interesting to test verb production related to cognitive functions in the following movement disorders:

Multiple system atrophy (MSA) is an adult-onset, sporadic, progressive neurodegenerative disease characterized by varying severity of Parkinsonian features, cerebellar ataxia, autonomic failure, urogenital dysfunction, and corticospinal disorders (Gilman et al., 2008). MSA is also accompanied by cognitive impairments associated with dysfunctional cortico-striato-cortical circuits (Herting et al., 2007).

PSP is a neurodegenerative disease characterized by defects in the vertical ocular gaze, bulbar dysfunction, increased frequency of falling, and akinetic-rigid features. In addition, cognitive impairments, in particular executive dysfunctions associated with alterations within the frontostriatal circuitry, occur (Millar et al., 2006).

CBD is characterized by slowly progressing, unilateral Parkinsonism with dystonia or myoclonus, unresponsiveness to Levodopa, and limb apraxia. Patients with CBD often demonstrate impairments in visuospatial processing and visuoconstruction (Tang-Wai et al., 2003) in combination with acalculia, dysexecutive symptoms and aphasia (McMonagle et al., 2006).

Thus far, only a few studies have investigated language processing in patients with atypical Parkinson syndromes, such as MSA (Apostolova et al., 2006), PSP and CBD (Josephs & Duffy, 2008; McMonagle et al., 2006).

6. Conclusion

This review highlights that the progressive degeneration of the cortico-striato-cortical circuits due to PD disturbs executive functioning and, thus contributes to deficits in language production and comprehension. One of the major conclusions based on this review is the importance of evaluating both the executive functions and modalities of language processing (i.e., comprehension and production) in patients with PD. This is not only crucial for our understanding of PD and for the relationship between languages and executive functions, but it is also particularly useful for efficiently identifying the needs for direct intervention

More research still needs to be done to illuminate further the impact of PD on language processing. Future research needs focus on the clinical implementation of evidence-based communication guidelines in order to guarantee a better quality of life for patients suffering from PD.

7. Acknowledgements

This chapter was written on the basis of Katrien Colman's PhD dissertation. Roelien Bastiaanse was the principal supervisor of the PhD project. This research project was funded by the Stichting Internationaal Parkinson Fonds (Hoofddorp, the Netherlands).

8. References

Aarsland, D., Andersen, K., Larsen, J. P., & Lolk, A. (2003). Prevalence and characteristics of dementia in parkinson disease: An 8-year prospective study. *Archives of Neurology, 60* (3), 387-392, ISSN-L 0003-9942.

Ackermann, H., & Ziegler, W. (1989). [Dysarthrophonia of parkinson syndrome]. *Fortschritte Der Neurologie-Psychiatrie, 57*(4), 149-160, ISSN 0720-4299.

Almor, A., Kempler, D., Andersen, E. S., Macdonald, M. C., Hayes, U. L., & Hintiryan, H. (2002). The production of regularly and irregularly inflected nouns and verbs in alzheimer and parkinson patients. *Brain and Language, 83*(1), 149-151, ISSN-L 0093-934X.

Angwin, A. J., Chenery, H. J., Copland, D. A., Murdoch, B. E., & Silburn, P. A. (2004). The time course of semantic activation in parkinson's disease. *Brain and Language, 91*(1), 145-146, ISSN-L 0093-934X.

Angwin, A. J., Chenery, H. J., Copland, D. A., Murdoch, B. E., & Silburn, P. A. (2005). Summation of semantic priming and complex sentence comprehension in parkinson's disease. *Cognitive Brain Research, 25*(1), 78-89, ISSN-L 0926-6410.

Angwin, A. J., Copland, D. A., Chenery, H. J., Murdoch, B. E., & Silburn, P. A. (2006). The influence of dopamine on semantic activation in parkinson's disease: Evidence from a multipriming task. *Neuropsychology, 20*(3), 299-306, ISSN-L 0894-4105.

Apostolova, L. G., Klement, I., Bronstein, Y., Vinters, H. V., & Cummings, J. L. (2006). Multiple system atrophy presenting with language impairment. *Neurology, 67*(4), 726-727, ISSN-L 0028-3878.

Auriacombe, S., Grossman, M., Carvell, S., Gollomp, S., Stern, M. B., & Hurtig, H. I. (1993). Verbal fluency deficits in parkinson's disease. *Neuropsychology, 7*(2), 182-192, ISSN-L 0894-4105.

Bartels, A. L., & Leenders, K. L. (2009). Parkinson's disease: The syndrome, the pathogenesis and pathophysiology. *Cortex, 45*(8), 915-921, ISSN-L 0010-9452.

Bastiaanse, R., & van Zonneveld, R. (2004). Broca's aphasia, verbs and the mental lexicon. *Brain and Language, 90*(1-3), 198-202, ISSN-L 0093-934X.

Benke, T., Hohenstein, C., Poewe, W., & Butterworth, B. (2000). Repetitive speech phenomena in parkinson's disease. *Journal of Neurology, Neurosurgery, and Psychiatry, 69*(3), 319-324, ISSN-L 0022-3050.

Berg, E., Bjornram, C., Hartelius, L., Laakso, K., & Johnels, B. (2003). High-level language difficulties in parkinson's disease. *Clinical Linguistics and Phonetics, 17*(1), 63-80, ISSN-L 0269-9206.

Bertella, L., Albani, G., Greco, E., Priano, L., Mauro, A., Marchi, S., . . . Semenza, C. (2002). Noun verb dissociation in parkinson's disease. *Brain and Cognition, 48*(2-3), 277-280, ISSN-L 0278-2626.

Bloom, L., & Lahey, M. (1978). *Language development and language disorders.* New York: John Wiley & Sons, ISBN 0-471-04438-5.

Botvinick, M. M., Braver, T. S., Barch, D. M., Carter, C. S., & Cohen, J. D. (2001). Conflict monitoring and cognitive control. *Psychological Review, 108*(3), 624-652, ISSN-L 0033-295X.

Boulenger, V., Mechtouff, L., Thobois, S., Broussolle, E., Jeannerod, M., & Nazir, T. A. (2008). Word processing in parkinson's disease is impaired for action verbs but not for concrete nouns. *Neuropsychologia, 46*(2), 743-756, ISSN-L 0028-3932.

Caplan, D., & Waters, G. S. (1999). Verbal working memory and sentence comprehension. *The Behavioral and Brain Sciences, 22*(1), 77-94, ISSN-L 0140-525X.

Castner, J. E., Copland, D. A., Silburn, P. A., Coyne, T. J., Sinclair, F., & Chenery, H. J. (2007). Lexical-semantic inhibitory mechanisms in parkinson's disease as a function of subthalamic stimulation. *Neuropsychologia, 45*(14), 3167-3177, ISSN-L 0028-3932.

Cheng, Y., & Martin, R. (2005). Selection demands vs. association strength in the verb generation task. *Brain and Language, 95*(1), 193-194, ISSN-L 0093-934X.

Cohen, H., Bouchard, S., Scherzer, P., & Whitaker, H. (1994). Language and verbal reasoning in parkinson's disease. *Neuropsychiatry, Neuropsychology, & Behavioral Neurology, 7*(3), 166-175, ISSN-L 0894-878X.

Colman, K., Koerts, J., van Beilen, M., Leenders, K. L., & Bastiaanse, R. (2006). The role of cognitive mechanisms in sentence comprehension in dutch speaking parkinson's disease patients: Preliminary data. *Brain and Language, 99*(1-2), 109-110, ISSN-L 0093-934X.

Colman, K. S. F. (2011). *Behavioral and neuroimaging studies on language processing in Dutch speakers with parkinson's disease.* (Unpublished PhD thesis). University of Groningen, Groningen, The Netherlands, ISBN (digital version) 9789036747530.

Colman, K. S. F., Koerts, J., van Beilen, M., Leenders, K. L., Post, W. J., & Bastiaanse, R. (2009). The impact of executive functions on verb production in patients with parkinson's disease. *Cortex, 45*(8), 930-942, ISSN-L 0010-9452.

Cools, R. (2006). Dopaminergic modulation of cognitive function-implications for L-DOPA treatment in parkinson's disease. *Neuroscience and Biobehavioral Reviews, 30*(1), 1-23, ISSN-L 0149-7634.

Copland, D. A., Chenery, H. J., & Murdoch, B. E. (2001). Discourse priming of homophones in individuals with dominant nonthalamic subcortical lesions, cortical lesions and parkinson's disease. *Journal of Clinical and Experimental Neuropsychology, 23*(4), 538-556, ISSN-L 1380-3395.

Copland, D. A. (2003). The basal ganglia and semantic engagement: Potential insights from semantic priming in individuals with subcortical vascular lesions, parkinson's disease, and cortical lesions. *Journal of the International Neuropsychological Society, 9*(7), 1041-1052, ISSN-L 1355-6177.

Cotelli, M., Borroni, B., Manenti, R., Alberici, A., Calabria, M., Agosti, C., . . . Cappa, S. F. (2006). Action and object naming in frontotemporal dementia, progressive supranuclear palsy, and corticobasal degeneration. *Neuropsychology, 20*(5), 558-565, ISSN-L 0894-4105.

Cotelli, M., Borroni, B., Manenti, R., Zanetti, M., Arévalo, A., Cappa, S. F., & Padovani, A. (2007). Action and object naming in parkinson's disease without dementia. *European Journal of Neurology, 14*(6), 632-637, ISSN-L 1351-5101.

Crescentini, C., Mondolo, F., Biasutti, E., & Shallice, T. (2008). Supervisory and routine processes in noun and verb generation in nondemented patients with parkinson's disease. *Neuropsychologia, 46*(2), 434-447, ISSN-L 0028-3932.

Dubois, B., & Pillon, B. (1995). Do cognitive changes of parkinson's disease result from dopamine depletion? *Journal of Neural Transmission. Supplementum, 45,* 27-34, ISSN-L 0303-6995.

Dubois, B., & Pillon, B. (1997). Cognitive deficits in parkinson's disease. *Journal of Neurology, 244*(1), 2-8, ISSN-L 0340-5354.

Ellis, C. (2006). *The contribution of the basal ganglia to expressive language performance.* (Unpublished PhD thesis), University of Florida, Gainesville, ISBN 9780542351716.

Ellis, C., okun, M. S., Gonzalez-Rothi, I. J., Crosson, B., Rogalski, Y., & Rosenbek, J. C. (2006). Expressive language after PD: Deficits in use but not form. *Movement Disorders, 21,* 897-898, ISSN-L 0885-3185.

Ellis, C., & Rosenbek, J. C. (2007). The basal ganglia and expressive language. A review and directions for research. *Communicative Disorders Review, 1*(1), 1-15, ISSN-L 1933-2831.

Engle, R. W., Cantor, J., & Carullo, J. J. (1992). Individual differences in working memory and comprehension: A test of four hypotheses. *Journal of Experimental Psychology. Learning, Memory, and Cognition, 18*(5), 972-992, ISSN-L 0278-7393.

Fahn, S., & Elton, R. (1987). Unified parkinson's disease rating scale. In: Fahn, S., Marsden, C. D., Calne, D. B., Goldstein, M. (Eds.), *Recent Developments in Parkinson's Disease, Volume 2,* (153-163), Florham Park, NJ. Macmillan Health Care Information.

Flowers, K. A., Robertson, C., & Sheridan, M. R. (1995). Some characteristics of word fluency in parkinson's disease. *Journal of Neurolinguistics, 9*(1), 33-46, ISSN-L 0911-6044.

Friederici, A. D., Kotz, S. A., Werheid, K., Hein, G., & von Cramon, D. Y. (2003). Syntactic comprehension in parkinson'd disease: Investigating early automatic and late integrational processes using event-related potentials. *Neuropsychology, 17*(1), 133-142, ISSN-L 0894-4105.

Friederici, A. D., & Mecklinger, A. (1996). Syntactic parsing as revealed by brain responses: First-pass and second-pass parsing processes. *Journal of Psycholinguistic Research, 25*(1), 157-176, ISSN-L 0090-6905.

Gernsbacher, M. A., Keysar, B., Robertson, R. R. W., & Werner, N. K. (2001). The role of suppression and enhancement in understanding metaphors. *Journal of Memory and Language, 45*(3), 433-450, ISSN-L 0749-596X.

Geyer, H. L., & Grossman, M. (1994). Investigating the basis for the sentence comprehension deficit in parkinson's disease. *Journal of Neurolinguistics, 8*(3), 191-205, ISSN-L 0911-6044.

Gilman, S., Wenning, G. K., Low, P. A., Brooks, D. J., Mathias, C. J., Trojanowski, J. Q., . . . Vidailhet, M. (2008). Second consensus statement on the diagnosis of multiple system atrophy. *Neurology, 71*(9), 670-676, ISSN-L 0028-3878.

Goodglass, H., & Kaplan, E. (1972). *The assessment of aphasia and related disorders.* Philadelphia: Lea & Febiger, ISBN 0812103572.

Grossman, M. (1999). Sentence processing in parkinson's disease. *Brain and Cognition, 40*(2), 387-413, ISSN-L 0278-2626.

Grossman, M., Carvell, S., Gollomp, S., Stern, M. B., Reivich, M., Morrison, D., . Hurtig, H. I. (1993). Cognitive and physiological substrates of impaired sentence processing in parkinson's disease. *Journal of Cognitive Neuroscience, 5*(4), 480-498, 1530-8898, ISSN 1530-8898.

Grossman, M., Carvell, S., Stern, M. B., Gollomp, S., & Hurtig, H. I. (1992). Sentence comprehension in parkinson's disease: The role of attention and memory. *Brain and Language, 42*(4), 347-384, ISSN-L 0093-934X.

Grossman, M., Cooke, A., DeVita, C., Lee, C., Alsop, D., Detre, J., . Hurtig, H. I. (2003). Grammatical and resource components of sentence processing in parkinson's disease: An fMRI study. *Neurology, 60*(5), 775-781, ISSN-L 0028-3878.

Grossman, M., Lee, C., Morris, J., Stern, M. B., & Hurtig, H. I. (2002). Assessing resource demands during sentence processing in parkinson's disease. *Brain and Language, 80*(3), 603-616, ISSN-L 0093-934X.

Grossman, M., Stern, M. B., Gollomp, S., Vernon, G., & Hurtig, H. I. (1994). Verb learning in parkinson's disease. *Neuropsychology, 8*(3), 413-423, ISSN-L 0894-4105.

Grossman, M., Zurif, E., Lee, C., Prather, P., Kalmanson, J., Stern, M. B., & Hurtig, H. I. (2002). Information processing speed and sentence comprehension in parkinson's disease. *Neuropsychology, 16*(2), 174-181, ISSN-L 0894-4105.

Gurd, J. M., & Ward, C. D. (1989). Retrieval from semantic and letter-initial categories in patients with parkinson's disease. *Neuropsychologia, 27*(5), 743-746, ISSN-L 0028-3932.

Henry, J. D., & Crawford, J. R. (2004). Verbal fluency deficits in parkinson's disease: A meta-analysis. *Journal of the International Neuropsychological Society, 10*(4), 608-622, ISSN-L 1355-6177.

Herting, B., Beuthien-Baumann, B., Pöttrich, K., Donix, M., Triemer, A., Lampe, J. B., . . . Holthoff, V. A. (2007). Prefrontal cortex dysfunction and depression in atypical parkinsonian syndromes. *Movement Disorders, 22*(4), 490-497, ISSN-L 0885-3185.

Hochstadt, J., Nakano, H., Lieberman, P., & Friedman, J. (2006). The roles of sequencing and verbal working memory in sentence comprehension deficits in parkinson's disease. *Brain and Language, 97*(3), 243-257, ISSN-L 0093-934X.

Hochstadt, J. (2009). Set-shifting and the on-line processing of relative clauses in parkinson's disease: Results from a novel eye-tracking method. *Cortex, 45*(8), 991-1011, ISSN-L 0010-9452.

Illes, J. (1989). Neurolinguistic features of spontaneous language production dissociate three forms of neurodegenerative disease: Alzheimer's, huntington's, and parkinson's. *Brain and Language, 37*(4), 628-642, ISSN-L 0093-934X.

Illes, J., Metter, E. J., Hanson, W. R., & Iritani, S. (1988). Language production in parkinson's disease: Acoustic and linguistic considerations. *Brain and Language, 33*(1), 146-160, ISSN-L 0093-934X.

Josephs, K. A., & Duffy, J. R. (2008). Apraxia of speech and nonfluent aphasia: A new clinical marker for corticobasal degeneration and progressive supranuclear palsy. *Current Opinion in Neurology, 21*(6), 688-692, ISSN-L 1080-8248.

Just, M. A., & Carpenter, P. A. (1992). A capacity theory of comprehension: Individual differences in working memory. *Psychological Review, 99*(1), 122-149, ISSN-L 0033-295X.

Just, M. A., Carpenter, P. A., & Keller, T. A. (1996). The capacity theory of comprehension: New frontiers of evidence and arguments. *Psychological Review, 103*(4), 773-780, ISSN-L 0033-295X.

Kaan, E., Harris, A., Gibson, E., & Holcomb, P. (2000). The P600 as an index of syntactic integration difficulty. *Language and Cognitive Processes, 15*(2), 159-201, ISSN-L 0169-0965.

Kaplan, E., Goodglass, H., & Weintraub, S. (1983). *The Boston naming test.* Philadelphia: Lea & Febiger, ISBN 9780812101003.

Kemmerer, D. (1999). Impaired comprehension of raising-to-subject constructions in parkinson's disease, *Brain and Language, 66*(3), 311-328, ISSN-L 0093-934X.

Kotz, S. A., Frisch, S., von Cramon, D. Y., & Friederici, A. D. (2003). Syntactic language processing: ERP lesion data on the role of the basal ganglia. *Journal of the International Neuropsychological Society, 9*(7), 1053-1060, ISSN-L 1355-6177.

Kotz, S. A., Frisch, S., Werheid, K., Hein, G., von Cramon, D. Y., & Friederici, A. D. (2002). The role of the basal ganglia in syntactic language processing: Event-related potential evidence from different patient populations and syntactic paradigms. *Brain and Language, 83*(1), 69-70, ISSN-L 0093-934X.

Kuperberg, G. R. (2007). Neural mechanisms of language comprehension: Challenges to syntax. *Brain Research, 1146*, 23-49, ISSN-L 0006-8993.

Kutas, M., & Van Petten, C. K. (1994). Psycholinguistics electrified: Event-related brain potential investigations. In M. A. Gernsbacher (Ed.), *Handbook of psycholinguistics* (83-143). San Diego: Academic Press, ISBN 0122808908.

Lee, C., Grossman, M., Morris, J., Stern, M. B., & Hurtig, H. I. (2003). Attentional resource and processing speed limitations during sentence processing in parkinson's disease. *Brain and Language, 85*(3), 347-356, ISSN-L 0093-934X.

Levelt, W. J. M. (1983). Monitoring and self-repair in speech. *Cognition, 14*(1), 41-104, ISSN-L 0010-0277.

Levelt, W. J. M. (1989). *Speaking: From intention to articulation.* Cambridge, MA: MIT Press, ISBN 0262121379.

Levelt, W. J. M., Schriefers, H., Vorberg, D., Meyer, A. S., Pechmann, T., & Havinga, J. (1991). The time course of lexical access in speech production: A study of picture naming. *Psychological Review, 98*(1), 122-142, ISSN-L 0033-295X.

Lieberman, P., Friedman, J., & Feldman, L. S. (1990). Syntax comprehension deficits in parkinson's disease. *The Journal of Nervous and Mental Disease, 178*(6), 360-365, ISSN-L 0022-3018.

Lieberman, P., Kako, E., Friedman, J., Tajchman, G., Feldman, L. S., & Jiminez, E. B. (1992). Speech production, syntax comprehension, and cognitive deficits in parkinson's disease. *Brain and Language, 43*(2), 169-189, ISSN-L 0093-934X.

Longworth, C. E., Keenan, S. E., Barker, R. A., Marslen-Wilson, W. D., & Tyler, L. K. (2005). The basal ganglia and rule-governed language use: Evidence from vascular and degenerative conditions. *Brain, 128*(3), 584-596, Online ISSN 1460-2156.

Longworth, C. E., Tyler, L. K., & Marslen-Wilson, W. D. (2003). Language deficits and basal ganglia lesions: The past tense. *Brain and Language, 87*(1), 7-8, ISSN-L 0093-934X.

Mari-Beffa, P., Hayes, A. E., Machado, L., & Hindle, J. V. (2005). Lack of inhibition in parkinson's disease: Evidence from a lexical decision task. *Neuropsychologia, 43*(4), 638-646, ISSN-L 0028-3932.

Martin, R. C., & Cheng, Y. (2006). Selection demands versus association strength in the verb generation task. *Psychonomic Bulletin and Review, 13*(3), 396-401, ISSN-L 1069-9384.

McDonald, C., Brown, G. G., & Gorell, J. M. (1996). Impaired set-shifting in parkinson's disease: New evidence from a lexical decision task. *Journal of Clinical and Experimental Neuropsychology, 18*(6), 793-809, ISSN-L 1380-3395.

McKinlay, A., Dalrymple-Alford, J. C., Grace, R. C., & Roger, D. (2009). The effect of attentional set-shifting, working memory, and processing speed on pragmatic language functioning in parkinson's disease. *European Journal of Cognitive Psychology, 21*(2), 330-346, ISSN-L 0954-1446.

McMonagle, P., Blair, M., & Kertesz, A. (2006). Corticobasal degeneration and progressive aphasia. *Neurology, 67*(8), 1444-1451, ISSN-L 0028-3878.

McNamara, P., & Durso, R. (2003). Pragmatic communication skills in patients with parkinson's disease. *Brain and Language, 84*(3), 414-423, ISSN-L 0093-934X.

McNamara, P., Obler, L. K., Au, R., Durso, R., & Albert, M. L. (1992). Speech monitoring skills in alzheimer's disease, parkinson's disease, and normal aging. *Brain and Language, 42*(1), 38-51, ISSN-L 0093-934X.

Millar, D., Griffiths, P., Zermansky, A. J., & Burn, D. J. (2006). Characterizing behavioral and cognitive dysexecutive changes in progressive supranuclear palsy. *Movement Disorders, 21*(2), 199-207, ISSN-L 0885-3185.

Miller, N., Noble, E., Jones, D., & Burn, D. J. (2006). Life with communication changes in parkinson's disease. *Age and Ageing, 35*(3), 235-239, ISSN-L 0002-0729.

Monetta, L., Grindrod, C. M., & Pell, M. D. (2008). Effects of working memory capacity on inference generation during story comprehension in adults with parkinson's disease. *Journal of Neurolinguistics, 21*(5), 400-417, ISSN-L 0911-6044.

Monetta, L., Grindrod, C. M., & Pell, M. D. (2009). Irony comprehension and theory of mind deficits in patients with parkinson's disease. *Cortex, 45*(8), 972-981, ISSN-L 0010-9452.

Monetta, L., & Pell, M. D. (2007). Effects of verbal working memory deficits on metaphor comprehension in patients with parkinson's disease. *Brain and Language, 101*(1), 80-89, ISSN-L 0093-934X.

Murray, L. L. (2000). Spoken language production in huntington's and parkinson's diseases. *Journal of Speech, Language, and Hearing Research, 43*(6), 1350-1366, ISSN-L 1092-4388.

Murray, L. L. (2008). Language and parkinson's disease. *Annual Review of Applied Linguistics, 28*(-1), 113-127, ISSN-L 0267-1905.

Murray, L. L., & Lenz, L. P. (2001). Productive syntax abilities in huntington's and parkinson's diseases. *Brain and Cognition, 46*(1-2), 213-219, ISSN-L 0278-2626.

Muslimović, D., Post, B., Speelman, J. D., & Schmand, B. (2005). Cognitive profile of patients with newly diagnosed parkinson disease. *Neurology, 65*(8), 1239-1245, ISSN-L 0028-3878.

Natsopoulos, D., Grouios, G., Bostantzopoulou, S., Mentenopoulos, G., Katsarou, Z., & Logothetis, J. (1993). Algorithmic and heuristic strategies in comprehension of complement clauses by patients with parkinson's disease. *Neuropsychologia, 31*(9), 951-964, ISSN-L 0028-3932.

Natsopoulos, D., Katsarou, Z., Bostantzopoulou, S., Grouios, G., Mentenopoulos, G., & Logothetis, J. (1991). Strategies in comprehension of relative clauses by parkinsonian patients. *Cortex, 27*(2), 255-268, ISSN-L 0010-9452.

Osterhout, L., & Holcomb, P. (1995). Event related potentials and language comprehension. In M. D. Rugg, & M. G. H. Coles (Eds.), *Electrophysiology of mind: Event-related brain potentials and cognition* (171-215). New York: Oxford University Press, ISBN 0198521359.

Pahwa, R., Paolo, A., Troster, A., & Koller, W. (1998). Cognitive impairment in parkinson's disease. *European Journal of Neurology, 5*(5), 431-441, ISSN-L 1351-5101.

Péran, P., Rascol, O., Demonet, J. F., Celsis, P., Nespoulous, J. L., Dubois, B., & Cardebat, D. (2003). Deficit of verb generation in nondemented patients with parkinson's disease. *Movement Disorders, 18*(2), 150-156, ISSN-L 0885-3185.

Péran, P., Cardebat, D., Cherubini, A., Piras, F., Luccichenti, G., Peppe, A., . . . Sabatini, U. (2009). Object naming and action-verb generation in parkinson's disease: A fMRI study. *Cortex, 45*(8), 960-971, ISSN-L 0010-9452.

Perkins, M. R. (2005). Pragmatic ability and disability as emergent phenomena. *Clinical Linguistics and Phonetics, 19*(5), 367-377, ISSN-L 0269-9206.

Piatt, A. L., Fields, J. A., Paolo, A. M., Koller, W. C., & Tröster, A. I. (1999a). Lexical, semantic, and action verbal fluency in parkinson's disease with and without dementia. *Journal of Clinical and Experimental Neuropsychology, 21*(4), 435-443, ISSN-L 1380-3395.

Piatt, A. L., Fields, J. A., Paolo, A. M., & Tröster, A. I. (1999b). Action (verb naming) fluency as an executive function measure: Convergent and divergent evidence of validity. *Neuropsychologia, 37*(13), 1499-1503, ISSN-L 0028-3932.

Pignatti, R., Ceriani, F., Bertella, L., Mori, I., & Semenza, C. (2006). Naming abilities in spontaneous speech in Parkinson's and Alzheimer's disease. *Brain and Language, 99*(1-2), 113-114, ISSN-L 0093-934X.

Portin, R., Laatu, S., Revonsuo, A., & Rinne, U. K. (2000). Impairment of semantic knowledge in parkinson disease. *Archives of Neurology, 57*(9), 1338-1343, ISSN-L 0003-9942.

Postma, A. (2000). Detection of errors during speech production: A review of speech monitoring models. *Cognition, 77*(2), 97-132, ISSN-L 0010-0277.

Prutting, C. A., & Kirchner, D. M. (1987). A clinical appraisal of the pragmatic aspects of language. *The Journal of Speech and Hearing Disorders, 52*(2), 105-119, ISSN-L 0022-4677.

Saling, L. L., & Phillips, J. G. (2007). Automatic behaviour: Efficient not mindless. *Brain Research Bulletin, 73*(1-3), 1-20, ISSN-L 0361-9230.

Signorini, M., & Volpato, C. (2006). Action fluency in parkinson's disease: A follow-up study. *Movement Disorders, 21*(4), 467-472, ISSN-L 0885-3185.

Spicer, K. B., Brown, G. G., & Gorell, J. M. (1994). Lexical decision in parkinson disease: Lack of evidence for generalized bradyphrenia. *Journal of Clinical and Experimental Neuropsychology, 16*(3), 457-471, ISSN-L 1380-3395.

Strauss, E., Sherman, E. M. S., & Spreen, O. (2006). *A compendium of neuropsychological tests: Administration, norms and commentary.* New York: Oxford University Press, ISBN 9780195159578.

Swinney, D., Zurif, E. B., Prather, P., & Love, T. (1996). Neurological distribution of processing resources underlying language comprehension. *Journal of Cognitive Neuroscience, 8,* 174-184, ISSN 1530-8898.

Tang-Wai, D. F., Josephs, K. A., Boeve, B. F., Dickson, D. W., Parisi, J. E., & Petersen, R. C. (2003). Pathologically confirmed corticobasal degeneration presenting with visuospatial dysfunction. *Neurology, 61*(8), 1134-1135, ISSN-L 0028-3878.

Thompson-Schill, S. L., & Botvinick, M. M. (2006). Resolving conflict: A response to martin and cheng (2006). *Psychonomic Bulletin and Review, 13*(3), 402-408, ISSN-L 1069-9384.

Ullman, M. T. (2001). A neurocognitive perspective on language: The declarative/procedural model. *Nature Reviews Neuroscience, 2*(10), 717-726, ISSN-L 1471-003X.

Ullman, M. T., Corkin, S., Coppola, M., Hickok, G., Growdon, J. H., Koroshetz, W. J., & Pinker, S. (1997). A neural dissociation within language: Evidence that the mental dictionary is part of declarative memory, and that grammatical rules are processed by the procedural system. *Journal of Cognitive Neuroscience, 9*(2), 266-276, ISSN 1530-8898.

van de Meerendonk, N., Kolk, H. H. J., Chwilla, D. J., & Vissers, C. T. W. M. (2009). Monitoring in language perception *Language and Linguistics Compass, 3*(5), 1211-1224, ISSN-L 1749-818X.

van Spaendonck, K. P. M., Berger, H. J. C., Horstink, M. W. I. M., Buytenhuijs, E. L., & Cools, A. R. (1996). Executive functions and disease characteristics in parkinson's disease. *Neuropsychologia, 34*(7), 617-626, ISSN-L 0028-3932.

van, Herten M. (2006). *Executive control of sentence perception: An electrophysiological investigation.* (Unpublished PhD thesis). Radbout Universiteit Nijmegen, the Netherlands, ISBN 9090208984.

van, Herten M., Chwilla, D. J., & Kolk, H. H. (2006). When heuristics clash with parsing routines: ERP evidence for conflict monitoring in sentence perception. *Journal of Cognitive Neuroscience, 18*(7), 1181-1197, ISSN 1530-8898.

Vissers, C. T. W. M. (2008). *Monitoring in language perception: An electrophysiological investigation.* (Unpublished PhD thesis). Radbout Universiteit Nijmegen, the Netherlands, ISBN 9789090230061.

Waters, G. S., & Caplan, D. (1996). The measurement of verbal working memory capacity and its relation to reading comprehension. *The Quarterly Journal of Experimental Psychology. A, 49*(1), 51-75, ISSN-L 0272-4987.

Whiting, E., Copland, D., & Angwin, A. (2005). Verb and context processing in parkinson's disease. *Journal of Neurolinguistics, 18*(3), 259-276, ISSN-L 0911-6044.

Wolters, E. C., & Bosboom, J. L. W. (2007). Parkinson's disease. In E. C. Wolters, T. van Laar & H. W. Berendse (Eds.), *Parkinsonism and related disorders.* Amsterdam: VU University Press, ISBN 9789086591503.

Zurif, E., Swinney, D., Prather, P., Solomon, J., & Bushell, C. (1993). An on-line analysis of syntactic processing in broca's and wernicke's aphasia. *Brain and Language, 45*(3), 448-464, ISSN-L 0093-934X.

Part 2

Novel Methods to Evaluate the Symptoms in Parkinson's Disease

9

Novel Methods to Evaluate Symptoms in Parkinson's Disease – Rigidity and Finger Tapping

Takuyuki Endo[1*], Masaru Yokoe[2*], Harutoshi Fujimura[1] and Saburo Sakoda[1†]

[1]*Toneyama National Hospital,*
[2]*Osaka University Graduate School of Medicine,*
Japan

1. Introduction

Parkinsonian symptoms such as tremor, rigidity, akinesia, and postural instability are perceived subjectively, and therefore understanding the degree of the symptoms varies depending on the neurologist. Sensing technologies and computer science have advanced and can now detect neurological symptoms and the detected data can be analyzed by software and described in a similar manner to how neurologists perceive those symptoms. This chapter discusses two popular neurological examinations in Parkinson's disease (PD); one is rigidity, which is representative of passive movement, and the other is finger tapping, which is representative of active movement.

Rigidity, a well known symptom of PD, is defined as increased muscle tone that is elicited when an examiner moves the patient's limbs, neck, or trunk, and this increased resistance to passive movement is equal in all directions (Fahn & Przedborski 2005). Many researchers have analyzed rigidity by applying biomedical engineering principles and electrophysiological techniques (Fung et al. 2000, Prochazka et al. 1997, Teravainen et al. 1989). However, we do not know exactly what we feel in muscle tone in PD.

Finger tapping, one of The Unified Parkinson's Disease Rating Scale (UPDRS) items, is commonly used in daily neurological examinations. Its evaluation includes velocity, amplitude, and rhythm. However, observation of these is subjective.

To evaluate rigidity and finger tapping, it is necessary to sense muscle tone and finger movement. We have previously developed novel methods to evaluate rigidity and finger tapping (Endo et al. 2009, Kandori et al., 2004). In this chapter, we showed the usefulness of these systems as objective markers of treatment.

2. Evaluating the effects of deep brain stimulation on rigidity and finger tapping

We evaluated the effects of deep brain stimulation (DBS) of the subthalamic nucleus (STN) on rigidity and finger tapping using our measuring materials. The preceded study of the

---

*equally contributed authors
†corresponding author

effects of STN-DBS revealed that rigidity responded immediately upon tuning DBS, while improvement of finger tapping needed longer time to manifest after tuning DBS. Thus, we analyzed Parkinsonian rigidity by comparing the DBS on state to the DBS off state and finger tapping by comparing pre-operation DBS to post-operation DBS in this study.

2.1 Subjects

Five patients in whom PD was diagnosed according to British Brain Bank clinical criteria (Gibb & Lees 1988) and who received STN-DBS were included in this study. Clinical details of patients with PD who participated in rigidity analysis are shown in Table 1, and those in finger tapping are shown in Table 2. Prior to measurement, patients with PD were assessed using the UPDRS Part III. In this examination, rigidity was scored using a five-point scale (0 = no rigidity, 1 = slight or detectable only when activated, 2 = mild to moderate, 3 = marked, and 4 = severe), and finger-tapping was also scored using the five-point scale (0 = normal; 1 = mild slowing and/or reduction in amplitude; 2 = moderately impaired, definite and early fatiguing, may have occasional arrests in movement; 3 = severely impaired, frequent hesitation in initiating movements or arrests in ongoing movement; and 4 = can barely perform the task). This study was approved by the Institutional Review Board of Osaka University Hospital and written informed consent was obtained from all subjects.

	Age (y)	Sex	Disease duration (y)	Duration after DBS	UPDRS score		
					Part III (*on)	Rigidity (Right)	Rigidity (Left)
pd1	73	M	5	One month	28	1/1(*on/off)	1/1(*on/off)
pd2	70	F	13	One month	8	1/2	1/1
pd3	60	F	11	One year	59	2/3	2/2
pd4	63	F	18	6 years	40	1/2	1/1
pd5	72	F	29	5 years	29	1/1	1/1

Table 1. Clinical details of patients who participated in rigidity analysis. * on/off; DBS-on/off

	Age (y)	Sex	Handed	Initially affected site	Evaluation interval between pre and post (month)	UPDRS PartIII		UPDRS PartIII Finger-tapping score	
						Pre	Post	Pre (L/R)	Post (L/R)
PD1	67	M	Right	Left	3	49	29	3/2	2/1
PD2	69	F	Right	Right	1	26	8	1/2	1/1
PD3	69	M	Right	Right	2	24	17	1/2	1/1
PD4	62	F	Right	Right	1	40	20	2/2	1/1
PD5	73	F	Right	Left	1	34	29	2/1	1/1

Table 2. Clinical details of patients who participated in finger tapping analysis

2.2 Sensing methods
2.2.1 Muscle tonus measurement device

Figure 1 shows a schematic diagram of the muscle tonus measurement system. Details of the device were described in a previous report (Endo et al. 2009). Briefly, elbow joint torque was estimated using the force along the Z-axis and the longitudinal length of the forearm. The elbow joint angle was calculated from the signal generated by the gyroscope. The EMG activity was recorded from surface electrodes attached to the *biceps brachii* and *triceps brachii*.

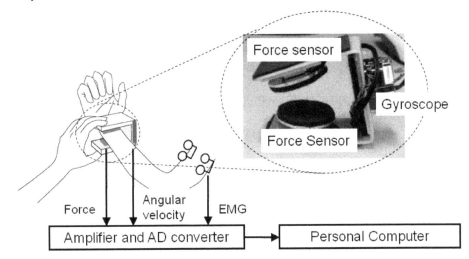

Fig. 1. Schematic diagram of the muscle tonus measurement system

2.2.2 Finger tapping measurement system

The basic method for sensing finger tap movement has been described previously (Kandori et al. 2003, Shima et al. 2008). The finger-tapping measurement system used in this study is shown in Figure 2. A magnetic sensor consisting of two coils is used to measure finger-tapping movement. The coil voltage depending on the distance between the two coils enables estimation of the distance between two fingertips. We calculated the rhythm, amplitude, and velocity of the finger-tapping movement.

2.3 Protocols
2.3.1 Protocols for measuring rigidity

Each subject with DBS-on state or DBS-off state was instructed to relax in a sitting position; the examiner applied the measuring device to the wrist joint of the subject and practiced passive flexion and extension movements at the elbow joint. The measurement of DBS-off state started at 1 min after DBS was turned off. The measurement was made by repeating the four phases of movement as described in a previous report (Endo et al. 2009): (1) holding the elbow at maximum extension for at least 3 s (Fig. 3A), (2) passive flexion for 2 s, (3) holding the elbow at maximum flexion for at least 3 s (Fig. 3B), and (4) passive extension for 2 s (ramp-and-hold). This measurement was repeated twice for each of the left and right upper limbs and the resulting values were averaged on each side independently. Two measurements each for left and right upper limbs were obtained per subject.

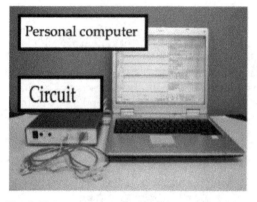
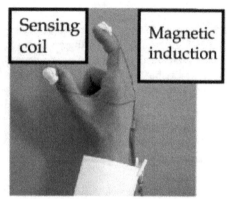

Fig. 2. Finger-tapping measurement system

Figure 4A and Figure 5A shows the typical longitudinal data extracted from the right upper limb of patient pd3 in Table 1 with a UPDRS rigidity score of 2/3 (DBS-on/off). Figure 4A represents the DBS-off state and Figure 5A represents the DBS-on state. Torque-angle characteristics in passive flexion and passive extension are also shown in Figure 4B (DBS-off state) and Figure 5B (DBS-on state).

2.3.2 Protocols for measuring finger tapping
Five patients with PD were evaluated 1 week before and 3 to 5 months after surgery. The magnetic sensors were worn on the subject's index finger and thumb. The subject practiced the finger tapping movement for about 10 s. The subject was asked to execute the finger tapping movements as quickly and widely as possible for 15 s. The finger-tapping wave of patient PD1 before and after intervention is shown in Figure 6.

2.4 Data analysis
2.4.1 Data analysis for rigidity
The resulting data were analyzed by extracting features from elbow joint torque-angle characteristics during passive flexion and extension as shown in Figure 7. The features used here were elastic coefficients in extension and flexion and the sum of the differences of averaged torque values. These were calculated as follows: for the elastic coefficients, the slopes of the regression lines for both flexion and extension were estimated based on the torque-angle data. The data from the start point to the last maximal extension phase were used to calculate the elastic coefficient, which included four to five cycles. At this time, torque values were adjusted for gravity using the mass of the forearms and hands as estimated from the subject's body weight (de Leva 1996). For the sum of the differences of averaged torque values, first we averaged the flexion torque values across four trials at a certain joint angle and also averaged the extension torque values similarly. Then, the differences of the averaged torque values at 30°, 60°, and 90° were calculated and the resulting values were summed.

These three features, that is, the elastic coefficients in extension and flexion and the sum of the differences of averaged torque values, were normalized using the mass of the subject's body weight, because these are dependent on the subject's muscle mass.

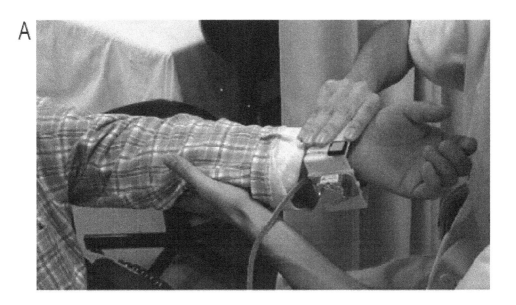

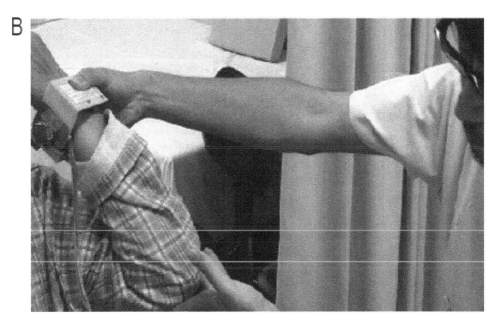

Fig. 3. Measuring protocol. A: holding the elbow at maximum extension. B: holding the elbow at maximum flexion

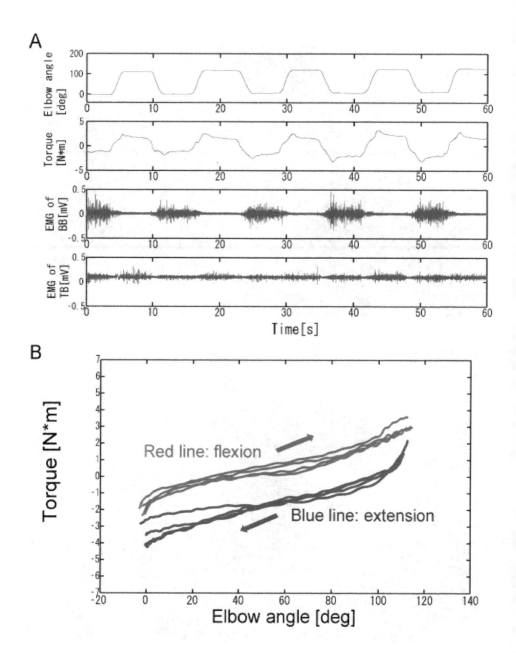

Fig. 4. Typical longitudinal data (A) and torque-angle characteristics (B) in passive flexion and passive extension (DBS-off state) obtained from the right upper limb of patient pd3 with UPDRS rigidity score 3.

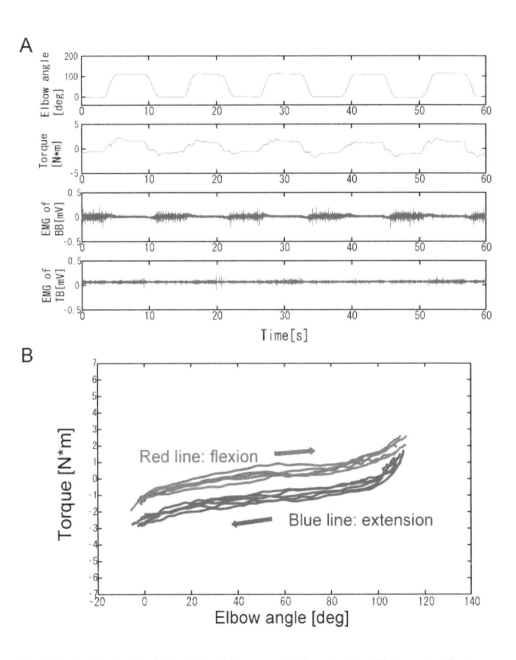

Fig. 5. Typical longitudinal data (A) and torque-angle characteristics (B) in passive flexion and passive extension (DBS-on state) obtained from the right upper limb of patient pd3 with UPDRS rigidity score 2.

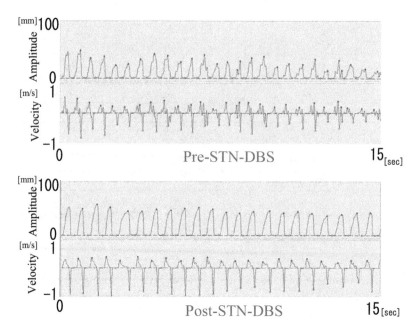

Fig. 6. The finger-tapping wave of patient PD1 before and after intervention

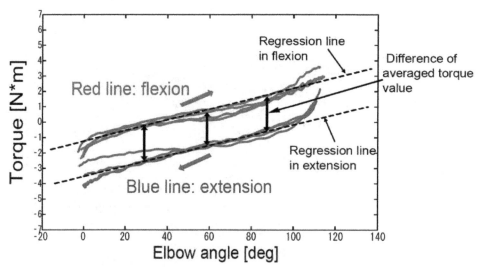

Fig. 7. Extracting features from torque-angle characteristics. Elastic coefficients in flexion
and extension were calculated by estimating the slopes of the regression lines for both
phases. Differences in the averaged torque values were calculated at 30°, 60°, and 90°.

2.4.2 Data analysis for finger tapping

We statistically analyzed five parameters of repetitive index finger-to-thumb oppositions for 15 seconds (Fig. 8). A single finger-tapping interval (FTI) was defined as the interval between the onset of a finger tap and the onset of the next finger tap. We measured the following: the maximum opening velocity (MoV) in a single finger-tapping movement; the maximum closing velocity (McV) in a single finger-tapping movement; the maximum amplitude (MA) during a single finger-tapping movement; and the standard deviation (SD) of FTI, the index of rhythm as the variation of finger-tapping coordination. The mean MA, MoV, and McV for 15 s were calculated. The frequency was the number of finger taps in 15 s (NFT).

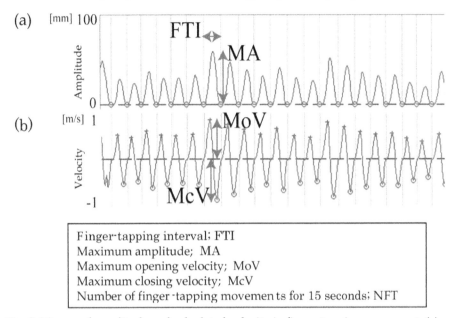

Finger-tapping interval; FTI
Maximum amplitude; MA
Maximum opening velocity; MoV
Maximum closing velocity; McV
Number of finger-tapping movements for 15 seconds; NFT

Fig. 8. Measured amplitude and calculated velocity in finger-tapping movement. (a) Measured amplitude, (b) Calculated velocity.

2.5 Results

Rigidity

Using the data obtained from both left and right upper limbs of five patients with PD, 10 data sets on muscle tonus were available for final analysis. The effects of STN-DBS on three parameters are shown in Figures 9, 10, and 11. Age-matched normal values of elastic coefficients in extension and flexion and the sum of the differences of averaged torque values from 20 control subjects were 1.0[N*m/rad*kg], 1.0[N*m/rad*kg], and 1.0[N*m/kg], respectively.

In the arms with a UPDRS rigidity score 2 or 3 in the DBS-off state, DBS-on improved their scores. Figures of elastic coefficients in extension and flexion and the sum of the differences of averaged torque values in this muscle tonus system supported UPDRS rigidity score improvement. In addition, these three parameters also showed improvement even in arms where the UPDRS rigidity scores did not improve in the DBS-on state. This result indicates that this muscle tonus measuring system is sensitive, objective, and precise. On the other hand, in arms with a UPDRS rigidity score of 1, which is a subtle change in muscle tonus, apparent improvement was not detected using this system. The difference of averaged torque values is the most sensitive among the three parameters.

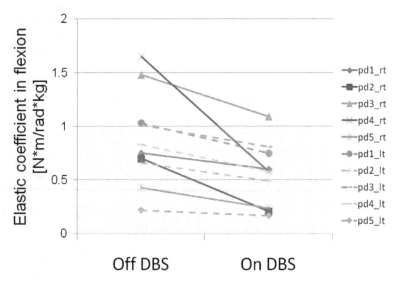

Fig. 9. Effects of deep brain stimulation on the elastic coefficient in flexion. The filled area (less than 1.0[N*m/rad*kg]) represents the normal region.

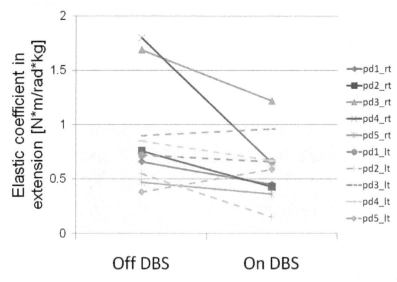

Fig. 10. Effects of deep brain stimulation on the elastic coefficient in extension. The filled area (less than 1.0[N*m/rad*kg]) represents the normal region.

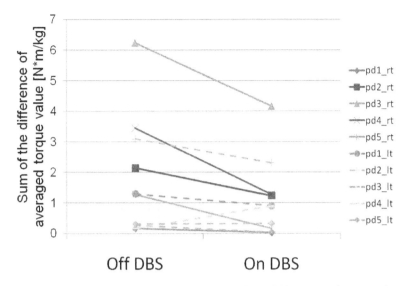

Fig. 11. Effects of deep brain stimulation on the sum of the differences of averaged torque values. The filled area (less than 1.0[N*m/kg]) represents the normal region.

Finger tapping

As shown in Table 2, improvement in UPDRS finger-tapping score after DBS was observed in PD1, PD2, and PD4. The finger-tapping wave of PD1 before and after intervention is shown in Figure 6. Irregular and disordered finger tapping changed to a smooth and correct performance after DBS. This system allows examiners to understand improvement at first sight. In the parameter analysis of finger-tapping movement, all patients with PD showed significant improvement after DBS in three parameters: mean of MoV, mean of McV, and mean of MA. However, it was not necessarily the case that STN-DBS improved the SD of FTI (Fig. 12). In summary, MoV, McV, and MA in PD1, PD2, and PD4 apparently improved, suggesting these are possible treatment markers.

3. Conclusion

We succeeded in showing the effects of DBS on rigidity and finger-tapping movement quantitatively using these instruments. The severity of symptoms obtained by these systems would not show much difference among examiners. Because neurologists could grasp subtle changes after not only DBS but also an increase in drug dose such as dopamine receptor agonists, these instruments would indicate treatment efficacy to neurologists before patients realized the improvement in their symptoms.

In the present analysis, rigidity was quantified by "work", in which the average work was done by the torque motor over one cycle (Shapiro et al. 2007). However, the concept of "work" views the flexion and extension movements as a single system, and strictly speaking, it is different from the sum of the differences of averaged torque values that we extracted. If one repeats sinusoidal flexion and extension movements as a measurement protocol, most features could not be properly evaluated at each phase because the stretch reflex has greater impact when the flexion phase is switched to the extension phase.

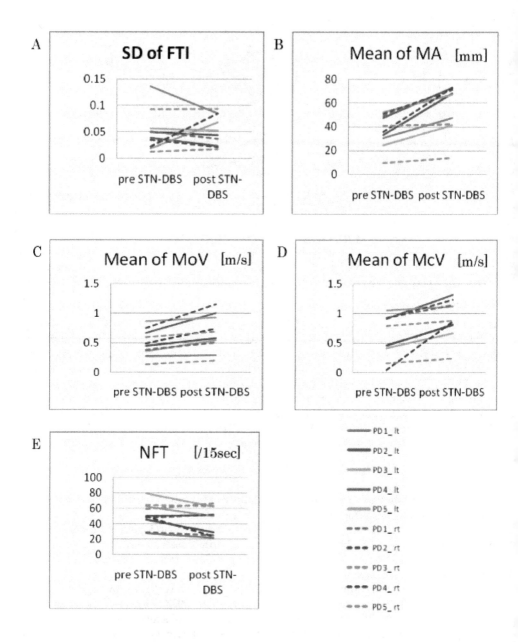

Fig. 12. Differences in five finger tapping parameters between before and after STN-DBS
(A)SD of FTI (B)Mean of MA (C)Mean of MoV (D)Mean of McV (E)NFT

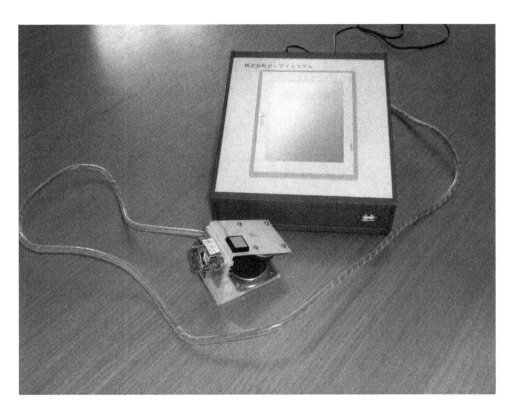

Fig. 13. Prototype of compact muscle tonus measurement system

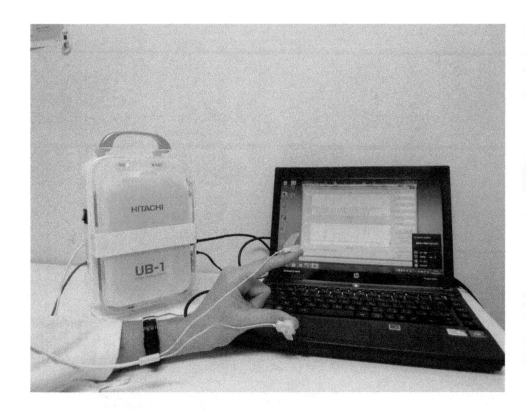

Fig. 14. New finger tapping analysis system by Hitachi Co. Ltd. (Hitachi Computer Peripherals Co. Ltd., Tokyo branch, 1-11-1, Ohmorikita, Ohta-ku, Tokyo, Zip.143-0016, JAPAN, TEL: +81-3-5753-6870, FAX: +81-3-5753-6872)

We previously reported that the muscle activity index in the static phase (EMG index) obtained for *biceps brachii* muscles, elastic coefficients, and sum of the differences of averaged torque values correlated well with the UPDRS score. Recently, we found that the EMG index is a good marker to distinguish a UPDRS rigidity score of 1 from the normal control (unpublished data). Because the elastic coefficients and the sum of the differences of averaged torque values seemed to be simple and better indicators of drug efficacy than the EMG index (unpublished data), we decided to use elastic coefficients and the sum of the differences of averaged torque values in this study. Rigidity is a clinical sign that gets worse immediately after DBS and therefore, this system is suitable for the tuning of DBS.

In finger tapping, we previously reported fourteen parameters of finger-tapping movement and a radar chart showed obvious differences in most of these parameters between normal controls and patients with PD (Yokoe et al. 2009). Principal component analysis showed that these parameters could be classified into three components: (1) mean of both amplitude and velocity, (2) number of finger tappings and mean FTI, and (3) SD of FTI. The first (velocity- and amplitude-related parameters) and third (rhythm-related parameters) components contributed to the discrimination of PD from normal controls. Regarding which component reflects treatment efficacy, parameters in the first component, including mean of MoV, mean of McV, and mean of MA, are good markers. The second component, including the number of finger tappings, does not reflect treatment efficacy. The third component, including the SD of FTI, depends on the patient. The left hand of PD1 showed improvement, although the right hand of PD2 worsened. However, both fingers moved faster and larger after DBS (Fig. 12). These results indicate that DBS works on the first component parameters rather than those of the third component.

These novel systems for testing muscle tonus and finger-tapping, which are compact, simple, and efficient, are very useful for daily neurological examinations. The muscle tonus measurement system was recently established, as shown in Figure 13 (product of PI System Co. Ltd, http://www.pis.co.jp), and the finger-tapping measurement system recently came on the market in Japan from Hitachi Co. Ltd. as shown in Figure 14.

These sensing systems identify rigidity or spasticity and the nature of abnormal finger tapping in PD and show Parkinsonian symptoms as a system error in software of repetitive movement.

4. Acknowledgment

We thank Dr. Kenzo Akazawa (Osaka Institute of Technology, Department of Biomedical Engineering), Dr. Ryuhei Okuno (Setsunan University, Department of Electrical and Electronic Engineering), Dr. Toshio Tsuji (Hiroshima University, Faculty of Engineering), Dr. Akihiko Kandori (Hitachi Co. Ltd., Advanced Research Laboratory) and Dr. Kei Fukada (Osaka General Medical Center) for their assistance during the design of this study. This study was supported by the Program for Promotion of Fundamental Studies in Health Sciences of the National Institute of Biomedical Innovation (NIBIO).

5. References

de Leva, P. (1996). Adjustments to Zatsiorsky-Seluyanov's segment inertia parameters. *Journal of Biomechanics* Vol.29, No.9, (September1996), pp.1223-1230, ISSN 0022-0949

Endo, T.; Okuno, R.; Yokoe, M.; Akazawa, K. & Sakoda, S. (2009). A Novel Method for Systematic Analysis of Rigidity in Parkinson's Disease. *Movement Disorders*, Vol.24, No.15, (November 2009), pp. 2218-2224, ISSN 0885-3185

Fahn, S.M.C.; Calne, D. & Goldstein, M. (1987). UPDRS Development Comittee. Unified Parkinson's disease rating scale, In: *Recent Developments in Parkinson's Disease*, Macmillan Healthcare Innformation, ISBN: 0-8816-7132-0, USA

Fahn, S. & Przedborski S. (2005). Parkinsonism, In: *Merritt's Neurology, eleventh edition*, Lewis P. Rawland, pp. 828-846, Lippincott Williams & Wilkins, ISBN 0-7817-5311-2, USA

Fung, V.S.; Burne, J.A. & Morris, J.G.(2000). Objective quantification of resting and activated parkinsonian rigidity: a comparison of angular impulse and work scores. *Movement Disorders*, Vol.15, No.1, (January 2000), pp.48-55, ISSN 0885-3185

Gibb, W.R. & Lees, A.J. (1988). The relevance of the Lewy body to the pathogenesis of idiopathic Parkinson's disease.*Journal of Neurology, Neurosurgery and Psychiatry*, Vol.51, No6, (June 1988), pp745-752, ISSN 0022-3050

Kandori, A.; Yokoe, M.; Sakoda, S.; Abe, K.; Miyashita, T.; Oe, H.; Naritomi, H.; Ogata, K. & Tsukada, K. (2004). Quantitative magnetic detection of finger movements in patients with Parkinson's disease, *Neuroscience Research*, Vol.49, No.2 (June 2004), pp.253-260, ISSN 0306-4552

Prochazka, A.; Bennett, D.J.; Stephens, M.J.; Patric, S.K.; Sears-Duru, R.; Roberts, T. & Jhamandas, J.H. (1997). Measurement of rigidity in Parkinson's disease. *Movement Disorders*, Vol.12, No.1, (January 1997), pp.24-32, ISSN 0885-3185

Shapiro, M. B.; Vaillancourt, D. E.; Sturman, M. M.; Metman, L. V.; Bakay, R. A. E.; & Corcos, D. M.(2007). Effects of STN DBS on Rigidity in Parkinson's Disease. *IEEE TRANSACTIONS ON NEURAL SYSTEMS AND REHABILITATION ENGINEERING*, Vol.15, No.2, (June 2007), pp. 173-181, ISSN 1534-4320

Shima, K.; Tsui, T.; Kan, E.; Kandori, A.; Yokoe, M. & Sakoda, S. (2008). Measurement and evaluation of finger tapping movements using magnetic sensors. *Conference Proceedings of IEEE Engineering in Medicine and Biology Society*, (August 2008), pp.5628-5631, ISBN 978-1-4244-1814-5

Teravainen, H.; Tsui, J.K.; Mak, E. & Calne, D.B. (1989). Optimal indices for testing parkinsonian rigidity. *Canadian Journal of Neurological Scieince*, Vol.16, No.2, (May1989), pp.180-183, ISSN:0317-1671

Yokoe, M.; Okuno, R.; Hamasaki, T.; Kurachi, Y.; Akazawa, K. & Sakoda, S. (2009). Opening velocity, a novel parameter, for finger tapping test in patients with Parkinson's disease, *Parkinsonism & Related Disorders*, Vol.15, No.6, (July 2009), pp.440-444, ISSN 1353-8020

10

Objective Evaluation of the Severity of Parkinsonism Using Power-Law Temporal Auto-Correlation of Activity

Weidong Pan[1,3], Yoshiharu Yamamoto[2] and Shin Kwak[1]
[1]Department of Neurology, Graduate School of Medicine, The University of Tokyo,
[2]Educational Physiology Laboratory, Graduate School of Education, The University of Tokyo,
[3]Department of Neurology, Shuguang Hospital Affiliated to Shanghai University of TCM,
[1,2]Japan,
[3]China

1. Introduction

Parkinson disease (PD) is a neurodegenerative disorder not only with motor symptoms, including resting tremor, rigidity, bradykinesia and postural instability, but also with non-motor symptoms, including autonomic disturbance, sleep disturbance and depression. Due to the lack of objective biomarkers like the blood glucose level for diabetes mellitus, severity of parkinsonism has been evaluated by using the symptom-based Unified Parkinson Disease Rating Scale (UPDRS) (Martinez-Martin et al., 1994) that covers the various aspects of symptoms in patients with PD. Although the UPDRS is the standard method for the assessment of parkinsonism and the evaluation of drug effects, the scoring is not free from inter-rater variance or the fluctuation of the symptoms.

Wearable accelerometers enable long-term recording of patient's movement during activities of daily living, and hence might be a suitable device for quantitative assessment of the disease severity and progression. Alterations in locomotor-activity levels and disturbances in rest-activity rhythms have long been recognized as integral signs of major psychiatric and neurological disorders (Teicher, 1995; Witting et al., 1990). Improvement of ambulatory activity monitors (actigraph) has enabled precise calibration and storage of thousands of activity measurements acquired at predetermined times, hence enabled long-term recording of patient's movement during ordinary daily living (Katayama, 2001; Korte et al., 2004; Mormont et al., 2000; Okawa et al., 1995; Teicher, 1995; Tuisku et al., 2003; van Someren et al., 1996). It has been demonstrated that use of these devices is useful for the quantitative estimation of human behavior properties in normal subjects and patients with a variety of diseases, including depression, pain syndrome, and PD (Jean-Louis et al., 2000; Korszun et al., 2002; Nakamura et al., 2007; Ohashi et al., 2003; Pan et al., 2007; van Someren et al., 1993; 1998; 2006). However, because the pattern of daily activity greatly influences the recording with accelerometers, recorded activity levels may not adequately reflect the disease severity (Fig 1). Therefore, reliable analytical methods of the body acceleration signal free from the level of activity are required to describe the characteristics of body activity during daily living. Recently, fractal analysis was shown to be a robust tool to disclose hidden auto-correlation patterns in biological data, such as heartbeat and limb movement (Ohashi et al., 2003; Pan et al., 2007; Peng et al., 1995; Sekine et al., 2004; Struzik et al., 2006). Power-law auto-correlation exponents for local maxima and minima of fluctuations of locomotor activity would be the most useful for our purpose, as they represent the level of persistency of movement patterns (Ohashi et al., 2003; Pan et al., 2007).

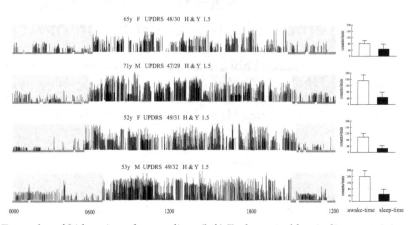

Fig. 1. Examples of 24 h actigraph recording. (left) Each vertical bar indicates activity counts per min. Sleep time is indicated in blue. Patients with approximately the same severity show different activity patterns and the activity counts (right: mean ± S.D.). UPDRS total/Part III.

In this review, we show how we can extract hidden autocorrelation patterns reflecting the severity of parkinsonism from the actigraph recording of patients' activity, and demonstrate that the analysis using power-law exponents is useful for the evaluation of effects of therapy on motor and non-motor symptoms of parkinsonism.

2. Analytical method of the motionlogger recordings for power-law auto-correlation exponents

We analyzed patients' physical activity records collected by an actigraph device using power-law exponents probing temporal auto-correlation of the activity counts. The power-law exponent for local maxima most sensitively and reliably reflects disability without being influenced by the presence of tremor or the patterns of daily living (Pan et al., 2007).

To examine temporal auto-correlation of the physical activity time series (i.e., *dynamic* aspects of physical activity), we used an extended, random-walk analysis, the detrended fluctuation analysis (DFA) (Peng et al., 1995), with a modification (Ohashi et al., 2003) for various "real-world" signals including activity time series. Briefly, a daytime physical activity time series was integrated, as in DFA, and wavelets with different time scales (S) were slid along the time series and correlated with the data to obtain the wavelet coefficients ($W(S)$) at each point. The third derivative of the Gaussian function was used as the so-called "mother wavelet":

$$\Psi(t) = t(3-t^2)e^{-0.5t^2},2$$

where t is time. This is equivalent to using the Gaussian second derivative (so-called "Mexican hat") wavelet to examine the raw signals (Fig. 2), though the integration approach automatically removes the local mean and the local linear trend, as in DFA. By changing the scale of the wavelet, this "hat-shaped" template dilates or contracts in time, probing transient increases or decreases in activity records in different time scales. The transient increases (low-high-low activity patterns) yield local maxima of the wavelet coefficients at their time points, while the decreases (high-low-high activity patterns) yield local minima of the wavelet coefficients (see Fig. 2). Next, the squared wavelet coefficients at the local maxima or minima were averaged for all the available days. As the coefficient gives the magnitude of local fluctuations matching the shape of $\psi(t)$ with different time scales, the squared $W(S)$ was used, again as in DFA. Finally, the power-law exponent (α) was obtained separately for local maxima and minima as the slope of a straight line fit in the double-logarithmic plot of S vs. $W(S)^2$. This method yields the same α–values as does DFA (Ohashi et al., 2003), but separately for periods with higher and lower activity levels. The power-law (scaling) exponent, α, reflects the probability of a simultaneous increase or decrease in the variability at two distant points in time in the time series, applied to all distances up to *long-range* time scales, thereby probing the nature of "switching'" patterns between high and low values in a statistical sense. Larger power-law exponents indicate positive temporal auto-correlation or *persistency* in the increase or decrease, and lower values correspond to negative auto-correlation or *anti-persistency* (Ohashi et al., 2003).

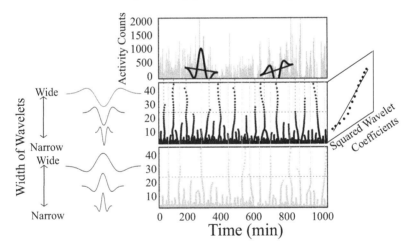

Fig. 2. Conceptual explanation of the method to obtain power-law exponents for local maxima and minima. (*top*) Various widths of hat-shaped wavelets are slid along the data to detect local minima (*middle*) and local maxima (*bottom*) of the wavelet coefficients. Note that the local minima and maxima appear at the transient decreases and increases of the activity, respectively. The power-law exponents are calculated from the slope of the log-log plot of squared wavelet coefficients vs. the scale for local minima and maxima. In the actual analysis, we used an integrated, rather than raw, time series and $\psi(t)$, i.e., the derivative of the "hat-shaped" wavelet. This yields the same power-law exponents as those obtained by the DFA method for the same local maxima and minima as obtained in this figure. Reprinted with permission from (Pan et al., 2007).

This method enables to evaluate relationships between time scales and magnitudes of fluctuation within each time scale, eliminating *non-stationarity* in the input data (i.e., changes in the baseline and trends within the data windows at different scales) that could affect calculation of the magnitudes of fluctuation. Therefore, this approach is suitable for the analysis of the long-term data collected in ambulatory settings (Pan et al., 2007).

3. Quantitative analysis of parkinsonism using power-law auto-correlation exponents

The data acquired during awake-time and sleep-time were separated with Action-W, Version 2 (Ambulatory Monitors Inc., Ardsley, NY) (Fig. 1) and the data during awake-time were used for analyses. Average wavelet coefficients for local maxima and minima of the severe and mild groups provided straight lines in the range of 8-35 min (Fig. 3A), indicative of very robust α-values. When the mean α-values for local maxima and minima were compared, they found a significantly lower α-value for local maxima in the mild group than in the severe group (Fig. 3B). All the patients (13 male and 9 female patients with Parkinson disease) in both the severe (Hoeh-Yahl score > 3.0; n=9)) and mild groups (H-Y score ≦ 3.0; n=10)) showed significantly lower α-values for local maxima on good-condition (GC) days than on bad-condition (BC) days that were classified according to diary scores, whereas there was no significant difference in the mean α-values for local minima (Fig. 3C).

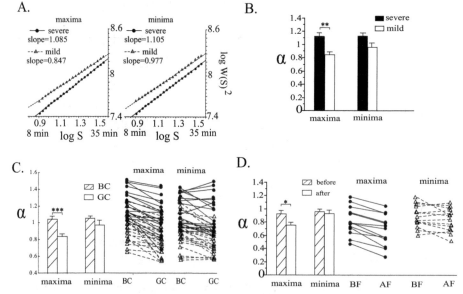

Fig. 3. Local maxima and minima of fluctuation of physical activity. (A) Average wavelet coefficients, as a function of the wavelet scale, for local maxima and minima. The slopes are power-law exponents, α. (B) Comparisons of the mean for the severe and the mild groups, (C) for BC and GC days and for individual patients, and (D) for days before and after antiparkinsonism medication and for each patient. *: $P < 0.05$, **: $P < 0.01$, and ***: $P < 0.001$. Reprinted with permission from (Pan et al., 2007).

When the effects of medication were examined, we found that all the patients who did not take any medication at the time of enrolement (n=6) showed lower α-values for local maxima on days more than three weeks after they received clinically effective anti-parkinsonism medication than on those before (Fig. 3D). Although presence of tremor significantly increased the activity counts in the arms with tremor as compared with those without tremor (Fig. 4A), power-law scaling of the records from arms with tremor showed a linear correlation between log S and log $W(S)^2$ in the range of 8 to 35 min (Fig. 4B) and α-values for local maxima were the same between the arms with tremor and those without tremor (Fig. 4B) with significantly higher α-values in patient arms than in control arms (Fig. 4C)

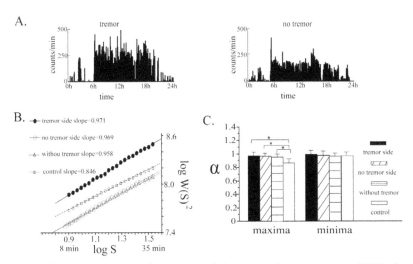

Fig. 4. Effects of tremor on actigraph counts and the power-law exponents. (A) Daily profiles of physical activity for the arm affected with tremor and that without tremor of a patient with unilaterally predominant parkinsonism with continuous tremor on one side. (B) Average wavelet coefficients for local maxima among arms with tremor (tremor) and without tremor (no tremor) of 6 patients with tremor, 26 arms of 13 patients without tremor (without tremor) and 20 arms of 10 control subjects (control). (C) The power-law exponents for local maxima and minima. *: $P < 0.05$. Reprinted with permission from (Pan et al., 2007).

Larger power-law exponents (α) indicate positive temporal auto-correlation, or *persistency*, in the increase or decrease in the variability of activity at two distant points in time in the time series, and lower values correspond to negative auto-correlation or *anti-persistency* (Ohashi et al., 2003). In other words, a lower α for local maxima or minima of activity records reflects more frequent switching behavior from low to high or high to low physical activity, respectively, and the switching behavior from lower to higher activity levels is considered to be related to akinesia in patients with parkinsonism. We found lower α-values for local maxima during GC days than during BC days, in the mild group than in the severe group, and before medication than after medication. Thus, these results demonstrate that the power-law analyses accurately describe the well known phenomenon that under these conditions patients switch their physical activity from lower to higher levels more easily, in other words they exhibit milder akinesia, when the parkinsonism is mild than when it is severe. It is worthy to note that lower α-values for local maxima were obtained for all the patients after medication than before, and when in good condition than in bad condition (Fig. 3C, D), thereby providing a temporal profile of parkinsonism in each individual patient.

These results thus suggest that analysis of power-law temporal auto-correlation of physical activity time series using the bi-directional extension (Ohashi et al., 2003) is applicable to patients with parkinsonism for the evaluation of motor dysfunction irrespective of the presence of tremor and may provide useful objective data necessary for the control of drug dosage in the out-patient clinic and also for the evaluation of new drugs for parkinsonism (Pan et al., 2007).

4. Evaluation of effects of traditional Chinese medicine on parkinsonian symptoms

Conventional antiparkinsonism drugs effectively ameliorate the symptoms of patients with PD during the initial several years of onset, but become increasingly less effective and induce motor fluctuations including wearing-off, on-off, dopa-induced dyskinesia, and agonist-induced sleep attack (Arnulf et al., 2002; Comella, 2002; Hobson et al., 2002; Ondo et al., 2001; Pahwa et al., 2006). PD patients not infrequently suffer from non-motor symptoms, such as neuropsychiatric symptoms, autonomic symptoms, gastrointestinal symptoms, sensory symptoms, non-motor fluctuations (autonomic symptoms, cognitive or psychiatric symptoms, sensory symptoms including pain), fatigue, and sleep disturbance (Chaudhuri& Schapira, 2009; Miyasaki et al., 2006; Park& Stacy, 2009), and these non-motor symptoms may be intrinsic to the disease pathology or may be the result of treatment with dopaminergic agents. Several studies have established that the non-motor symptoms of PD are common, occur across all stages of PD, and are a key determinant of quality of life (Chaudhuri& Schapira, 2009).

Herbal remedies have a long history of use (particularly in East Asian countries) for alleviating various symptoms and have been increasingly used as alternative medicines worldwide, including the United States (De Smet, 2002). Traditional Chinese medicines (TCM) ameliorate various symptoms, particularly the ageing-related symptoms, and hence are likely to be beneficial for chronic diseases such as PD (Iwasaki et al., 2004; 2005a; 2005b). Good compliance for long-term use with few side effects may be another merit of TCM suitable for patients with PD (Lian& Luo, 2007; Zhao et al., 2007).

In order to evaluate the effects of TCM on symptoms of parkinsonism, we evaluated the effects of Zeng-xiao An-shen Zhi-chan 2 (ZAZ2) on patients with PD using this method together with conventional scales for parkinsonism (Pan et al., 2011a). ZAZ2 granule is made up of 14 kinds of herbs; *Uncaria rhynchophylla* 10 g, *Rehmanniae radix* 10 g, *Cornus officinalis* 8 g, *Asnaragus cochinchinensic* 10 g, *Paeonia lactiflora* 10 g, *Desertliving cistanche* 10 g, *Puerariae radix* 10 g, *Arisaema consanguineum Schott* 10 g, *Salviae Miltiorrhizae radix* 10 g, *Acorus tatarinowii* 10 g, *Curcuma longa Linn* 12 g, *Morindae officinalis radix* 10 g, *Rhizoma gastrodiae* 10 g, and*Rhizoma chuanxiong* 10 g. One hundred and fifteen patients with idiopathic PD took 8 g of either ZAZ2 granule or placebo granule that was not distinguished by appearance or taste for 13 weeks. Patients were randomly assigned to the ZAZ2 group (n=59) or placebo group (n=56). There was no difference in the mean age, gender ratio or disease duration between the ZAZ2 and placebo groups, and the post hoc test revealed no significant baseline (week 0) differences in UPDRS scores, Hoehn & Yahr stages, mean counts, power-law temporal exponent α values, or in the dosage of antiparkinonian drugs between the two groups. All the patients were evaluated at week 0, week 1, and week 13 for the actigraph recording, UPDRS and Secondary Symptom Score, which is conventionally used in China to evaluate the effects of antiparkinsonism drugs and consists of 8 parts, including the assessments of non-fluent speech, vertigo, insomnia/nightmares, headache, sweating or night sweats, tiredness, sense of cold, and dysuria (Long, 1992). The awake-time and sleep-time actigraph data were used separately for the power-law temporal analyses.

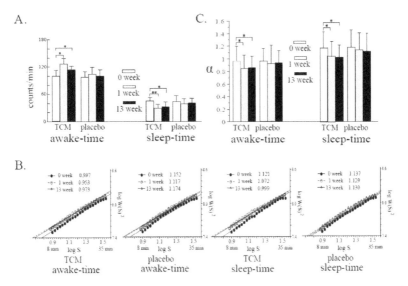

Fig. 5. Effects of TCM and placebo granules on actigraph recondings. (A) Counts of physical activity (mean ± S.D.). (B) Average wavelet coefficients, as a function of the wavelet scale for awake-time and sleep-time. The slopes are power-law exponents α. (C) Power-law exponents α (mean ± S.D.). *: $P < 0.05$, **: $P < 0.01$. (Pan et al., 2011a)

The local power-law exponent α values during both awake-time and sleep-time were significantly decreased after taking ZAZ2 granule, but not after taking placebo granule (Table 1, Fig 5). The average wavelet coefficients exhibited linear relationships in the range of scales from 8 min to 35 min both for the ZAZ2 and placebo groups (Fig. 5B). The local power-law exponent α values during both awake-time and sleep-time were significantly decreased both week 1 and 13 in the ZAZ2 group, but not in the placebo group (Table 1 and Fig 5C, P<0.01; Bonferroni test). The beneficial effects of ZAZ2 were shown with UPDRS scores, as well; significant and persistent improvements were found in the scores of Part II, Part II + Part III, and Part IV (Table 1). These scores at week 13 were significantly different between the ZAZ2 group and the placebo group. As the exploratory outcome of this study, most of the secondary symptoms were improved after taking ZAZ2 granule, whereas only a few symptoms were transiently improved in the placebo group (Table 2).

We evaluated the beneficial effects of TCM specifically on sleep disturbance of patients with parkinsonism. We used placebo-controlled, randomized study design, in which 48 patients

	Placebo（n = 54）			TCM（n = 56）		
	Week 0	Week 1	Week 13	Week 0	Week 1	Week 13
UPDRS total score	46.6 ± 16.3	44.7 ± 15.3	45.9 ± 18.1	46.3 ± 17.1	37.1 ± 11.2*##	40.7 ± 15.1*#
UPDRS I	2.5 ± 0.7	2.3 ± 1.1	2.4 ± 1.2	2.6 ± 0.8	2.1 ± 0.7*	2.3 ± 0.9
UPDRS II	15.7 ± 9.3	14.8 ± 11.2	15.3 ± 11.6	15.9 ± 11.3	12.5 ± 4.6*#	13.4 ± 9.8*#
UPDRS III	25.5 ± 12.9	23.8 ± 10.6*	24.9 ± 12.7	25.4 ± 10.1	19.3 ± 9.8*#	21.6 ± 10.4*
UPDRS IV	3.1 ± 1.1	2.9 ± 1.6	3.0 ± 1.4	3.2 ± 1.4	2.6 ± 0.8*#	2.7±1.3*#
Awake-time (counts/min)	98.5 ± 14.1	102.6 ± 18.9	100.7 ± 16.9	99.8 ± 17.8	126.7 ± 13.4*##	118.4 ± 11.8*##
Sleep-time (counts/min)	42.9 ± 17.1	38.8 ± 15.6*	40.1 ± 14.8	43.2 ± 11.6	35.6 ± 13.6*#	32.8 ± 13.6*#
α(awake-time)	0.97 ± 0.21	0.95 ± 0.28	0.96 ± 0.18	0.97 ± 0.24	0.88 ± 0.21*#	0.86 ± 0.19*##
α(sleep-time)	1.19 ± 0.28	1.16 ± 0.27	1.15 ± 0.29	1.18 ± 0.26	1.04 ± 0.22*#	1.02 ± 0.18*##

Data presented are mean ± SD.*:$P < 0.05$; **:$P < 0.01$ compared to week 0 (Repeated-measure ANOVAs).
#$P < 0.05$; ##:$P < 0.01$ compared to placebo (Bonferroni test). UPDRS: Unified Parkinson's Disease Rating Scale.
α: power-law exponent.

Table 1. Measurements before and after taking test granules. (Pan et al., 2011a)

Group	Time	Non-fluent speech	Vertigo	Insomnia/ nightmare	Headache	Sweating or night sweats	Tiredness	Sense of cold	Dysuria
	week 0	1.08 ± 0.74	1.33 ± 0.83	2.77 ± 0.98	0.92 ± 0.56	2.11 ± 0.68	1.66 ± 0.57	1.90 ± 0.67	2.23 ± 0.69
TCM	week 1	0.56 ± 0.28*	0.84 ± 0.26*#	2.03 ± 0.78*	0.64 ± 0.28*##	1.38 ± 0.69*#	1.21 ± 0.46*	1.48 ± 0.57*	1.43 ± 0.31*#
	week 13	0.65 ± 0.33*##	0.95 ± 0.37*	1.73 ± 0.38*#	0.63 ±0.19*#	1.48 ± 0.28*##	1.27 ± 0.51*#	1.58 ± 0.61	1.46 ± 0.36*##
	week 0	1.12 ± 0.59	1.31 ± 0.97	2.67 ± 0.87	1.03 ± 0.75	2.13 ± 1.32	1.70 ± 0.97	1.78 ± 0.39	2.29 ± 1.02
Placebo	week 1	0.69 ± 0.32*	1.12 ± 0.69	2.40 ± 0.69*	0.96 ± 0.36*	1.87 ± 0.58	1.35 ± 0.69*	1.39 ± 0.81	1.69 ± 0.92*
	week 13	1.02 ± 0.36	1.28 ± 0.53	2.45 ± 0.38	0.99 ± 0.65	2.18 ± 0.56	1.58 ± 0.66	1.64 ± 0.58	2.18 ± 1.30

Data presented are mean ± SD.*: $P < 0.05$, **: $P < 0.01$ compared with 0 weeks (Repeated-measure ANOVAs).
#:$P < 0.05$, ##:$P < 0.01$ compared to placebo (Bonferroni test).

Table 2. Secondary symptom scores before and after taking test granules. (Pan et al., 2011a)

with idiopathic PD who had at least three awakenings per night occurring at least 3 nights per week participated. Patients wore the actigraph on the wrist of their non-dominant hand for seven consecutive days twice at week 0 (before) and week 6 of taking either one of the granule. For control, age-matched 25 patients with non-neurological diseases who had neither sleep disturbance nor parkinsonism wore the actigraph for seven consecutive days. Daily profiles of activity counts clearly demonstrated an improvement of the biological rhythm after the additional treatment in the TCM group but not in the placebo group (Fig. 6A). After treatment, sleep latency, median sleep efficiency and the median 5 least active hour, all of which were the parameters specifically reflected sleep disturbance (Pan et al., 2011b), shifted towards the values of the control group in the TCM group, but not in the placebo group (Fig 6B).

Scores in UPDRS Part II reflects the long-term outcome of the patients (Harrison et al., 2009). That both α-values for local maxima and the scores in UPDRS Part II, Part II + Part III and Part IV improved after TCM suggested that α-values for local maxima reflected patients' overall ADL, including motor symptoms and non-motor symptoms. Therefore, it is likely that analysis of the α-values is useful for the evaluation of drug effects on the long-term outcome of patient with PD (Pan et al., 2011a; 2011b).

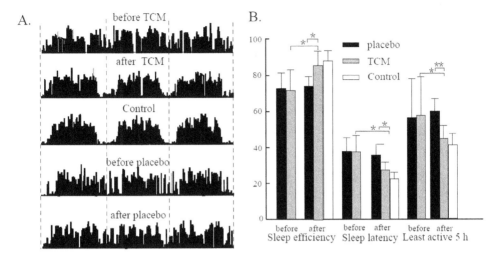

Fig. 6. Effects of cerebral granule (TCM). (A) Daily profiles of actigraph count for three consecutive days before and after taking TCM. Dashed line: midnight. (B) Changes from baseline in actigraph counts. Columns and bars (mean ± S.D.) indicate sleep efficiency (%), sleep latency (min) and the 5 least active hours (counts/min). *: $p < 0.05$; **: $p < 0.01$. Reprinted with permission from (Pan et al., 2011b).

5. Assessment for effects of GVS for ameliorating parkinsonism

Enhancing neuronal transmission is a possible non-pharmacological therapeutic strategy for neurological diseases. The cranial nerves send direct inputs to the brain, and their stimulation may lead to alterations in various central functions. Such stimulation may potentially be a therapeutic strategy for brain disorders due to the low invasiveness as compared to deep brain stimulation. Considering its central connections, the vestibular nerve can influence limbic-to-motor functions, and we applied non-invasive and non-nociceptive noisy galvanic vestibular stimulation (GVS) to the patients with parkinsonism. We successfully improved parkinsonian symptoms by using noisy GVS at a low-frequency range targeting the vestibular nerves of patients with levodopa responsive PD and levodopa unresponsive parkinsonism (Yamamoto et al., 2005). This effect is presumably through the demonstrated vestibule-cerebellar connections, and input noise played the beneficial role in sensitizing neural systems, possibly through a mechanism known as stochastic resonance, a basic physical mechanism underlying noise-enhanced responses of nonlinear systems to weak signals. It is hypothesized that a central circuit signaling the onset of movement of which the threshold is relatively increased due to the diseases may benefit from noisy emulation of the afferent firing rates. We analyzed whether the beneficial effects of GVS on parkinsonism was reflected in a decrease of the α-value for local maxima.

As previously described (Yamamoto et al., 2005), a portable GVS device was used to deliver currents using a bilateral unipolar configuration, in which electrodes were placed over the patient's bilateral mastoid processes with the reference electrodes placed on the forehead. The waveform, a zero-mean, linearly detrended noisy current with a 1/f-type power spectrum (Struzik et al., 2006) within a range of 0.01-2.0 Hz or a constant zero current for control, with a duration of 300 sec was continuously repeated during the tests. The magnitude of noisy GVS was set to 60% of each subject's nociceptive threshold (0.29 ± 0.20 mA). Then either the noisy GVS or the control zero current was continuously applied for the first 24 hours, and then switched to the counter-part and applied for another 24 hours, while the patients' wrist activity was monitored continuously for 48 hours. The order of noisy GVS and the control zero current was determined for each patient by random selection.

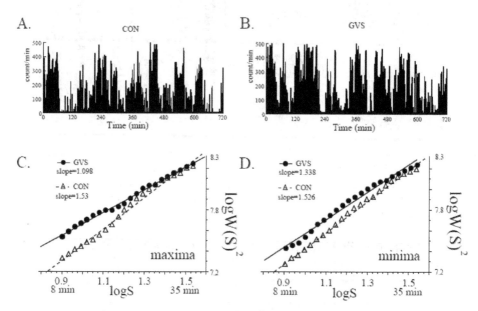

Fig. 7. Illustrative examples of wrist activity data of a PD patient during the control (CON) period (A) and during GVS application (B). The wavelet coefficients ($W(S)$) of these data, as a function of the wavelet scale (S) are shown for local maxima (C) and minima (D). The slopes are power-law exponents α. Reprinted with permission from (Pan et al., 2008).

The representative wrist activity data of a PD patient during the control period and during the application of GVS were shown in Fig. 7A, B. Compared to control, GVS was associated with more frequent switching between higher and lower levels of activity. This resulted in a higher wavelet power ($W(S)^2$) with GVS (Fig. 7C, D), particularly at smaller scales (S), or higher frequencies, for local maxima (Fig.7C). The power-law exponent α, given by the slope of the log S vs. Log $W(S)^2$ relationship and characterizing the nature of switching patterns between high and low values in a statistical sense, was smaller with GVS than with control stimulation, especially for the local maxima (Fig. 7C,D).

The group average wavelet coefficients exhibited linear relationships in the range of scales (S) from 8 min to 35 min both for local maxima and minima and for GVS and control conditions (Fig. 8A, B). The slope for local maxima with noisy GVS was substantially less than that with control stimulation. For local maxima, the mean power-law exponent was significantly smaller for GVS than for the control (Fig. 8C). The difference in the mean α for local minima was much less than that for the local maxima. When the mean α-values for the

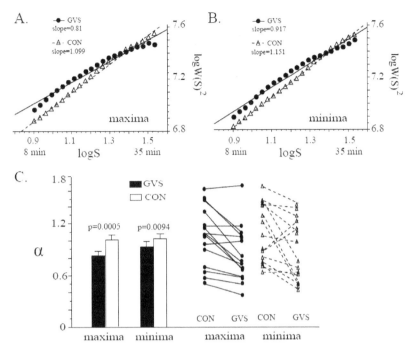

Fig. 8. The group average wavelet coefficients for local maxima (A) and minima (B) for GVS and control (CON) conditions. (C) Comparisons of the mean α for GVS and CON (left) and the within-individual differences (right). The error bars represent SEM. Reprinted with permission from (Pan et al., 2008).

first and the second days were compared, significant differences were not observed either for local maxima or minima, suggesting that the above differences were due to the GVS application itself, not to an order effect.

We confirmed that measurement of the mean α for local maxima detected the improvement of parkinsonism during GVS with sufficient sensitivity (Pan et al., 2008).

6. Conclusion

Analysis of patients' physical activity records collected by an actigraph device using power-law exponents probing temporal autocorrelation of the activity counts provides methods for the evaluation of disability resulting from motor and non-motor parkinsonism without being influenced by the presence of tremor or different patterns of daily living (Pan et al., 2007). Sufficient sensitivity and reliability of this method warrants the objectivity in the evaluation of symptom severity (Pan et al., 2008; Pan et al., 2011a) , hence this method may be useful for the evaluation of disease progression and efficacy of new drug.

7. Acknowledgement

This study was supported in part by Grants-in-Aid for Scientific Research from the Ministry of Health, Labor, and Welfare of Japan to S.K.

8. References

Arnulf, I., Konofal, E., Merino-Andreu, M., Houeto, J.L., Mesnage, V., Welter, M.L., Lacomblez, L., Golmard, J.L., Derenne, J.P. & Agid, Y. (2002). Parkinson's disease and sleepiness: an integral part of PD. *Neurology*, Vol. 58, No. 7, (Apr 2002), pp. 1019-1024, ISSN 0028-3878

Chaudhuri, K.R. & Schapira, A.H. (2009). Non-motor symptoms of Parkinson's disease: dopaminergic pathophysiology and treatment. *Lancet Neurol*, Vol. 8, No. 5, (May 2009), pp. 464-474, ISSN 1474-4422

Comella, C.L. (2002). Daytime sleepiness, agonist therapy, and driving in Parkinson disease. *JAMA*, Vol. 287, No. 4, (Jan 2002), pp. 509-511, ISSN 0098-7484

Comella, C.L., Morrissey, M. & Janko, K. (2005). Nocturnal activity with nighttime pergolide in Parkinson disease: a controlled study using actigraphy. *Neurology*, Vol. 64, No. 8, (Apr 2005), pp. 1450-1451, ISSN 1526-632X

De Smet, P.A. (2002). Herbal remedies. *N Engl J Med*, Vol. 347, No. 25, (Dec 2002), pp. 2046-2056, ISSN 1533-4406

Harrison, M.B., Wylie, S.A., Frysinger, R.C., Patrie, J.T., Huss, D.S., Currie, L.J. & Wooten, G.F. (2009). UPDRS activity of daily living score as a marker of Parkinson's disease progression. *Mov Disord*, Vol. 24, No. 2, (Jan 2009), pp. 224-230, ISSN 1531-8257

Hobson, D.E., Lang, A.E., Martin, W.R., Razmy, A., Rivest, J. & Fleming, J. (2002). Excessive daytime sleepiness and sudden-onset sleep in Parkinson disease: a survey by the Canadian Movement Disorders Group. *JAMA*, Vol. 287, No. 4, (Jan 2002), pp. 455-463, ISSN 0098-7484

Iwasaki, K., Kobayashi, S., Chimura, Y., Taguchi, M., Inoue, K., Cho, S., Akiba, T., Arai, H., Cyong, J.C. & Sasaki, H. (2004). A randomized, double-blind, placebo-controlled clinical trial of the Chinese herbal medicine "ba wei di huang wan" in the treatment of dementia. *J Am Geriatr Soc*, Vol. 52, No. 9, (Sep 2004), pp. 1518-1521, ISSN 0002-8614

Iwasaki, K., Maruyama, M., Tomita, N., Furukawa, K., Nemoto, M., Fujiwara, H., Seki, T., Fujii, M., Kodama, M. & Arai, H. (2005a). Effects of the traditional Chinese herbal medicine Yi-Gan San for cholinesterase inhibitor-resistant visual hallucinations and neuropsychiatric symptoms in patients with dementia with Lewy bodies. *J Clin Psychiatry*, Vol. 66, No. 12, (Dec 2005), pp. 1612-1613, ISSN 0160-6689

Iwasaki, K., Satoh-Nakagawa, T., Maruyama, M., Monma, Y., Nemoto, M., Tomita, N., Tanji, H., Fujiwara, H., Seki, T., Fujii, M., Arai, H. & Sasaki, H. (2005b). A randomized, observer-blind, controlled trial of the traditional Chinese medicine Yi-Gan San for improvement of behavioral and psychological symptoms and activities of daily living in dementia patients. *J Clin Psychiatry*, Vol. 66, No. 2, (Feb 2005), pp. 248-252, ISSN 0160-6689

Jean-Louis, G., Mendlowicz, M.V., Gillin, J.C., Rapaport, M.H., Kelsoe, J.R., Zizi, F., Landolt, H. & von Gizycki, H. (2000). Sleep estimation from wrist activity in patients with major depression. *Physiol Behav*, Vol. 70, No. 1-2, (Jul 2000), pp. 49-53, ISSN 0031-9384

Katayama, S. (2001). Actigraph analysis of diurnal motor fluctuations during dopamine agonist therapy. *Eur Neurol*, Vol. 46, No. Suppl 1, (2001), pp. 11-17, ISSN 0014-3022

Korszun, A., Young, E.A., Engleberg, N.C., Brucksch, C.B., Greden, J.F. & Crofford, L.A. (2002). Use of actigraphy for monitoring sleep and activity levels in patients with fibromyalgia and depression. *J Psychosom Res*, Vol. 52, No. 6, (Jun 2002), pp. 439-443, ISSN 0022-3999

Korte, J., Hoehn, T. & Siegmund, R. (2004). Actigraphic recordings of activity-rest rhythms of neonates born by different delivery modes. *Chronobiol Int*, Vol. 21, No. 1, (Jan 2004), pp. 95-106, ISSN 0742-0528

Lian, X.F. & Luo, X.D. (2007). [Effect of TCM treatment according to syndrome differentiation in enhancing curative effect and reducing side-effect of madopa]. *Zhongguo Zhong Xi Yi Jie He Za Zhi*, Vol. 27, No. 9, (Sep 2007), pp. 796-799, ISSN 1003-5370

Long, C. (1992). Definition and evaluation of parkinsonism in TCM. *Journal of Beijing University of Traditional Chinese Medicine* Vol. 4, No. 15, (1992), pp. 39.

Martinez-Martin, P., Gil-Nagel, A., Gracia, L.M., Gomez, J.B., Martinez-Sarries, J. & Bermejo, F. (1994). Unified Parkinson's Disease Rating Scale characteristics and structure. The Cooperative Multicentric Group. *Mov Disord*, Vol. 9, No. 1, (Jan 1994), pp. 76-83, ISSN 0885-3185

Miyasaki, J.M., Shannon, K., Voon, V., Ravina, B., Kleiner-Fisman, G., Anderson, K., Shulman, L.M., Gronseth, G. & Weiner, W.J. (2006). Practice Parameter: evaluation and treatment of depression, psychosis, and dementia in Parkinson disease (an evidence-based review): report of the Quality Standards Subcommittee of the American Academy of Neurology. *Neurology*, Vol. 66, No. 7, (Apr 2006), pp. 996-1002, ISSN 1526-632X

Mormont, M.C., Waterhouse, J., Bleuzen, P., Giacchetti, S., Jami, A., Bogdan, A., Lellouch, J., Misset, J.L., Touitou, Y. & Levi, F. (2000). Marked 24-h rest/activity rhythms are associated with better quality of life, better response, and longer survival in patients with metastatic colorectal cancer and good performance status. *Clin Cancer Res*, Vol. 6, No. 8, (Aug 2000), pp. 3038-3045, ISSN 1078-0432

Nakamura, T., Kiyono, K., Yoshiuchi, K., Nakahara, R., Struzik, Z.R. & Yamamoto, Y. (2007). Universal scaling law in human behavioral organization. *Phys Rev Lett*, Vol. 99, No. 13, (Sep 2007), pp. 138103, ISSN 0031-9007

Ohashi, K., Nunes Amaral, L.A., Natelson, B.H. & Yamamoto, Y. (2003). Asymmetrical singularities in real-world signals. *Phys Rev E Stat Nonlin Soft Matter Phys*, Vol. 68, No. 6 Pt 2, (Dec 2003), pp. 065204, ISSN 1539-3755

Okawa, M., Mishima, K., Hishikawa, Y. & Hozumi, S. (1995). [Rest-activity and body-temperature rhythm disorders in elderly patients with dementia--senile dementia of Alzheimer's type and multi-infarct dementia]. *Rinsho Shinkeigaku*, Vol. 35, No. 1, (Jan 1995), pp. 18-23, ISSN 0009-918X

Ondo, W.G., Dat Vuong, K., Khan, H., Atassi, F., Kwak, C. & Jankovic, J. (2001). Daytime sleepiness and other sleep disorders in Parkinson's disease. *Neurology*, Vol. 57, No. 8, (Oct 2001), pp. 1392-1396, ISSN 0028-3878

Pahwa, R., Factor, S.A., Lyons, K.E., Ondo, W.G., Gronseth, G., Bronte-Stewart, H., Hallett, M., Miyasaki, J., Stevens, J. & Weiner, W.J. (2006). Practice Parameter: treatment of Parkinson disease with motor fluctuations and dyskinesia (an evidence-based review): report of the Quality Standards Subcommittee of the American Academy of Neurology. *Neurology*, Vol. 66, No. 7, (Apr 2006), pp. 983-995, ISSN 1526-632X

Pan, W., Kwak, S., Liu, Y., Sun, Y., Fang, Z., Qin, B. & Yamamoto, Y. (2011a). Traditional Chinese medicine improves nocturnal activity in Parkinson's disease. *Parkinson's disease*, in press. doi:10.4061/2011/789506,ISSN 2042-0080

Pan, W., Liu, Y., Fang, Z., Zhu, X., Kwak, S. & Yamamoto, Y. (2011b). A compound belonging to traditional Chinese medicine improves nocturnal activity in Parkinson's disease. *Sleep Med*, Vol. 12, No. 3, (Mar 2011), pp. 307-308, ISSN 1878-5506

Pan, W., Ohashi, K., Yamamoto, Y. & Kwak, S. (2007). Power-law temporal autocorrelation of activity reflects severity of parkinsonism. *Mov Disord*, Vol. 22, No. 9, (Jul 2007), pp.1308-1313, ISSN 1531-8257

Pan, W., Soma, R., Kwak, S. & Yamamoto, Y. (2008). Improvement of motor functions by noisy vestibular stimulation in central neurodegenerative disorders. *J Neurol*, Vol. 255, No. 11, (Nov 2008), pp. 1657-1661, ISSN 0340-5354

Park, A. & Stacy, M. (2009). Non-motor symptoms in Parkinson's disease. *J Neurol*, Vol. 256, No. Suppl 3, (Aug 2009), pp. 293-298, ISSN 1432-1459

Peng, C.K., Havlin, S., Stanley, H.E. & Goldberger, A.L. (1995). Quantification of scaling exponents and crossover phenomena in nonstationary heartbeat time series. *Chaos*, Vol. 5, No. 1, (1995), pp. 82-87, ISSN 1054-1500

Sekine, M., Akay, M., Tamura, T., Higashi, Y. & Fujimoto, T. (2004). Fractal dynamics of body motion in patients with Parkinson's disease. *J Neural Eng*, Vol. 1, No. 1, (Mar 2004), pp. 8-15, ISSN 1741-2560

Struzik, Z.R., Hayano, J., Sakata, S., Kwak, S. & Yamamoto, Y. (2004). 1/f scaling in heart rate requires antagonistic autonomic control. *Phys Rev E Stat Nonlin Soft Matter Phys*, Vol. 70, No. 5, (Nov 2004), pp. 050901, ISSN 1539-3755

Struzik, Z.R., Hayano, J., Soma, R., Kwak, S. & Yamamoto, Y. (2006). Aging of complex heart rate dynamics. *IEEE Trans Biomed Eng*, Vol. 53, No. 1, (Jan 2006), pp. 89-94, ISSN 0018-9294

Teicher, M.H. (1995). Actigraphy and motion analysis: new tools for psychiatry. *Harv Rev Psychiatry*, Vol. 3, No. 1, (May-Jun 1995), pp. 18-35, ISSN 1067-3229)

Tuisku, K., Holi, M.M., Wahlbeck, K., Ahlgren, A.J. & Lauerma, H. (2003). Quantitative rest activity in ambulatory monitoring as a physiological marker of restless legs syndrome: a controlled study. *Mov Disord*, Vol. 18, No. 4, (Apr 2003), pp. 442-448, ISSN 0885-3185

van Someren, E.J., Hagebeuk, E.E., Lijzenga, C., Scheltens, P., de Rooij, S.E., Jonker, C., Pot, A.M., Mirmiran, M. & Swaab, D.F. (1996). Circadian rest-activity rhythm disturbances in Alzheimer's disease. *Biol Psychiatry*, Vol. 40, No. 4, (Aug 1996), pp. 259-270, ISSN 0006-3223

van Someren, E.J., Pticek, M.D., Speelman, J.D., Schuurman, P.R., Esselink, R. & Swaab, D.F. (2006). New actigraph for long-term tremor recording. *Mov Disord*, Vol. 21, No. 8, (Aug 2006), pp. 1136-1143, ISSN 0885-3185

van Someren, E.J., van Gool, W.A., Vonk, B.F., Mirmiran, M., Speelman, J.D., Bosch, D.A. & Swaab, D.F. (1993). Ambulatory monitoring of tremor and other movements before and after thalamotomy: a new quantitative technique. *J Neurol Sci*, Vol. 117, No. 1-2, (Jul 1993), pp. 16-23, ISSN 0022-510X

van Someren, E.J., Vonk, B.F., Thijssen, W.A., Speelman, J.D., Schuurman, P.R., Mirmiran, M. & Swaab, D.F. (1998). A new actigraph for long-term registration of the duration and intensity of tremor and movement. *IEEE Trans Biomed Eng*, Vol. 45, No. 3, (Mar 1998), pp. 386-395, ISSN 0018-9294

Witting, W., Kwa, I.H., Eikelenboom, P., Mirmiran, M. & Swaab, D.F. (1990). Alterations in the circadian rest-activity rhythm in aging and Alzheimer's disease. *Biol Psychiatry*, Vol. 27, No. 6, (Mar 1990), pp. 563-572, ISSN 0006-3223

Yamamoto, Y., Struzik, Z.R., Soma, R., Ohashi, K. & Kwak, S. (2005). Noisy vestibular stimulation improves autonomic and motor responsiveness in central neurodegenerative disorders. *Ann Neurol*, Vol. 58, No. 2, (Aug 2005), pp. 175-181, ISSN 0364-5134

Zhao, H., Li, W.W. & Gao, J.P. (2007). [Clinical trial on treatment of Parkinson's disease of Gan-Shen yin deficiency type by recipe for nourishing Gan-Shen]. *Zhongguo Zhong Xi Yi Jie He Za Zhi*, Vol. 27, No. 9, (Sep 2007), pp. 780-784, ISSN 1003-5370

11

Relevance of Aerodynamic Evaluation in Parkinsonian Dysarthria

Sarr Mamadou Moustapha[1], Ghio Alain[2], Espesser Robert[2],
Teston Bernard[2], Dramé Moustapha[3] and Viallet François[2,4]
[1]UFR Santé- Université deThiès
[2]Laboratoire Parole et Langage-Aix-en-Provence
[3]Université de Reims
[4]Service de Neurologie du Centre Hospitalier du Pays d'Aix- Aix-en-Provence
[1]Sénégal
[2,3,4]France

1. Introduction

Parkinsonian dysarthria is generally known under the name of hypokinetic dysarthria. Dysarthria, according to Darley et al (1969), is characterized by all speech disorders related to disturbances of muscular control of the speech organs, whose origin is a central or peripheral nervous system injury. So we must understand by dysarthria all failures related to either different levels of speech production (respiratory, phonatory, articulatory and even prosodic). Parkinsonian dysarthria, meanwhile, is mainly based on rigidity and hypokinesia. That's why it is considered as « hypokinetic » (Darley et al., 1975; Gentil et al., 1995). This term refers not only to reduction of articulatory movements but also to decreasing of speech prosody modulation described as monotonic (Viallet & Teston, 2007). Parkinsonian dysarthria arises, like other signs of Parkinson's disease, the depletion of dopamine in charge of phonatory incompetence by muscular hypokinesia. It is a major handicap factor that may compromise in long-term oral communication of the patient, as worsening over the course of the disease, responding less well to treatment and thereby posing additional difficulties in support. So we thought to better assess this dysarthria in order to gain a better understanding and improve management. This assessment can be done by perceptual analysis. She could also be done by various instrumental methods (acoustic and physiological) focusing on one of the speech production levels mentioned above. Such studies are numerous in literature and we will report some examples in this chapter. What is more rare in literature is assessment of parkinsonian dysarthria in study combined several levels as might allow, for example, the dual approach appealing to physiology of speech production with firstly an aerodynamic component related to pneumophonic coordination (respiratory and phonatory levels) and, secondly, an acoustic component in relation to phonoarticulatory coordination (phonatory and articulatory levels). Through this chapter we want show that it is possible to assess appropriately parkinsonian dysarthria by using aerodynamic parameters that combine respiratory and phonatory levels, so such an experiment that we report in this chapter after having reviewed main methods of evaluation.

2. Perceptual analysis

Perceptual analysis is subject to a large degree of subjectivity and inter or intra individual differences. However it can capture all functions involved in speech production system and is main foundation of parkinsonian dysarthria evaluation. On perceptual side, major disorder of parkinsonian speech is dysprosody. Prosody is defined as using of three vocal parameters (pitch, intensity and duration) which variations contribute to emotional and linguistic information. Parkinsonian voice is often described as low, monotonous, altered in timbre, too slow with hoarse character and difficult starting (Hartelius & Svensson, 1994). In addition articulations'problems were reported including a certain loss of identity of phonemes, the most suitable example being realization of plosives (/ t /, / d /) as fricatives (/ s /, / z /) due to insufficient closure of vocal tract (Robert & Spezza, 2005). These disorders can occur very early during disease's course, perhaps as early as the clinical onset of it even at the presymptomatic stage (Harel et al., 2004). Dysphonia is first manifestation that appears early. It is secondarily complemented by articulatory disorders and airflow dysfunctions (Ho et al. 1998; Logeman et al., 1978). However articulatory disorders and airflow dysfunctions alter intelligibility more than dysphonia. Chronological order of disorders appearing suggests abnormalities progression down to up of the vocal tract during disease's course. Disorders begin at laryngeal level and end with bilabial constriction via lingual and palate constriction also. In all cases, perceptual marks of parkinsonian dysarthria were well reported by Selby (1968). Points of emphasis disappear, voice volume decreases, while consonants pronunciation is deteriorating and sentence ends in a whisper. At clinical onset of parkinsonian dysarthria, voice is low, monotonous (no variation in height). After, progressive worsening of dysarthria leads to inaudible and unintelligible diction. In some cases general slowness of movement is also reflected in speech rate. In others cases patients talk quickly, tangle words and sometimes carry words acceleration until sentence ending, imitating feast walking. Perceptual disturbances of Parkinsonian speech could also be summarized by identifying two clusters. On the one hand, a main cluster of prosodic insufficiency that combines monotony of pitch and intensity, accent reduction, quick acceleration, variable flow and consonants imprecision. On the other hand, an accessory cluster of phonatory incompetence that is related to voice disturbances.

Despite large amount of information it provides, perceptual analysis must be supplemented by more objective methods of assessment.

3. Acoustic analysis

Instrumental methods are generally limited in their analysis field. Despite this limitation, they allow, from quantified data, complex functions evaluation and objective comparisons between patients and normal subjects.

On acoustic side, perceptual impressions physical basis of Parkinsonian dysarthria have been studied by measuring several parameters.

3.1 Fundamental frequency

Measurements of voice fundamental frequency (F0) reported mixed results. However, most studies concluded that a F0 average increase in PD patients during sustained vowel, text reading or spontaneous speech (Flint et al. 1992; Hertrich & Ackermann, 1993; Robert & Spezza, 2005). For example, Ludlow and Bassich (1984) found a F0 average of 165.8 Hz for

PD patients while F0 average value for control subject apparied in age and sex was 143.2 Hz. As well Canter (1963) found F0 average values of 129 Hz for patients and 106 Hz for normal subjects. F0 increased with disease severity (Metter & Hanson, 1986). Nevertheless, other studies have clearly demonstrated a F0 average reduction (Jankowski et al., 2004; Sanabria et al. 2001; Viallet et al., 2002,). It is therefore logical to agree on a certain diversity of trends in F0 that can be either lowered or increased or unchanged. F0 trends diversity could be due to biases related to patient age, gender, disease duration, variability of performance inter- and intra-individual as well as heterogeneity of measurement or evaluation methods. Regarding F0 variability in sentences production, it is reported much lower values in PD patients than normal subjects. Thus Canter (1963) noted frequency variations between 0.15 and 0.59 octaves for PD patients against 0.60 and 1.64 octaves for normal subjects. This limited variability observed in PD may be related to laryngeal rigidity that induces insufficient contraction including lack of crico-thyroid muscle which is mainly responsible for F0 increase. In sustained vowel task, there is disclosed an increase in F0 variability from cycle to cycle (Jitter) in patients, indicating an alteration of pneumophonic control stability (Jankowski et al, 2004).

3.2 Intensity
Regarding the vocal intensity, the results of perceptual analysis and acoustic measurements are not always consistent. For example, Fox and Ramig (1997) reported that the sonorous volume of PD patients was significantly lower than control subjects, around 2 to 4 decibels during speech production or other speech tasks such as sustained vowel. This result demonstrates clearly the hypophonic caracter of parkinsonian dysarthria. The results of other acoustic studies showed no significant differences between PD patients and normal subjects (Canter, 1963; Metter & Hanson, 1986). The alteration or no of the sonorous volume rather depend on the degree of severity of illness (Ludlow & Bassich, 1984). Despite these mixed results, however, there would be leaning towards a small reduction of mean intensity which falls within the phonatory incompetence associated with the subglottic pressure decreasing. The shimmer is for intensity what the jitter is for frequency, and it reflects intensity variability of sound vibration from cycle to cycle. A shimmer increasing in the task of sustained vowel has been reported in Parkinson's disease (PD) patients compared with control subjects, indicating an alteration of laryngeal stability control (Jimenez et al., 1997). These findings suggest that a reflex part of speech production control appears to be intact, contrary to the dysfunction of voluntary control directly induced by the disease.

3.3 Abnormalities of vocal timbre
Acoustic measurements during sustained vowel confirmed the perceptual abnormalities of timbre (blown, frayed or tremulous character) in addition to showing F0 and intensity increasing variability from cycle to cycle, changes longer term due mainly to the tremor, with a reduction of signal/noise ratio (Viallet & Teston, 2007).

3.4 Speed of speech
The speed of speech of PD patients is highly variable from one subject to another (Darley et al, 1975). Some studies showed no significant difference between parkinsonian and normal subjects (Ackermann & Ziegler, 1991; Ludlow et al. 1987). Other studies have reported a

faster speech rate in PD patients (Weismes, 1984). Finally, the speech speed can also be slower (Volkmann et al., 1992). These differences reflect not only the variability between subjects, but also the possible variation of results depending on the task (Ho et al., 1998). In all cases, Parkinsonian speech is marked by abnormalities which are described a long time and may impact on speed: festination, palilalia and pseudo-stuttering with dysfluences (Monfrais-Pfauwadel, 2005). What is more, the fine analysis of the acoustic signal from read speech extracts with attentive listening has led to a better study of the Parkinsonian speech temporal organization: the speed of speech tends to be slower. This slowness seems correlated with a longer pause time, duration of breaks was found significantly higher in PD patients compared with control subjects (Duez, 2005). In addition breaks inside of words have been observed in PD patients and not in controls subjects. Finally many dysfluences, such as omissions, repetitions and false starts, were found almost exclusively in PD patients. Numerous breaks and dysfluences not only slow the speed of speech, but also deconstruct the language units, disrupt perceptive waiting of listeners and finally degrade intelligibility.

3.5 Imprecise consonants
The most typical perceptual error articulatory in Parkinsonian dysarthria, namely the realization of consonants as fricatives was also confirmed by the acoustic analysis. In effect during these tests, it is found, instead of a silence due to normally carried out occlusion, a signal corresponding to a low intensity friction noise due to air passage and defined as the spirantisation phenomenon. Similarly, the lack of acoustic contrasts reflecting a lack of articulation is a common feature of parkinsonian speech spectrograms (Kent & Rosenbek, 1982).

3.6 Other anomalies
Finally, other deviations were reported always in acoustic studies: the reduced duration of formant transitions (Connor et al. 1989; Forrest et al., 1989), the voicing of voiceless consonants assigned to the rigidity of the larynx, a control loss of voice onset time (VOT), that is to say, the time between the release of the consonant and the beginning of voicing, resulting in a lack of coordination between the larynx and articulatory organs (Forrest et al., 1989; Lieberman et al., 1992).

4. Physiological analysis

It essentially uses electromyographic methods, vidéocinematographic, kinematic and aerodynamic. It provides quantitative data on respiratory plans, phonatory and articulatory (Teston, 2007).

4.1. Respiratory system
Kinematic studies have measured the thoracic and abdominal movements. The spirometric measurements allowed to assess the volumes of mobilized air during inspiration and expiration. At rest PD patients respiration is characterized by a shortening of respiratory cycle at the expense of expiration and, moreover, a relative decline of thoracic participation in respiratory movement. During speech production, it was noted in PD patients an inspiratory volume reduction of the thoracic cage, and an increase in inspiratory abdominal volume, which suggests an alteration of expiratory airflow necessary to set the appropriate contribution of laryngeal vibrator (Solomon & Hixon, 1993).

4.2 Phonatory system

The rigidity of the laryngeal musculature is a major determinant of hypophonia associated with parkinsonian dysarthria. It has been demonstrated by studies in laryngoscopy which provided direct light on the anomalies of the larynx. Larynx anomalies include glottal gap by chord adherence default, sometimes hypertonia of ventricular bands and tremor which can be localized at chordal level or above glottal part of vocal tract (Jiang et al., 1999; Yuceturk et al., 2002). Laryngeal rigidity induces a particularly curved form of vocal cords responsible for the unusually large and constant aperture of the vocal tract (Smith et al., 1995).

4.3 Articulatory system

On physiological side it is mainly explored by electromyographic and kinematic methods. In fact electromyographic and kinematic methods permit to analyze strenght and movement of articulatory organs in order to better understand the motor speech disorders

4.3.1 Articulatory organs movement

The mobility of articulatory organs of speech, like other movements, is disturbed by two major symptoms of Parkinson's disease: rigidity and hypokinesia.

The rigidity incrimination has been strengthened on the basis of certain works. For example Hunker et al. (1982) were able to evaluate a coefficient of rigidity by applying known forces on labial muscles and observing the resulting displacement. The lower lip of PD patients showed a significantly higher rigidity than control subjects, whereas for the upper lip, there was no significant difference between the two groups. Moreover a correlation between the degree of rigidity and the movements' reduction was observed by recording the lips movement with a strain- gauge system in connection with the muscular activities of inferior orbicularis and mentalis, (Barlow et al., 1983). However, this rigidity is not expressed identically on all articulatory organs, affecting preferentially muscles which are poor in neuro-muscular spindles and without stretch reflex such as the tongue comparatively to other muscles which are richer in neuro-muscular spindles and with monosynaptic reflex activity such as the jaw elevators (Abbs et al., 1987).

The hypokinetic character of some articulatory movements during parkinsonian speech is reported in particular by Ackermann et al. (1993). In this study recording the lips and tongue movements with an electromagnetic system during the repetition of syllables [pa] and [ta], there was an increased frequency and decreased amplitude of articulatory movements during the repetition of the syllable [ta] and no anomaly was found during the repetition of the syllable [pa]. This result suggests that there may be different mechanical properties between the tongue and lips. Kinematic studies also showed that hypokinesia of muscles, thus the nature of motor performance, may depend on factors such as familiarity of the task, the existence of visual guidance (Connor and Abbs, 1991) or even speed of speech (Caligiuri, 1989). Finally the kinematic studies have also confirmed, in PD patients, lack of coordination between different muscles involved in the complex activity that is speech production. Indeed the kinematic analysis of jaw, upper and lower lip showed a different motor behavior of these three structures. The lower lip was working normally when the upper lip and jaw had velocity peaks and/or reduced amplitude of movement (Connor et al., 1989).

4.3.2 The articulatory organs forces

It is usually assessed by using force transducers (Barlow et al., 1983). Muscle abnormalities are also detectable by using electromyographic explorations (Leanderson et al., 1971). The latter, despite their relative inaccessibility to non-medical researchers and the difficulties attached to their technical realization and interpretation, can provide a wealth of information on the chronology of muscular events and agonist-antagonists relation (Teston, 2007). It has been noted in parkinsonian dysarthria abnormal electromyographic signal during the study of orbicularis upper lip activity in repetition of the syllable [pa]. Indeed, in PD patients comparatively with control subjects and during repetition, the short bursts of muscle activity associated with each syllable had duration of shorter and shorter with an associated reduction in their amplitude (Netsel et al., 1975).

These physiological analysis concerning only one level of peripheral production of speech should be more and more replaced by the combined study of at least two levels; example of such a combined analysis is provided by the study of pneumophonic coordination.

4.4 The pneumophonic coordination

It reflects the synergy of action that must exist during speech production between respiratory and laryngeal levels. The measurement of subglottic pressure (SGP) is a good indicator of this pneumophonic coordination. Indeed, the SGP is evaluable indirectly via the intraoral pressure (IOP) during the production of plosives and depends on both the expiratory airflow and laryngeal resistance. In other words, SGP results from a dynamic conflict between air thrust forces and laryngeal resistance, so the evaluation of its trend in a group of breath can give a powerful index of the speaker pneumophonic coordination (Teston, 2007). So such a parameter, related to the aerodynamic side of speech production with in addition its non-invasive character, can be relevant in the assessment of parkinsonian dysarthria.

5. Relevance of the evaluation of aerodynamic parameters

Our research team has experience of using aerodynamic parameters in the assessment of parkinsonian dysarthria. The measurement of such parameters has been performed in PD patients and control subjects by using the voice evaluation system Eva 2 of SQ LAB society in Aix-En-Provence.

5.1 Used parameters

We worked primarily on three parameters: the intra-oral pressure (IOP), the mean oral airflow (MOAF) and laryngeal resistance (LR).

IOP is an indirect reflection of subglottic pressure which is itself nothing other than the pressure exerted by the expiratory air column on the vocal cords. Subglottic pressure is an important aerodynamic parameter and could allow a better understanding of some dysfunctions in speech production system (Baken & Orlikoff, 2000).

The MOAF is another important aerodynamic parameter associated with the laryngeal function and speech production. MOAF and subglottic pressure allow together a better description of the aerodynamic component of speech production.

Finally, the LR is the ratio of IOP on the MOAF and should be able to give an idea about the functioning level of laryngeal stage.

5.2 Equipement and measurement technique
5.2.1 Equipement

We used in this study the vocal evaluation system EVA 2 developed by the Laboratory of Speech and Language and sold by SQ-Lab society. EVA 2 operates as a workstation PC in the Windows environment (**See Figures 1 and 2**) with different software applications dedicated to acoustic and aerodynamic analysis of speech production.

The recording device includes an acoustic channel and two aerodynamic channels: one for measurement of mean oral airflow (MOAF), the other for the IOP measurement. It is thus possible to measure IOP during holding of a voiceless plosive. As a reminder, IOP is the estimated subglottic pressure.

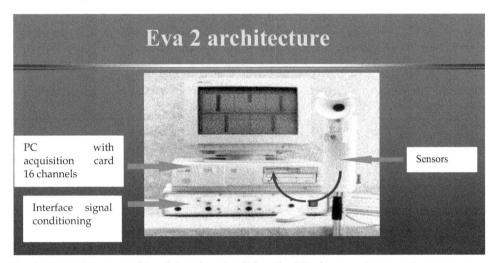

Fig. 1. General Feature of Eva 2 (workstation PC in the Windows environment)

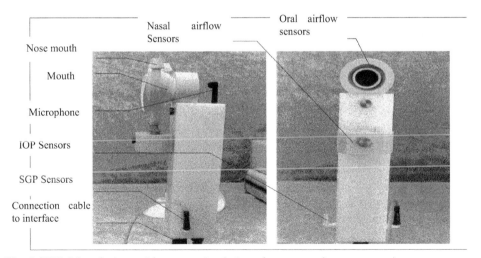

Fig. 2. EVA 2 hand piece with accessories (microphone, mouth, sensors etc.)

5.2.2 Technique

The measurement technique derives from the general theory of fluids dynamic applied to the airway. According to this theory it is possible by adjustments of valves to estimate pressure-flow upstream from the direct measurement of pressure-flow downstream of the target site. The adjustments of valves in question occur naturally during the pronunciation of certain sounds. For example, during production of the consonant / p / the lips are closed while the glottis is open. In contrary during pronunciation of the vowel / a / the lips are open while the glottis is closed. The different conformation of these examples of valves located on the airway (glottis and lips) has a physical impact on the pressure and flow dynamics prevailing inside airway. So during the realization of a voiceless plosive (/ p /), there is a momentary equilibration of intra-oral and subglottic pressures. This equilibration allows indirect assessment of SGP (upstream) via the direct measurement of IOP (downstream). The momentary equilibration of subglottic and intra-oral pressures occurs when holding the voiceless plosive because at this moment there is no phonation, the lips are closed and the glottis is open. Thus the peak pressure generated by holding a voiceless plosive may be considered as a "snapshot" of the subglottic pressure immediately preceding phonation. Similarly during the realization of the vowel (/ a /) following a voiceless plosive (lips are open and glottis is closed), it is possible to consider the oral airflow as a snapshot of translaryngeal airflow because of continuity of flow through the upper airway when the mouth is open. Once we got the two parameters, it suffices to calculate the ratio of intra-oral pressure on the oral airflow to determine the laryngeal resistance (Smitheran & Hixon, 1981; Demolin et al, 1997) (**See Figure 3**).

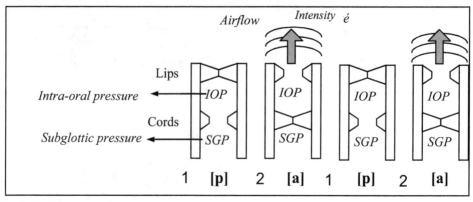

Fig. 3. Evaluation of the subglottic pressure.

Intraoral pressure (IOP) is equivalent to the subglottic pressure (PSG) during the labial occlusion of phoneme "p". Subglottic pressure is estimated indirectly by "Interrupted Airway Method" (Smitheran & Hixon, 1981), method validated notably by Demolin et al. (1997).

Measurements were performed while the subject produced at a constant rate the sentence "Papa ne m'a pas parlé de beau-papa" (Daddy did not speak to me about daddy-in-law). During this production, oral mouth was firmly against the underside of the face to minimize air leakage (**see Figure 4**). Taking IOP is performed using a disposable suction catheter approximately 4 mm (**See Figure 5**). The probe was placed between the incisors and should not be crushed between the teeth or be obstructed by saliva.

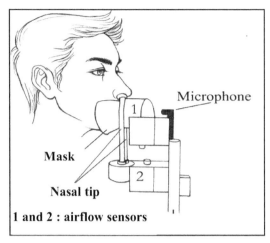

Fig. 4. Oral mouth firmly against the underside of the face

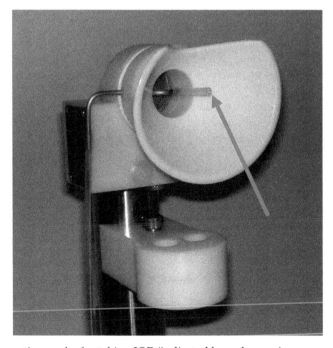

Fig. 5. Note the suction probe for taking IOP (indicated by red arrow)

5.3 Patients and control subjects
The study included 24 subjects with PD who had an average age of 59 years (SD = 5.65) with a mean duration of disease about 9, 9 years (SD = 3.27). Patients were recorded after withdrawal of L-dopa for at least 12 h (condition called OFF DOPA).

50 healthy subjects served as controls. They had an average age of 61 years (SD = 10, 5).

5.4 Statistical analysis

Statistical comparisons between groups (CTRL vs. OFF DOPA) were conducted on the basis of a linear mixed model (software "R" version 2.6.2, http://www.r-project.org). This model emerged as best suited to the analysis of grouped data. Indeed, the repeated measurements, longitudinal studies are data that are presenting a group structure. And in our case, a single individual is undergoing multiple measures, and structured data in this way no longer meet one of the fundamental prerequisites for the validity of a classical linear model, namely the independence of measures. We set our statistical comparisons as follows: measurements of aerodynamic parameters (IOP, MOAF and LR) accounted for the numerical factor of the model, the group (CTRL, OFF DOPA), the position of the consonant / p / in the sentence produced (P1, P2, P3, P4, P5, P6) and the subject (patients, controls) were the three factors model variability.

A p-value less than 0.05 was accepted as statistical significance.

5.5 Results

In a study that involved 20 male patients registered in terms ON / OFF STIM and 11 control subjects, measurement of IOP showed a statistically significant fall of this parameter in OFF STIM patients compared to controls. The stimulation of Subthalamic nucleus (STN) improved partially IOP with a statistically significant difference at the first two measurement points whereas there was an effect of convergence on the third point (Sarr et al., 2009).

In another study that focused on 24 patients registered in OFF DOPA condition and compared with 50 control subjects, three parameters (IOP, MOAF and LR) were measured on six / P / (P1 to P6) of the sentence « Papa ne m'a pas parlé de beau papa » that subjects pronounced at a constant rate.

Here too, there was, as regards the IOP, a statistically significant decrease in patients compared to controls (p = 0.0001) (**See Table 1 and Figure 6**).

	P1	P2	P3	P4	P5	P6
OFF DOPA	3,84 (1,9)	6,22 (2,2)	4,46 (1,8)	4,7 (1,9)	4,49 (1,9)	4,26 (1,7)
CTRL	5,23 (2,00)	6,97 (2,15)	5,73 (1,90)	5,9 (1,93)	6,06 (1,98)	5,67 (2,00)

Table 1. Average of intraoral pressure (IOP) in control subjects (CTRL) and OFF DOPA patients at six measurement points. Standard deviations are in parentheses.

Concerning mean oral airflow (MOAF) the curve of mean values at six points of measurement in control subjects (CTRL) and OFF DOPA patients showed an convergent aspect at extremities so that P1 and P6 while at the other measurement points (P2 to P5), the two curves were clearly separated: that of control subjects remain above that of OFF DOPA patients (**see Table 2 and Figure 7**). The comparison between the two groups was statistically significant (p = 0.001).

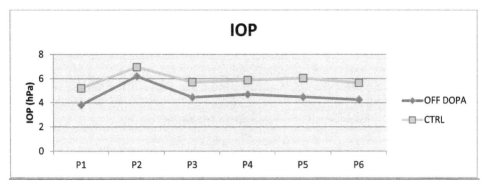

Fig. 6. Curve of the intra-oral pressure (IOP) in control subjects (CTRL) and OFF DOPA patients at six measurement points.

	DAOM 1	DAOM 2	DAOM 3	DAOM 4	DAOM 5	DAOM 6
OFF	0,2	0,16	0,17	0,17	0,19	0,2
DOPA	(0,09)	(0,08)	(0,08)	(0,08)	(0,07)	(0,08)
CTRL	0,2	0,21	0,21	0,20	0,21	0,2
	(0,08)	(0,07)	(0,07)	(0,08)	(0,06)	(0,06)

Table 2. Average of mean oral airflow (MOAF) in control subjects (CTRL) and OFF DOPA patients at six measurement points. Standard deviations are in parentheses.

NB: DAOM is the french abbreviation of mean oral air flow (MOAF)

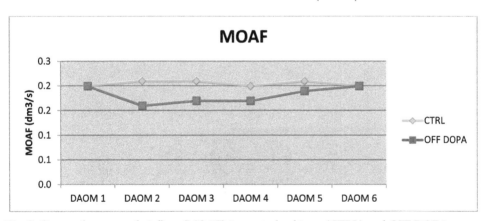

Fig. 7. Curve of mean oral airflow (MOAF) in control subjects (CTRL) and OFF DOPA patients at six measurement points.

Finally for the LR, the graphical representation of mean values at six points of measurement in control subjects (CTRL) and OFF DOPA patients showed on one hand a more linear overall appearance of the control-subjects 'curve, on the other hand, a curve of OFF Dopa patients above that of control subjects from P1 to P4 and then, below, beyond P4. In addition standard deviations were significantly larger in OFF DOPA patients than in control subjects (**See Table 3 and Figure 8**). The comparison between the two groups was statistically significant (p <0.05).

	RL 1	RL 2	RL 3	RL 4	RL 5	RL 6
OFF	28,05	51,22	33,77	33,99	27,09	29,21
DOPA	(20,50)	(40,14)	(23,1)	(21,97)	(16,27)	(26,74)
CTRL	25,75	35,38	30,81	33,40	30,84	33,64
	(16,92)	(13,54)	(11,83)	(14,09)	(11,64)	(13,51)

Table 3. Mean of laryngeal resistance in control subjects (CTRL) and OFF DOPA patients at six measurement points. Standard deviations are in parentheses.

NB: RL is the french abbreviation of laryngeal resistance (LR)

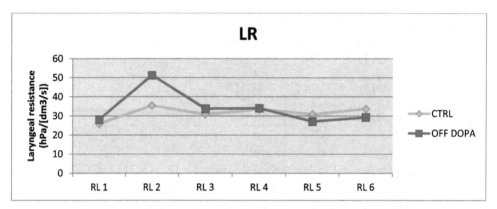

Fig. 8. Curve of mean values of laryngeal resistance (LR) in control subjects (CTRL) and OFF DOPA patients at six measurement points.

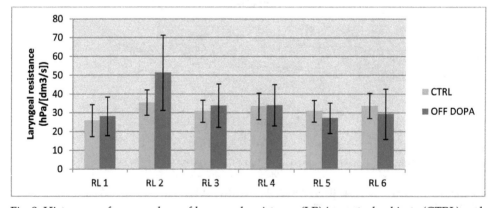

Fig. 9. Histogram of mean values of laryngeal resistance (LR) in control subjects (CTRL) and patients OFF DOPA at six measurement points, with standard deviations. The histogram allows to better see the standard deviations significantly larger in patients.

5.6 Discussions

This new study that examined 24 patients and 50 control subjects confirms the decrease of IOP on all six measurement points of the sentence when comparing patients with control subjects. The decrease of IOP, found in a previous study (Sarr et al., 2009), seems to confirm definitively the alteration of this parameter in parkinsonian dysarthria. The decrease of IOP in patients is due to dopamine deficiency inherent in PD. Dopamine deficiency induces a dysfunction of the respiratory muscles that is partly responsible for the dysarthria (Murdoch et al., 1989). Indeed there are, within overall poor control of expiratory airflow, an alteration of the air quantity needed for the vibration of vocal cords (Jiang et al., 1999a ; Solomon & Hixon, 1993). However, the SGP is the result of a surge in air column by the pressure of lung with laryngeal resistance (Crevier-Buchman, 2007; Solomon, 2007). In the particular context of this study, when measuring IOP via the GSP, the glottis is open, at that time so it's a pressure gradient which is measured and not a static value. This gradient is the result of coordinated action between the respiratory muscles and laryngeal floor, so it indicates pneumophonic coordination quality. In PD, the fall in pulmonary pressure associated with hypokinetic movements of laryngeal muscles induced an alteration of the SGP. So we have shown in this study that it is possible to consider the GSP, or IOP, as a strong indicator of Parkinsonian dysarthria in general and its pneumophonic side particularly. We confirm in same time the results already published in a preliminary study (Sarr et al., 2009). Therefore, the measurement of IOP may allow together, comparing OFF DOPA patients and control subjects, assessment of the disease impact on speech disorders and contribution to evaluation of somes therapies such as L-dopa and subthalamic nucleus stimulation on parkinsonian dysarthria. As a reminder in our study (Sarr et al., 2009), STN stimulation improves IOP significantly in the initial part of the expiratory phase.

Regarding the mean oral airflow (MOAF), no difference was found between patients in OFF DOPA and control subjects at the first and last measurement point (P1 and P6). That means patients and control subjects would develop the same speed to start and finish the sentence « Papa ne m'a pas parlé de beau-papa ». Difference between the two groups was only noted during the course of sentence production. Indeed at other measurement points (P2 to P5), the curve of control subjects is well above that of patients in OFF DOPA, the difference between the two groups was significant (p = 0.001). It is also found that the curve of control subjects had a more stable pace with its roughly more linear shape **(See figure 7)**. This could reflect a greater mastery of oral airflow by control subjects. In other words, the relatively greater irregularity of the curve of average values of MOAF in patients could reinforce the idea of a less good control of the MOAF. The reported decrease of MOAF could merely be a consequence of the fall in IOP. For example, assuming that laryngeal resistance is constant, the drop in IOP is necessarily associated with diminution in MOAF. However it seems exist in this study a large variability in laryngeal resistance in patients, as an overview was provided us in the morphological analysis of their value curves. This suggests a relatively fluctuating fall in MOAF which may also be related to tissue properties, configuration of the glottis and impedance of the vocal apparatus (Jiang & Tao, 2007). It is reported more generally in extrapyramidal syndromes glottic and supraglottic disorders such as movement disorders. These disorders can obstruct completely or partially the upper airway to induce sometimes severe airflow decrease (Vincken et al., 1984). The MOAF decline during speech production of PD patients could also be explained by similar mechanisms, among others.

Finally for the laryngeal resistance (LR), Parkinson's disease could induce a greater variability of this parameter in patients compared to control subjects, as evidenced by the general morphology of control subjects and OFF DOPA patients' curves. In other words, control subjects would have more stable values of LR, which would mean that Parkinson's disease induces instability of laryngeal resistance. The values of standard deviations significantly larger in OFF DOPA patients than control subjects, again reflecting greater variability in the values of LR at all measurement points, seem to confirm this trend (**See Figure 9**). The study of LR values distribution histogram in the two groups seems to be in the same direction. Indeed, the histogram shows a fairly symmetrical distribution for control subjects where OFF DOPA patients have more skewed distributions, with thus a tendency to give most often higher LR values compared to control subjects (**See Figure 10**).

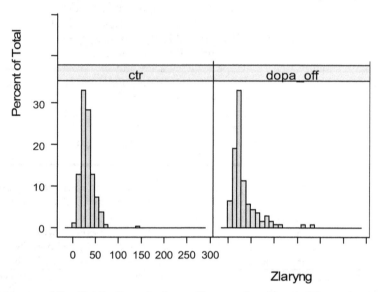

Fig. 10. Histogram of the distribution of values of laryngeal resistance (Zlaryng). There is a fairly symmetrical distribution for control subjects, while values distributions are more skewed in OFF DOPA patients.

Laryngeal resistance is equal to the ratio of IOP on MOAF; its greater constancy among control subjects may indicate a more perfect mastery of these two parameters. Besides this relative constancy of laryngeal resistance in control subjects was found in the measures performed by Smitheran and Hixon (1981). Smitheran and Hixon measurements were performed to compare laryngeal resistance values in non-invasive technique of measurement with those of invasive procedures. The mean laryngeal resistance in their patients was 35.7 + / - 3.3 cm H20/LPS (all measurements are between 30 and 43, 1). Blosser et al. (1992) reported similar values with a mean of 38.4 + / - 7.43 cm H20/LPS. In addition laryngeal resistance may reflect the larynx subject behavior. This has been demonstrated in a canine animal model which is able of maintaining, like humans, a constant subglottic pressure during phonation. In this model it was found a significant rise in laryngeal resistance when increasing the recurrent laryngeal nerve stimulation while the same nerve paralysis induced a significant drop of laryngeal resistance (Nasri et al., 1994). This significant rise in LR was also found in other disease involving larynx impairment with patients 'average to 65 + / - 8.15 cm H20/LPS (Blosser et al., 1992). We can therefore assume that the instability of laryngeal resistance in OFF DOPA patients reflects a more variable behavior of their larynx, but also a greater fluctuation in IOP and MOAF. We know, as seen previously, that patients have IOP lower than those of control subjects at all measurement points. So the important rise of patients' laryngeal resistance in the first half of the sentence, beyond the intrinsic behavior of larynx, may result from a larger drop of their airflow as we had also seen. Therefore the decline in patients' IOP in the second half of the sentence would induce the consequent decline of their laryngeal resistance. That's why the global evolutionary pace of patients' curve shows increased laryngeal resistance in the first half of the sentence and significant drop in the second half. These high laryngeal resistances in the beginning of the sentence could be related to a lack of pneumophonic coordination, that is to say a kind of phase shift between the air expiratory thrust and resistance state of the larynx. Everything would go as if, when the expiratory air exerts its thrust, the larynx is still at resistance level higher than normal. The larynx would amount only to a resistance normal level later, which would explain the decrease of laryngeal resistance in the second half of the sentence. In short, this phenomenon simply imitate, but this time at the pneumophonic floor, the mechanism of control loss of voice onset time (VOT) which reflects a lack of coordination between the larynx and articulatory organs (Forrest et al. 1989; Lieberman et al., 1992).

It thus appears that there is in Parkinson's disease pneumophonic coordination impairments which are evidenced by the fall in IOP and that of MOAF in patients compared with control subjects. And it follows from the alteration of these two parameters a greater instability of laryngeal resistance which is none other than ratio of two above mentioned parameters. For didactic sake, we attempted to separately discuss the different parameters (IOP, MOAF and LR). However it should be borne in mind that these parameters are closely related functionally, and that any change in one inevitably has repercussions on the other two. Indeed, the SGP (reflected here by the IOP) depends on the air expiratory column thrust and laryngeal resistance (LR) while translaryngeal airflow (reflected here by the MOAF) is merely the result of the conflict between expiratory thrust forces (SGP) and laryngeal resistance (LR) forces (Crevier-Buchman, 2007; Solomon, 2007). Reported disturbances in the three parameters pose the problem of events' real chronology because of parameters' correlation. Is it the increase in LR at the beginning of the sentence which induces a fall in MOAF or, conversely, would it fall in MOAF resulting of expiratory thrust poor dynamic that would cause the increase in LR? It could probably be a simultaneous mechanism combining both alteration of expiratory dynamic (leading to fall in IOP and MOAF) and elevated laryngeal resistance notably at sentence beginning (reinforcing the fall in MOAF). Such a mechanism would both explain decrease in IOP and initial elevation of laryngeal resistance which both lead to a decline in MOAF that patients would be tempted to correct by vocal abuse. Finally, such a mechanism would fit perfectly to a lack of pneumophonic coordination imitating, as we noted above, the lack of coordination in phono-articulatory stage which induces the voice onset time (VOT).

6. Conclusion

Parkinson's disease, given the study of these three parameters, likely induces an alteration of pneumophonic coordination involving a decrease in IOP, a decrease in MOAF and instability of the LR. So the measurements of these three aerodynamics parameters, by reflecting the dysfunction induced by disease, may well be relevant factors in parkinsonian dysarthria evaluation. These parameters can also be valuable in evaluation of several therapies used in Parkinson's disease treatment in general and dysarthria in particular. A limit of the present work is the lack of acoustic parameters assessment. In fact we thought that the sentence "Papa ne m'a pas parlé de beau-papa" is less appropriate than other tasks such as sustained vowel for evaluation of acoustic parameters. In any case, increasingly, methods for assessing parkinsonian dysarthria should be larger, including both central and peripheral levels of speech production. Future research to better understand and assess parkinsonian dysarthria would benefit from taking more account of a more global study of dysarthria contours.

7. References

Abbs JH, Hartman DE, Vishwanat B. *Orofacial motor control impairment in Parkinson's disease.* Neurology 1987, 37: 394-398.

Ackermann H, Grone BF, Hoch G, Schonle PW. *Speech freezing in Parkinson's disease: a kinematic analysis of orofacial movement by means of electromyographic articulography.* Folia phoniat 1993, 45: 84-89.

Ackermann H, Ziegler W. *Articulatory deficits in parkinsonian dysarthria: an acoustic analysis.* Journal of Neurology, Neurosurgery, and Psychiatry 1991, 54: 1093-1098.

Baken RJ and Orlikoff RF (2000). *Clinical Measurement of Speech and Voice*, 2nd ed. (Singular, Thomson Learning, San Diego).

Barlow SM, Abbs JH. *Force transducers for the evaluation of labial, lingual, and mandibular motor impairments.* Journal of Speech and Hearing Research 1983, 26: 616-621.

Blosser S, Wigley FM, Wise RA. *Increase in translaryngeal resistance during phonation in rheumatoid arthritis.* Chest 1992, 102(2):387-90.

Caligiuri M. *The influence of speaking rate on articulatory hypokinesia in parkinsonian dysarthria.* Brain lang 1989, 36: 493-502.

Canter GJ. *Speech characteristics of patients with Parkinson's disease: I Intensity, pitch and duration.* J Speech Hearing Dis 1963, 28: 221-229.

Connor NP, Abbs JH. *Task-dependent variations in parkinsonian motor impairment.* Brain 1991, 114: 321-332.

Connor NP, Abbs JH, Cole KJ, Gracco VL. *Parkinsonian deficits in serial multiarticulate movements for speech.* Brain 1989, 112: 997-1009.

Crevier-Buchman L. *Modélisation du fonctionnement laryngé.* In Auzou P, Monnoury-Rolland V, Pinto S, Özsancak C (eds),Les dysarthries. Solal. Marseille. 2007 pp 91-100.

Darley FL, Aronson AE, Brown JR. *Differential diagnostic patterns of dysarthria.* Journal of Speech and Hearing Research 1969, 12: 246-269.

Darley FL, Aronson AE, Brown JR. (1975). *Motor speech disorders*, pp. 171-197. Saunders WB, Philadelphia.

Demolin D, Giovanni A, Hassid S, Heim C, Lecuit V, Socquet A (1997). *"Direct and indirect measurements of subglottic pressure"*, Proc. Larynx 97, Marseille, p.69-72.

Duez D. *Organisation temporelle de la parole et dysarthrie parkinsonienne.* In Özsancak C, Auzou P (ed). Les troubles de la parole et de la déglutition dans la maladie de Parkinson. Solal. Marseille. 2005, pp 195-211.

Flint AJ, Black SE, Campbell-Taylor I, Gailey GF, Levinton C. *Acoustic analysis in the differentiation of Parkinson's disease and major depression.* Journal of Psycholinguistic Research 1992, 21: 383-389.

Forrest K, Weismer G, Turner GS. *Kinematic, acoustic and perceptual analyses of connected speech produced by parkinsonian and normal geriatric adults.* J Acoust Soc Am 1989, 85: 2608-2622.

Fox C, Ramig LO. *Vocal sound pressure level and self-perception of speech and voice in men and women with idiopathic Parkinson disease.* American Journal of Speech-Language Pathology 1997, 6: 85-94.

Gentil M, Pollak P, Perret J. *La dysarthrie parkinsonienne.* Rev. Neurol. (Paris) 1995, 151, 2, 105-112.

Harel B, Cannizzaro M, Snyder PJ. *Variability in fundamental frequency during speech in prodromal and incipient Parkinson's disease: a longitudinal case study.* Brain Cognition 2004, 56: 24-29.

Hartelius L, Svensson P. *Speech and swallowing symptoms associated with Parkinson's disease and Multiple sclerosis : A survey.* Folia Phoniatr Logop 1994, 46: 9-17.

Hertrich I, Ackermann H. *Acoustic analysis of speech prosody in Huntington's and Parkinson's disease: a preliminary report.* Clin Ling Phonetics 1993, 7:285-297.

Ho AK, Iansek R, Bradshaw JL. *Regulation of parkinsonian speech volume: the effect of interlocutor distance.* J Neurol Neurosurg Psychiatry 1999, 67 :199-202.

Ho AK, Iansek R, Marigliani C, Bradshaw JL, Gates S. *Speech impairment in a large sample of patients with Parkinson's disease.* Behav Neurol 1998, 11: 131-137.

Hunker CJ, Abbs JH, Barlow SM. *The relationship between parkinsonian rigidity and hypokinesia in the oro-facial system: a quantitative analysis.* Neurology 1982, 32: 749-754.

Jankowski L, Purson A, Teston B, Viallet F. *Effets de la L-Dopa sur la dysprosodie et le fonctionnement laryngien de patients parkinsoniens.* Actes des XXVèmes journées d'études sur la parole, Fès, Maroc, 19-22 avril 2004.

Jiang J, Tao C. *The minimum glottal airflow to initiate vocal fold oscillation.* J Acoust Soc Am 2007, 121(5):2873-81.

Jiang J, Lin E, Wang J, Hanson DG. *Glottographic measures before and after Levodopa treament in Parkinson's disease.* Laryngoscope 1999, 109: 1287-1294.

Jiang J, O'Mara T, Chen HJ, Stern JI, Vlagos D, Hanson D. *Aerodynamic measurements of patients with Parkinson's desease.* J Voice 1999a, 13:583-591.

Jimenez-Jimenez FJ, Gamboa J, Nieto A, Guerrero J, Orti-Pareja M, Molina JA, Garcia-Albea E, Cobeta I. *Acoustic voice analysis in untreated patients with Parkinson's disease.* Parkinsonism & Related Disorders 1997, 3: 111-116.

Kent RD, Rosenbek JC. *Prosodic disturbance and neurologic lesions.* Brain Lang 1982, 15: 259-291.

Leanderson R, Persson A, Ohman S. *Electromyographic studies of facial muscle activity in speech.* Acta Oto-laryngologica 1971, 72: 361-369.

Lieberman P, Kako E, Friedman J, Tajchman G, Feldman LS, Jiminez EB. *Speech production, syntax comprehension and cognitive deficits in Parkinson's disease.* Brain Lang 1992, 43: 169-189.

Logemann JA, Fisher HB, Boshes B, Blonsky ER. *Frequency and cooccurrence of vocal tract dysfunctions in the speech of a large sample of Parkinson patients.* J Speech Hear Dis 1978, 43: 47-57.

Ludlow CL, Connor NP, Bassich CJ. *Speech timing in Parkinson's and Huntington's disease.* Brain and Language 1987, 32: 195-214.

Ludlow CL, Bassich CJ. (1984). *Relationship between perceptual ratings and acoustic measures of hypokinetic speech.* In: McNeil M, Rosenbek JC, Aronson AE (eds), The dysarthrias : Physiology, acoustic, perception, management, pp. 163-196. College Hill Press, San Diego.

Metter EJ, Hanson WR. *Clinical and acoustical variability in hypokinetic dysarthria.* J Comm Disorders 1986, 19: 347-366.

Monfrais-Pfauwadel MC. *Palilalies et pseudobégaiements*. In Özsancak C, Auzou P (eds). Les troubles de la parole et de la déglutition dans la maladie de Parkinson. Solal. Marseille. 2005, pp 213-222.

Murdoch BE, Chenery HJ, Bowler S, Ingram JC. *Respiratory function in parkinson's subjects exhibiting a perceptible speech deficit: a kinematic and spirometric analysis.* J Speech Hear Dis 1989, 54:610-626.

Nasri S, Namazie A, Kreiman J, Sercarz JA, Gerrat BR, Berke GS. *A pressure-regulated model of normal and pathologic phonation.* Otolaryngol Head Neck Surg. 1994, 111 (6):807-15.

Netsell R, Daniel B, Celesia GG. *Acceleration and weakness in parkinsonian dysarthria.* J Speech Hearing Dis 1975, 40: 170-178.

Robert D, Spezza C. *La dysphonie parkinsonienne et les troubles articulatoires dans la dysarthrie parkinsonienne.* In Özsancak C, Auzou P (eds). Les troubles de la parole et de la déglutition dans la maladie de Parkinson. Solal. Marseille. 2005, pp 131-159.

Sanabria J, Garcia Ruiz P, Guttierez R. *The effect of Levodopa on vocal function in Parkinson's disease.* Clin Neuropharmacol 2001, 24: 99-102.

Sarr MM, Pinto S, Jankowski L, Teston B, Purson A, Ghio A, Régis J, Peragut JC, Viallet F. *Contribution de la mesure de la pression intra-orale pour la compréhension des troubles de la coordination pneumophonique dans la dysarthrie parkinsonienne.* Rev Neurol 2009, 165: 1055 – 1061.

Selby G. (1968). *Parkinson's disease.* In: PJ Winken & GW Bruyn, Handbook of clinical neurology, pp. 173-211. North Holland Publishing Company, Amsterdam.

Smith ME, Ramig LO, Dromey C, Perez KS, Samandari R. *Intensive voice treatment in Parkinson disease: laryngostroboscopic finding.* Journal of Voice 1995, 9: 453-459.

Smitheran J., Hixon T. *A Clinical method for estimating laryngeal airway resistance during vowel production.* J Speech Hear Dis 1981, 46:138-146.

Solomon NP. *La fonction respiratoire dans la production de parole.* In Auzou P, Monnoury-Rolland V, Pinto S, Özsancak C (eds),Les dysarthries. Solal. Marseille. 2007 pp 44-55.

Solomon NP, Hixton TJ. *Speech breathing in Parkinson's disease.* Journal of Speech and Hearing Research 1993, 36: 294-310.

Teston B. *L'étude instrumentale des gestes dans la production de la parole : Importance de l'aérophonométrie.* In Auzou P, Monnoury-Rolland V, Pinto S, Özsancak C (eds),Les dysarthries. Solal. Marseille. 2007 pp 248-258.

Viallet F, Teston B. *La dysarthrie dans la maladie de Parkinson.* In Auzou P, Monnoury-Rolland V, Pinto S, Özsancak C (eds),Les dysarthries. Solal. Marseille. 2007 pp 375-382.

Viallet F, Teston B, Jankowski L, Purson A, Peragut J, Régis J, Witgas T. *Effects of pharmacological versus electrophysical treatements on parkinsonian dysprosody.* In : Speech prosody, pp 679-682. Aix-en-Provence (2002)

Vincken WG, Gauthier SG, Dollfuss RE, Hanson RE, Darauay CM, Cosio MG. *Involvement of upper-airway muscles in extrapyramidal disorders. A cause of airflow limitation.* N Engl J Med. 1984, 311(7):438-42.

Volkmann J, Hefter H, Lange HW, Freund HJ. *Impairment of temporal organization of speech in basal ganglion diseases.* Brain Lang 1992, 43: 386-399.

Weismer G. (1984) *Articulatory characteristics of parkinsonian dysarthria.* In: The dysarthrias: Physiology, acoustics, perception, management (McNeil M, Rosenbek J, Aronson AE, eds), pp 101-130. San Diego: College Hill Press.

Yuceturk AV, Yilmaz H, Egrilmez M, Karaca S. *Voice analysis and videolaryngostroboscopy in patients with Parkinson's disease.* Eur Arch Otorhinolaryngol 2002, 259: 290-293.

12

Postural Control While Sitting and Its Association with Risk of Falls in Patients with Parkinson's Disease

Ryoichi Hayashi[1], Takeshi Hayashi[2], Junpei Aizawa[3],
Hiroaki Nagase[4] and Shinji Ohara[5]
[1]*Department of Neurology, Okaya City Hospital,*
[2]*Department of Computer Science and Systems Engineering,*
Graduate School of Engineering Kobe University
[3]*Department of Material Technology, Nagano Prefecture*
General Industrial Technology Center,
[4]*Department of Information Technology, Nagano Prefecture*
General Industrial Technology Center
[5]*Department of Neurology, Matsumoto Medical Center*
Japan

1. Introduction

Abnormal postures and falls in patients with Parkinson's disease (PD) have been well recognized from the time of its earliest clinical description (Parkinson, 1817). Abnormal postures in PD are observed in the entire body, including flexion to the anterior, lateral, or anterolateral direction of the trunk, neck flexion, flexion of the extremities, and abnormal postures of the hands, fingers, and toes. A lateral deviation of the spine and a corresponding tendency to lean to one side was reported (Duvoisin and Marsden 1975; Hayashi et al., 2010). These postural abnormalities cause postural instability and falls. In a recent study, approximately 50% of the PD patients had fallen, compared to about 15% of healthy elderly subjects, and approximately 75% of falls in PD patients occurred during activities associated with daily living, such as turning around, standing up, and bending forward (Bloem et al., 2001). Postural instability is caused by an inability to adjust the center of gravity quickly enough to account for perturbations in the environment (Shivitz et al., 2006). Maki and colleagues (1994) have suggested that increased lateral sway is associated with increased risk of falling in elderly persons. Several studies have quantified postural stability during quiet stance in patients with PD and revealed that PD patients have more difficulty in controlling lateral postural sway than anteroposterior sway (Mitchell et al., 1995; Rocchi et al., 2002).

In the standing position, postural adjustments can be accomplished with responses at the ankle, knee, hip, and trunk joints, independently or combined (Hodges et al., 2002; Krishnamoorthy et al., 2005) and these complex structures consisting of multiple linked segments must be maintained in a stable position on a relatively narrow support base formed by the feet. Lee and coworkers (1995) studied preparatory postural adjustments associated with a lateral leg-raising task in parkinsonian patients with postural instability. In the sitting position, the influence of hip joints and lower extremities can be minimized to study the postural control of the trunk. Van der Burg and coworkers (2006) studied the postural control of the trunk during unstable sitting in PD patients and revealed that PD patients showed difficulty in truncal control. They suggested that these changes may be related to postural instability and fall risk.

In this study, the body movement in PD patients during sitting was investigated by measuring center of pressure (COP) excursions and trunk deviations under two conditions: 1) sitting at rest for two minutes, 2) raising his/her arm laterally to 90 degrees. An additional aim was to study differences in trunk control between patients who had a history of falling (fallers) and patients who did not have a history of falling (non-fallers). The aim of this study is also to test the hypothesis that postural abnormality in a lateral direction may, or would be a high risk factor for falling during the daily activities of PD patients and further attempts to formulate the pattern of muscle tone abnormalities that may underline this disturbance.

2. Patients and methods

2.1 Patients

17 consecutive idiopathic PD patients and 8 age-matched normal controls were studied. These 17 patients received regular outpatient treatment every month over the course of a one-year follow-up period. All patients satisfied the following inclusion criteria: Hoehn and Yahr stage II or higher while off medication (II=1, III=11, IV=5), a clear history of significant responsiveness to levodopa and an absence of other neurologic diseases including significant dementia or autonomic dysfunction. The patients' clinical data are given in Table 1. All patients (mean age ± sd: 72±6 years) did not have any neurological or other diseases that might affect their postural stability or ability to perform the experimental tasks.

Patient	Sex	Age (years)	Hoehn & Yahr	Duration (years)	Number of falls (per year)
1	F	70	3	12	more than 5
2	F	65	3	12	under 5
3	M	65	4	8	under 5
4	F	77	3	7	more than 5
5	F	64	3	11	0
6	M	75	3	6	under 5
7	F	67	3	11	0
8	M	78	3	13	under 5
9	F	75	2	4	0
10	F	75	4	11	under 5
11	M	71	3	6	0
12	M	75	4	8	under 5
13	F	81	3	6	0
14	F	79	4	11	more than 5
15	F	62	3	25	0
16	M	78	4	6	more than 5
17	F	69	3	11	more than 5

Table 1. Clinical characteristics of PD patient

This study was approved by the Okaya City Hospital Committee for Research on Human Subjects, and informed consent was obtained from all test subjects.

2.2 Experimental setup and procedure

A stable stool was placed on a force platform (Kistler platform type 9281CA, Winterthur, Switzerland). The stool was high enough so that each subject's legs could hang down without touching the platform (Fig. 1). Subjects sat on the stool at ease. At that time, if subjects presented a tilt of the trunk away from the vertical position, they were not asked to correct their trunk to the vertical position. Subjects were asked to maintain a sitting posture on the stool for 1) 2 minutes at rest, and 2) 30 seconds with a lateral arm raised alternatively up to 90 degrees with their legs hanging down and their hand placed on each thigh except for a raising arm. Subjects were also asked to keep their eyes open and to focus on the target point in front of them.

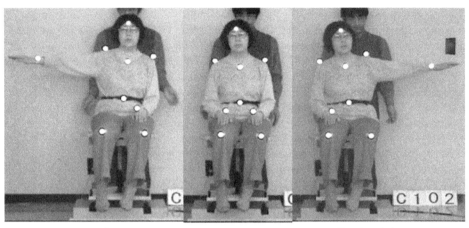

| Raising right arm | At rest | Raising left arm |

Fig. 1. Example of postural changes both during sitting on a stool at resting posture and during the raising of each arm.

Using the forced plate with a sampling frequency of 500Hz, the excursion of the centre of pressure (COP) was measured. The position of the body segments was also measured using a video image processing system, with the images being developed in our laboratory. Nine reflective markers (1 cm in diameter) were placed on the forehead, the upper part of the sternum, shoulders, wrists, knees, and the level of the umbilicus, and reflections from the markers were recorded with a sampling rate of 30 Hz.

2.3 Evaluation of truncal inclination at rest

Both COP excursions and the body-marker displacement were recorded simultaneously for 2 minutes. Values for the initial 10 seconds and the last 10 seconds were averaged, and the difference was calculated for each trial. The values obtained by the two trials for each subject were averaged.

2.4 Evaluation of truncal inclination while raising arm

After evaluation of truncal inclination at rest, the patient was studied when each of their arms were raised laterally up to 90 degrees two times in the following sequence: at rest for

30 seconds, raising the right arm for 30 seconds, at rest for 30 seconds, then raising the left arm for 30 seconds.

2.5 Statistical analysis
For each posturographic parameter and clinical measurement, Student's t-test or an analysis of variance (ANOVA) was used to compare group means between normal controls and PD patients. Correlation between the degree of COP displacement and the degree of body displacement was evaluated with Spearman's rank correlation coefficient.

3. Results

3.1 Clinical features
On examination, in all 17 patients, the side of initial symptoms was also the side of dominant clinical signs. Over the one-year follow-up period, 6 of 17 patients (35%) experienced no falls. The remaining 11 patients (65%) fell at least two times. Five of patients experienced more than 5 falls during the one-year follow-up, and these patients were described as "frequent fallers" in this paper. Patients who experienced less than 5 falls were described as a "less frequent fallers." This study found a strong correlation between disease severity and frequency of falls. The mean value with standard deviation of the Hoehn and Yahr stage in non-fallers and "less frequent fallers" was 2.8 ± 0.4, and that of the "frequent fallers" was 3.5 ± 0.5 ($p<0.02$). There was no significant difference between "frequent fallers" and "non-fallers" and "less frequent fallers" in age or duration of illness (73.3 ± 5.2 years versus 70.0 ± 7.0 years, $p=0.3$ in age; 9.5 ± 2.6 years versus 10.5 ± 7.7 years, $p=0.7$ in duration).

3.2 Body inclination during sitting
A consistency in lateral displacement was observed in all 17 patients. Table 2 shows the values of two parameters of body inclination in each group. There was a tendency toward increased values of both lateral COP displacement and trunk displacement in a group of PD patients compared with controls. However, there was no significant difference in these parameters between that of the control group and the PD-patient group. When each parameter obtained by "frequent fallers" is compared with controls, there was a significant difference in each parameter (lateral COP displacement $p=0.01$, trunk displacement $p=0.01$).

	Control	PD		
		all	non-fallers & fallers (under 5)	Fallers (more than 5)
	n=8	n=17	n=12	n=5
Lateral COP displacement	2.0 ± 1.7	6.2 ± 7.0 (p=0.11)	3.5 ± 2.5 (p=0.16)	12.9 ± 12.9 (p=0.01)
Trunk displacement	7.1 ± 4.8	17.3 ± 18.2 (p=0.14)	10.1 ± 7.7 (p=0.35)	34.5 ± 34.5 (p=0.01)

unit: mm

Table 2. This data represents the mean value with one standard deviation of each parameter of body inclination in control subjects and in PD patients at rest for 2 minutes. Each mean value was calculated using an absolute value of each parameter obtained from each subject.

Fig. 2 shows the relationship between changes of lateral COP displacement and trunk displacement obtained from all 17 patients. The amount of lateral COP displacement was correlated significantly with that of trunk displacement ($r=0.94$, $p<0.0001$).

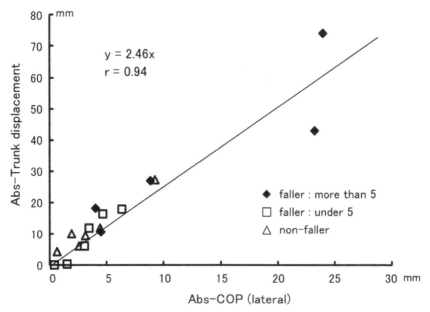

Fig. 2. The relationship between the absolute value of lateral COP displacement (Abs-COP) and the absolute value of trunk displacement (Abs- trunk displacement) obtained from 17 patients at rest.

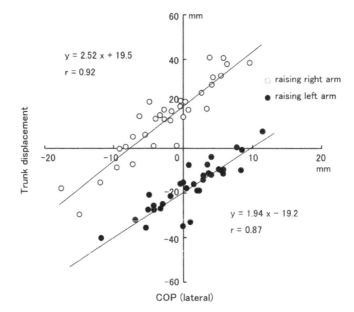

Fig. 3. The relationship between the value of lateral COP displacement (COP) and the value of trunk displacement obtained from 17 patients during arm-raising examination.

3.3 Postural change during arm raising

Two patients, who were "frequent fallers" and showed a large lateral inclination, had difficulty in keeping their sitting posture for more than 10 seconds and had to be supported by experimenters to prevent them from falling during arm-raising test. Therefore, the following was analyzed: 1) the relationship between the lateral COP displacement and the trunk displacement using the value observed at 1 second after raising the arm to 90 degrees for all 17 patients, and 2) changes of the body axis during the arm-raising for 15 patients.

A postural change observed from one patient during the arm-raising test is shown in Figure 1. When the patient raised her arm laterally up to 90 degrees, the trunk marker shifted to the opposite side. In Figure 3, the relationship between the lateral COP displacement and the trunk displacement obtained from all 17 patients is shown.

| | Control | PD | | |
	n=8	all n=17	non-fallers & fallers (under 5) n=12	Fallers (more than 5) n=3
Raising right arm	4.4 ± 1.6	4.5 ± 2.1 (p=0.5)	4.3 ± 2.0 (p=0.9)	5.1 ± 2.8 (p=0.6)
Raising leftt arm	3.7 ± 0.9	5.3 ± 2.7 (p=0.2)	4.4 ± 2.3 (p=0.4)	5.3 ± 1.5 (p=0.3)

unit: degree

Table 3. The absolute mean value with one standard deviation of each change of body inclination in control subjects and in PD patients when each subject raised each arm 90 degrees.

A positive relationship with a high correlation coefficient was observed, which was the same as the relationship observed during maintaining sitting posture at rest, only the shift of the initial position of the trunk marker. Table 3 shows the change of body axis associated with the arm-raising in each group. There was no significant difference between both the control group and the PD patient group, or between the control group and the "frequent faller" PD patient group.

In this test, R was defined as the following equation under a hypothesis that the relationship between the lateral COP displacement (ΔG) and the trunk displacement (ΔL) obtained during the sitting condition also applied to the lateral arm raising condition. In the sitting test, the relationship between ΔL and ΔG is expressed as following equation; $\Delta L = 2.46 * \Delta G$ (cf. Figure 2).

$$R = \Delta L - 2.46 * \Delta G$$

Figure 4 shows each parameter obtained from one subject during the arm raising test and the calculated results applied using the equation above. The calculated data showed a square change during the arm-raising phase (Figure 4B). The square change associated with the arm raising was observed in all patients except two patients who had fallen.

3.4 Estimation of trunk muscle tone

In this paper, we proposed a simulation model (cf. Figure 7) and an estimation of trunk muscle tone was made using patient's data under following conditions: 1) to mimic a sitting posture at rest and 2) to mimic a sitting posture with an arm raising. A detail of the model and a calculation procedure are described in the Appendix of this paper. Each body segment

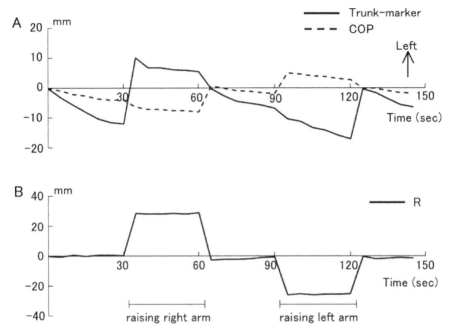

Fig. 4. A: A sequential change of lateral COP displacement (COP) and the value of trunk displacement (Trunk-marker) when one patient raised her arm alternatively. B: The R value change, which was calculated by our proposed equation (see Text).

Patient	Weight (kg)	Sitting height (cm)	Shoulder biacromial breadth (cm)	Bicristal breadth (cm)	Arm length (cm)	Torque (Nm) at rest	Torque (Nm) arm raising
1	46.0	70.0	32.9	23.6	55.0	5.87	39.1
2	60.0	73.6	32.9	26.4	62.9	5.02	44.4
3	44.0	73.6	33.6	28.6	61.4	3.54	42.4
4	37.5	64.3	28.6	25.7	54.3	3.13	37.8
5	48.0	72.9	32.1	28.6	60.0	2.37	42.4
6	61.0	72.9	33.6	25.7	64.3	0.11	43.6
7	43.0	74.3	32.1	26.4	62.1	0.94	43.8
8	60.0	70.0	30.7	25.7	62.9	0.05	43.4
9	44.0	72.9	29.3	25.7	61.4	1.31	43.3
10	47.0	64.3	30.7	27.1	61.4	1.22	43.3
11	57.0	73.6	38.6	27.9	55.7	2.65	38.7
12	54.0	70.0	37.9	27.9	62.9	2.89	43.2
13	44.0	64.3	27.9	26.4	62.1	2.23	43.8
14	34.0	64.3	30.7	21.4	58.6	1.68	41.7
15	51.6	67.9	34.3	26.4	60.7	6.33	45.3
16	45.0	76.4	31.4	27.1	62.1	9.78	42.8
17	65.0	72.9	32.1	27.1	58.6	22.51	41.5

Table 4. Each body segment size or body weight, which were used to estimate the torque, and the estimated value of torque both at rest and arm-raising.

size or body weight, which was used to estimate the torque, is shown in Table 4. There was a tendency toward increased value of the torque in PD patients who experienced falling frequently. The mean value with standard deviation of the torque at rest in non-fallers and less frequent fallers was 2.4 Nm±1.9 Nm, and that of the frequent fallers was 8.6 Nm±8.4 Nm (p<0.03). In Figure 5, the relationship between the value of trunk displacement and the estimated torque for each patient is shown. An estimated torque value was calculated using an averaged data value of all 17 patients when our model leaned. The data suggested that the trunk muscle tone was larger in the patients with high falling risk than the patients with less falling risk. In a simulation of the arm-raising, there was no significant difference between the non-fallers (42.9±2.3 Nm) and the fallers (42.1±2.0 Nm) (p>0.47).

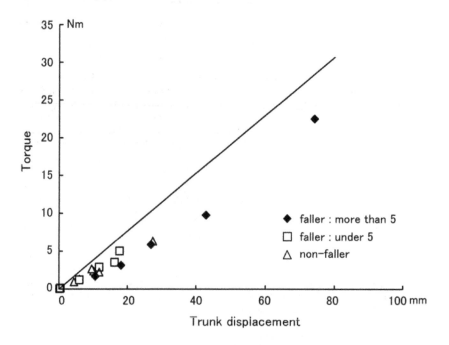

Fig. 5. Relationship between the value of trunk displacement and the estimated torque for each patient. An estimated torque value to the trunk displacement is shown as a straight line: a simulation was conducted using each of the following parameters calculated by averaging the data obtained from each of our 17 patients; body weight (except legs): 49.5 kg; arm weight 3.2 kg; sitting height 70.5 cm; shoulder biacromial breadth 32.3 cm; bicristal breadth 26.3 cm; arm length 60.4 cm.

In Figure 6, both the trunk displacement and the COP displacement were shown when the arm segment of the model was raised up to 90 degrees. Although we observed a transient response when the arm segment moved from a resting posture to a 90-degree arm raising posture or when the arm segment moved from the 90-degree position to the initial position, a constant value was observed when the arm segment was held at the 90-degree position or at the rest position.

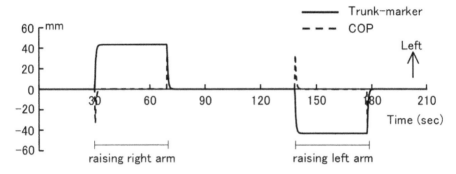

Fig. 6. Simulation representing an arm-raising test. A sequential change of lateral COP displacement and the value of trunk displacement when the model raised an arm alternately. A simulation was conducted using each of the following parameters calculated by averaging the data obtained from each of our 17 patients; body weight (except legs): 49.5 kg; arm weight 3.2 kg; sitting height 70.5 cm; shoulder biacromial breadth 32.3 cm; bicristal breadth 26.3 cm; arm length 60.4 cm.

4. Discussion

In this study, we demonstrated that PD patients who fell frequently tended to have 1) a value of lateral COP displacement greater than the value of control subjects, 2) a geometrical relationship between the arm and the trunk was preserved in PD patients, the same as in control subjects, and 3) a significant difference in postural muscle tone between frequent fallers and non-fallers or less frequent fallers. These results suggest that the measurement of both lateral COP displacement during sitting and arm-raising would be useful in predicting the risk of falling and predicting the trunk rigidity in PD patients.

4.1 Body inclination during sitting and in relation to falling frequency

Postural instability is one of the major symptoms of Parkinson's disease, and the instability in the control of upright stance and posture in PD often results in falling (Bloem et al., 2001; Wood et al., 2002; Grimbergen et al., 2004; Bloem et al., 2006). Several studies reported that postural sway patterns during quiet stance in PD patients are different compared to those of healthy elderly subjects, with PD patients displaying larger lateral excursion compared with anteroposterior excursion (Mitchell et al., 1995; Morris et al., 2000; Van Wegen et al., 2001; Van der Burg et al., 2006). In our study, the same tendency of postural sway pattern during sitting was observed and the excursions in the lateral direction in PD patients were larger than those of control subjects. Regarding postural control during standing, several authors suggested that instability in the anterior-posterior direction was compensated for by increasing excursion in the lateral direction in PD patients (Schieppati et al., 1994; Mitchell et al., 1995; Van Wegen et al., 2001). These mechanisms might be working during sitting and would have eventually increased the lateral inclination. Van Emmerik et al. (1999) also suggested that lateral impairment in postural control in patients with PD might be a reflection of axial rigidity.

Several studies suggested that increased lateral sway is associated with increased risk of falling in both elderly subjects (Maki et al., 1994) and patients with PD (Mitchell et al., 1995; Rocchi et al., 2002). Our study also showed that the degree of lateral inclination during sitting was significantly larger in PD patients with history of falls than PD patients without history.

Based on these results, we suggest the risk of falls would increase when compensation in the anterior-posterior body sway with the lateral body sway is difficult. Measurement of postural change in the lateral direction during sitting for a relatively long time, 2 minutes in this study, is a simple and effective method that can be used in daily clinical examinations to evaluate the risk of falling.

4.2 Postural change associated with a lateral arm-raising task

A large number of human motor actions cause potential displacement of the body center of gravity (COP) and it is well known that voluntary movement is preceded and accompanied by postural muscular activities. Several studies which fall into this category include activation of posterior trunk and leg muscles when the arms are raised in front of the body (Traub et al., 1980; Zattare & Bouisset, 1988) or when a leg is raised while standing (Lee et al., 1995).

There are several reports that postural adjustments of the upper extremities may also be disrupted in Parkinson's disease. Abnormalities in the timing or amplitude of anticipatory postural adjustments, which occur when rapid voluntary arm movements are made while in the standing position, have been reported in parkinsonian subjects (Dick et al., 1986). Lee and coworkers (1995) studied the preparatory postural adjustments associate with a lateral leg raising task in parkinsonian patients and described the amplitude of the initial displacement of COP was markedly reduced and the interval between the earliest force changes and the onset of leg elevation was prolonged. These authors focused on the initial phase of the preparatory postural adjustments in parkinsonian patients with postural instability. On the other hand, in our study, the postural change after elevating and holding the arm was examined. We found no significant difference in the trunk inclination, associated with arm-raising between normal controls and PD patients, or between raising the right arm and the left arm test in PD patients. These test results indicated that the postural controls during the arm raising were preserved in PD patients we studied.

Adopting an appropriate body orientation, and maintaining this posture to the displacing effects of gravity or external forces is essential for postural control. Patients with Parkinson's disease had difficulty in postural control, especially the control of body vertically (Vaugoyeau et al., 2007; Hayashi et al., 2010). Steiger et al. (1996) reported that PD patients had difficulty in coordinating the orientation of the axial segments along the spinal axis. Several investigators also reported that the proprioceptive feedback information to the static position and movement perception processing decreased in PD patients (Zia et al., 2002; Keijsers et al., 2005; Vaugoyeau et al., 2007). In this study, the body inclination was observed during the arm-raising test, and the R-value was constant. These results suggested that a geometric relationship between the raised arm and the trunk was preserved during the arm-raising phase even though the trunk inclined.

4.3 Estimation of postural muscle tone in the body axis

Rigidity is a continuous and uniform increase in muscle tone, felt as a constant resistance throughout the range of passive movement of a limb or a neck, and is a cardinal symptom of Parkinson's disease. Clinically, rigidity is usually assessed by passively flexing and extending a patient's limb. Objectively, most previous investigators examined rigidity in the muscles in PD patients, using either torque motor or isokinetic dynamometer (Nuyens et al., 2000; Hayashi et al., 2001). A few studies have done quantitatively to measure of postural muscle tone in the body axis of healthy test subjects (Kumar 2004; Gurfinkel et al., 2006) or to measure of trunk rigidity in parkinsonian patients (Mak et al., 2007). In these studies, the measurement procedures were different; each estimated value of muscle tone was close. Gurfinkel et al. (2006) reported that the value was 2 Nm to 9 Nm in standing, 40 Nm to 80 Nm in sitting (Kumar, 2004). Mak and coworkers (2007) reported PD patients had a significantly higher trunk muscle tone when compared with normal controls in the standing position, in both passive trunk flexion (17-22 Nm · deg in the control group, 27-40 Nm · deg in PD patients) and passive trunk extension (21-26 Nm · deg in the control group, 28-45 Nm · deg in PD patients).

In this paper, we estimated the postural muscle tone in the body axis based on our model and showed that the positive relationship between the trunk displacement and the estimated torque value at rest condition. The estimated torque value in the high risk PD patients for falls was larger than that of lower risk PD patients. These results were consistent with that reported by Mak and coworkers (2007). In their study, it was reported that unstable PD patients had a tendency to have high trunk muscle tone.

5. Conclusion

Based on these results, we conclude that a measurement of body inclination for an extended period of 2 minutes as in this study is a valuable predictor for the risk of falling and is a simple and easy method to estimate the trunk muscle tone. This study also demonstrates that even PD patients with high falling risk are capable of controlling their postural geometry between the raised arm and the trunk.

6. Appendix

The proposed model, which simplified a sitting posture on a chair, was developed using an ODE (Open Dynamic Engine) simulator. This model is composed of the following 7 parts, including the upper part of the trunk, arm part, shoulder hinge joint, impedance joint set under the upper part, waist hinge joint, lower part of the trunk and the hip hinge joint. Body segment parameters used at the simulator are given by general physical data obtained from our patients, and an estimation value of each body segment was made based on the previous reports (Jensen et al., 1994, Okada et al., 1996).

The unique point of our model is using an "impedance joint", which consist of two parts: "elastic property" and "viscous properties" to artificially reproduce the muscles encompassing the waist.

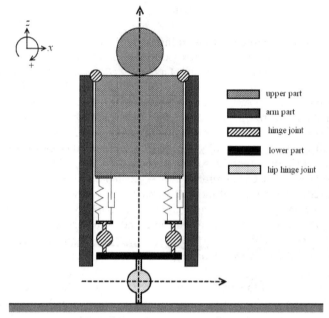

Fig. 7. A proposed model

The mathematical expression of the each impedance joint is shown as:

$$I\ddot{\theta} = \tau - d\dot{\theta} - k\theta$$

where I is the fictitious force, θ is the angle of the joint, τ is the muscle torque around the waist, d is the elastic property and k is the viscous property. By using this impedance joint, it becomes very easy to simulate the behavior of the body. The hinge joints work as an actuator, rotation sprig or a torque motor; which are used in the shoulder, waist and hip joint. It is also possible to obtain the data of each part and the whole body's barycentric coordinates using this simulator.

The procedure of the simulation is thus illustrated as follows: first, each parameter of the model such as weight or height et al. was estimated based on the previous Japanese reports (Okada et al., 1996) and our patients (cf. Table 4). Then a condition was imposed on the model to remain stable while a small disturbance to the body was applied. During this procedure the torque exerted on each of the joints was calculated, and using this data we were able to calculate the optimal solution of the stiffness for each joint.

At the next step, a stiffness condition was imposed on the model, which was evaluated from the previous simulation and then, set the same condition for the model to stay stable. This time, instead of applying a small disturbance, we requested the model to raise their arm up to the 90-degree position in 1 second. Through simulation, we gave careful consideration of the body sway by using the impedance joint and the hinge joints. Tuning the two impedance joints and the stiffness joints through the numerical simulations, we estimated an identified torque, which is needed to maintain posture maintenance.

Winter et al. (1998) reported that a relationship between COP and COM (center of mass or barycenter) was expressed in the following equation in a stiffness control of balance in the quiet standing position.

$$COP - COM = -\frac{I}{mgh}\ddot{x}$$

Where I is the inertial around the mass, m is the mass of the object, g is the acceleration due to gravity, h is the length from the origin coordinates and $\ddot{x}$ is the second derivative of COM. At this simulation, thereafter the arm is raised up to the 90-degree position, the body will be stationary; thereby we can consider $\ddot{x} = 0$.

The barycentric coordinate of the full body (P_{tx}, P_{tz}) will be expression as:

$$P_{tx} = (M_{un} \cdot P_{un\_x} + M_{up} \cdot P_{up\_x} + M_{la} \cdot P_{la\_x} + M_{ra} \cdot P_{ra\_x}) / (M_{un} + M_{up} + M_{la} + M_{ra})$$
$$P_{tz} = (M_{un} \cdot P_{un\_z} + M_{up} \cdot P_{up\_z} + M_{la} \cdot P_{la\_z} + M_{ra} \cdot P_{ra\_z}) / (M_{un} + M_{up} + M_{la} + M_{ra})$$

Where $M_{un}, M_{up}, M_{la}, M_{ra}$ is the mathamatical representation of "lower part of the trunk (21.5% of body weight)", "upper part of the trunk (28.5% of body weight)", "left arm (6.5% of body weight)", "right arm (6.5% of body weight)", and $P_{un\_x}, P_{up\_x}, P_{la\_x}, P_{ra\_x}, P_{un\_z}, P_{up\_z}, P_{la\_z}, P_{ra\_z}$ is the barycentric position of each part where x and z represent the horizontal component and the vertical component, respectively. The angle between "barycentric position" and "hip hinge joint" will be expression as:

$$angle = \arctan(P_{tx} / (P_{tz} - P_h)).$$

Where P_h is the length from the home position.
1. to mimic a sitting posture at rest
   The torque applied to the hip hinge joint will be express as:

$$torque_h = G_{Dh}(0 - R_{Vh}) + G_{Ph}(0 - R_{Ah}),$$

   where G_{Dh}, G_{Ph} are a derivative gain and a proportional gain of the torque.
   And R_{Vh}, R_{Ah} are a displacement and an angular rate of the body.
2. to mimic a sitting posture with the right arm raising, we used the right arm hinge torque and the hip hinge torque.
   Right arm hinge torque can be represented excellently by:

$$torque_{ra} = -G_{Da}(B_{Va} - R_{Va}) - G_{Pa}(B_{Aa} - R_{Aa})$$

   where G_{Da}, G_{Pa} are a derivative gain and a proportional gain of the torque.
   And R_{Va}, R_{Aa} are a displacement and an angular rate and B_{Va}, B_{Aa} are the target trajectories of the arm.

7. References

Bloem, BR., Grimbergen, YAM., Cramer, M., Willemsen, M., Zwinderman, AH. Prospective assessment of falls in Parkinson's disease. *J Neurol.* 248, 2001, pp 950-8.

Bloem, BR., Grimbergen, YAM., van Dijk, JG., Munneke, M. The "posture second" strategy: a review of wrong priorities in Parkinson's disease. *J Neurol Sci.* 248, 2006, pp 196-204.

Dick, JP., Rothwell, JC., Berardelli, A., Thompson, PD., Gioux, M., Benecke, R., Day, BL., Marsden, CD. Associated postural adjustments in Parkinson's disease. *J Neurol Neurosurg Psychiatry.* 49, 1986, pp 1378-85.

Duvoisin, RC., Marsden, CD. Note on the scoliosis of Parkinsonism. *J Neurol Neurosurg Psychiatry.* 38, 1975, pp 787-93.

Grimbergen, YAM., Munneke, M., Bloem, BR. Falls in Parkinson's disease. *Curr Opin Neurol.* 17, 2004, pp 405-15.

Gurfinkel, V., Cacciatore, TW., Cordo, P., Horak, F., Nutt, J., Skoss, R. Postural muscle tone in the body axis of healthy humans. *J Neurophysiol.* 96, 2006, pp 2678-87.

Hayashi, R., Hashimoto, T., Tada, T., Ikeda, S. Relation between changes in long-latency stretch reflexes and muscle stiffness in Parkinson's disease comparison before and after unilateral pallidotomy. *Clin Neurophysiol.* 112, 2001, pp 1814-21.

Hayashi, R., Aizawa, J., Nagase, H., Ohara, S. Lateral inclination of the trunk and falling frequency in Parkinson's disease patients. *Electromyogr Clin Neurophysiol.* 50, 2010, pp 195-202.

Hodges, PW., Gurfinkel, VS., Brumagne, S., Smith, TC., Cordo, PC. Coexistence of stability and mobility in postural control: evidence from postural compensation for respiration. *Exp Brain Res.* 144, 2002, pp 293-302.

Jensen, RK., Fletcher, P. Distribution of mass to the segments of elderly males and females. J Biomech. 27,1994, pp 89-96.

Keijsers, NL., Admiraal, MA., Cools, AR., Bloem, BR., Gielen, CC. Differential progression of proprioceptive and visual information processing deficits in Parkinson's disease. *Eur J Neurosci.* 21, 2005, pp 239-48.

Kumar, S. Ergonomics and biology of spinal rotation. *Ergonomics.* 47, 2004, pp 370-415.

Krishnamoorthy, V., Yang, JF., Scholz, JP. Joint coordination during quiet stance: effects of vision. *Exp Brain Res.* 164, 2005, pp 1-17.

Lee, RG., Tonolli, I., Viallet, F., Aurenty, R., Massion, J. Preparatory postural adjustments in parkinsonian patients with postural instability. *Can J Neurol Sci.* 22, 1995, pp 126-35.

Mak, MK., Wong, EC., Hui-Chan, CW. Quantitative measurement of trunk rigidity in parkinsonian patients. *J Neurol.* 254, 2007, pp 202-9.

Maki, BE., Holliday, PJ., Topper, AK. A prospective study of postural balance and risk of falling in an ambulatory and independent elderly population. *J Gerontol.* 49, 1994, pp M72-84.

Mitchell. SL., Collins, JJ., De Luca, CJ., Burrows, A., Lipsitz, LA. Open-loop and closed-loop postural control mechanisms in Parkinson's disease: increased mediolateral activity during quiet standing. *Neurosci Lett.* 197, 1995, pp 133-6.

Morris, M., Iansek, R., Smithson, F., Huxham, F. Postural insatiability in Parkinson's disease: a comparison with and without a concurrent task. *Gait Posture.* 12, 2000, pp 205-16.

Nuyens, G., De Weerdt, W., Dom, R., Nieuwboer, A., Spaepen, A. Torque variations during repeated passive isokinetic movements of the knee in subjects with Parkinson's disease and healthy control subjects. *Parkinsonism Relat Disord.* 6, 2000, pp87-93.

Okada, H., Ae, M., Fujii, N., Morioka, Y. Body segment inertia properties of Japanese elderly. *Biomechanisms* Vol.13, 1996, pp 125-139. The Society of Biomechanisms. ISBN 4-13-060134-3, Japan

Parkinson, J. (1817). *An essay on the shaking palsy.* Sherwood, Neely, and Jones, London.

Rocchi, L., Chiari, L., Horak, FB. Effects of deep brain stimulation and levodopa on postural sway in Parkinson's disease. *J Neurol Neurosurg Psychiatry.* 73, 2002, pp 267-74.

Schieppati, M., Hugon, M., Grasso, M., Nardone, A., Galante, M. The limits of equilibrium in young and elderly normal subjects and in parkinsonians. *Electroencephalogr Clin Neurophysiol.* 93, 1994, pp 286-98.

Shivitz, N., Koop, MM., Fahimi, J., Heit, G, Bronte-Stewart HM. Bilateral subthalamic nucleus deep brain stimulation improves certain aspects of postural control in Parkinson's disease, whereas medication does not. *Mov Disord.* 21, 2006, pp 1088-97.

Steiger, MJ., Thompson, PD., Marsden, CD. Disordered axial movement in Parkinson's disease. *J Neurol Neurosurg Psychiatry.* 61, 1996, pp 645-8.

Traub, MM., Rothwell, JC., Marsden, CD. Anticipatory postural reflexes in Parkinson's disease and other akinetic-rigid syndromes and in cerebellar ataxia. *Brain.* 103, 1980, pp 393-412.

Van der Burg, JCE., van Wegen, EEH., Rietberg, MB., Kwakkel, G., van Dieën, JH. Postural control of the trunk during unstable sitting in Parkinson's disease. *Parkinsonism Relat Disord.* 12, 2006, pp 492-8.

Van Emmerik, REA., Wagenaar, RC., Winogrodzka, A., Wolters, EC. Identification of axial rigidity during locomotion in Parkinson disease. *Arch Phys Med Rehabil.* 80, 1999, pp186-91.

Van Wegen, EEH., van Emmerik, REA., Wagenaar, RC., Ellis, T. Stability boundaries and lateral postural control in Parknson's disease. *Motor Control.* 3, 2001, pp 254-69.

Vaugoyeau, M., Viel, S., Assaiante, C., Amblard, B., Azulay, JP. Impaired vertical postural control and proprioceptive integration deficits in Parkinson's disease. *Neuroscience.* 146, 2007, pp 852-63.

Winter, DA., Patla, AE., Prince, F., Ishac, M., Gielo-Perczak K. Stiffness control of balance in quiet standing. *J Neurophysiol.* 80, 1998, pp-1211-21.

Wood, BH., Bilclough, JA., Bowron, A., Walker, RW. Incidence and prediction of falls in Parkinson's disease: a prospective multidisciplinary study. *J Neurol Neurosurg Psychiatry.* 72, 2002, pp 721-5.

Zattara, M., Bouisset, S. Posturo-kinetic organisation during the early phase of voluntary upper limb movement. 1. Normal subjects. *J Neurol Neurosurg Psychiatry*. 51, 1988, pp 956-65.

Zia, S., Cody, FW., O'Boyle, DJ. Identification of unilateral elbow-joint position is impaired by Parkinson's disease. *Clin Anat*. 15, 2002, pp 23-3.

Permissions

The contributors of this book come from diverse backgrounds, making this book a truly international effort. This book will bring forth new frontiers with its revolutionizing research information and detailed analysis of the nascent developments around the world.

We would like to thank Dr. Juliana Dushanova, for lending her expertise to make the book truly unique. She has played a crucial role in the development of this book. Without her invaluable contribution this book wouldn't have been possible. She has made vital efforts to compile up to date information on the varied aspects of this subject to make this book a valuable addition to the collection of many professionals and students.

This book was conceptualized with the vision of imparting up-to-date information and advanced data in this field. To ensure the same, a matchless editorial board was set up. Every individual on the board went through rigorous rounds of assessment to prove their worth. After which they invested a large part of their time researching and compiling the most relevant data for our readers. Conferences and sessions were held from time to time between the editorial board and the contributing authors to present the data in the most comprehensible form. The editorial team has worked tirelessly to provide valuable and valid information to help people across the globe.

Every chapter published in this book has been scrutinized by our experts. Their significance has been extensively debated. The topics covered herein carry significant findings which will fuel the growth of the discipline. They may even be implemented as practical applications or may be referred to as a beginning point for another development. Chapters in this book were first published by InTech; hereby published with permission under the Creative Commons Attribution License or equivalent.

The editorial board has been involved in producing this book since its inception. They have spent rigorous hours researching and exploring the diverse topics which have resulted in the successful publishing of this book. They have passed on their knowledge of decades through this book. To expedite this challenging task, the publisher supported the team at every step. A small team of assistant editors was also appointed to further simplify the editing procedure and attain best results for the readers.

Our editorial team has been hand-picked from every corner of the world. Their multi-ethnicity adds dynamic inputs to the discussions which result in innovative outcomes. These outcomes are then further discussed with the researchers and contributors who give their valuable feedback and opinion regarding the same. The feedback is then collaborated with the researches and they are edited in a comprehensive manner to aid the understanding of the subject.

Apart from the editorial board, the designing team has also invested a significant amount of their time in understanding the subject and creating the most relevant covers. They scrutinized every image to scout for the most suitable representation of the subject and create an appropriate cover for the book.

The publishing team has been involved in this book since its early stages. They were actively engaged in every process, be it collecting the data, connecting with the contributors or procuring relevant information. The team has been an ardent support to the editorial, designing and production team. Their endless efforts to recruit the best for this project, has resulted in the accomplishment of this book. They are a veteran in the field of academics and their pool of knowledge is as vast as their experience in printing. Their expertise and guidance has proved useful at every step. Their uncompromising quality standards have made this book an exceptional effort. Their encouragement from time to time has been an inspiration for everyone.

The publisher and the editorial board hope that this book will prove to be a valuable piece of knowledge for researchers, students, practitioners and scholars across the globe.

List of Contributors

Elena Lukhanina, Irina Karaban and Natalia Berezetskaya
Department of Brain Physiology, A.A. Bogomoletz Institute of Physiology, Parkinson's Disease Treatment Centre, Institute of Gerontology, Kiev, Ukraine

Silvia Marino, Pietro Lanzafame, Silvia Guerrera, Rosella Ciurleo and Placido Bramanti
IRCCS Centro Neurolesi "Bonino-Pulejo", Messina, Italy

Juliana Dushanova
Institute of Neurobiology, Bulgarian Academy of Sciences, Bulgaria

Jorge E. Quintero and Zhiming Zhang
Department of Anatomy and Neurobiology, Morris K. Udall Parkinson's Disease Research Center of Excellence, USA

Zhiming Zhang
Magnetic Resonance Imaging and Spectroscopy Center, University of Kentucky Chandler Medical Center, Lexington, USA

Xiaomin Wang
Department of Physiology, Key Laboratory for Neurodegenerative Disorders of the Ministry Education, Capital Medical University, Beijing, PR of China

Yangho Kim
Department of Occupational and Environmental Medicine, Ulsan University Hospital, University of Ulsan College of Medicine, Ulsan, Korea

Po-Lei Lee
Department of Electrical Engineering, National Central University, Taiwan
Center for Dynamical Biomarkers and Translational Medicine, National Central University, Taiwan

Po-Lei Lee, Yu-Te Wu and Jen-Chuen Hsieh
Institute of Brain Science, National Yang-Ming University, Taiwan

Margherita Speziali
CNR-IENI (Institute for Energetics and Interphases), Department of Pavia, University of Pavia, Pavia, Italy

Michela Di Casa
Department of Chemistry, University of Pavia, Pavia, Italy

Katrien Colman and Roelien Bastiaanse
University of Groningen, The Netherlands

Takuyuki Endo, Harutoshi Fujimura and Saburo Sakoda
Toneyama National Hospital, Japan

Masaru Yokoe
Osaka University Graduate School of Medicine, Japan

Weidong Pan and Shin Kwak
Department of Neurology, Graduate School of Medicine, The University of Tokyo, Japan

Yoshiharu Yamamoto
Educational Physiology Laboratory, Graduate School of Education, The University of Tokyo, Japan

Weidong Pan
Department of Neurology, Shuguang Hospital Affiliated to Shanghai University of TCM, China

Sarr Mamadou Moustapha
UFR Santé- Université deThiès, Sénégal

Ghio Alain, Espesser Robert, Teston Bernard and Viallet François
Laboratoire Parole et Langage-Aix-en-Provence, France

Dramé Moustapha
Université de Reims, France

Viallet François
Service de Neurologie du Centre Hospitalier du Pays d'Aix- Aix-en-Provence, France

Ryoichi Hayashi
Department of Neurology, Okaya City Hospital, Japan

Takeshi Hayashi
Department of Computer Science and Systems Engineering, Graduate School of Engineering Kobe University, Japan

Junpei Aizawa
Department of Material Technology, Nagano Prefecture General Industrial Technology Center, Japan

Hiroaki Nagase
Department of Information Technology, Nagano Prefecture General Industrial Technology Center, Japan

Shinji Ohara
Department of Neurology, Matsumoto Medical Center, Japan

Printed in the USA
CPSIA information can be obtained
at www.ICGtesting.com
JSHW011442221024
72173JS00004B/904